Mariani Foundation Paediatric Neurology Series
Editorial Board

Giuliano Avanzini, Milan, Italy
Philippe Evrard, Paris, France
Raoul Hennekam, Amsterdam, The Netherlands
Eugenio Mercuri, Rome, Italy
Fabio Sereni, Milan, Italy
Lawrence Wrabetz, Buffalo, NY, USA

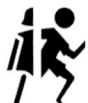

Fondazione Pierfranco e Luisa Mariani
Viale Bianca Maria 28
20129 Milan, Italy

Telephone: +39 02 795458
Fax: +39 02 76009582
e-mail: publications@fondazione-mariani.org
www.fondazione-mariani.org

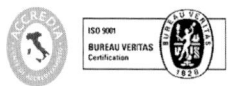

Fondazione con SGQ certificato

Progressive Myoclonus Epilepsies
State of the Art

Edited by

Berge A. Minassian, Pasquale Striano and Giuliano Avanzini

Preface by

Antonio V. Delgado-Escueta

Mariani Foundation Paediatric Neurology Series: 30
Series Founder: Maria Majno
Associate Editor: Valeria Basilico

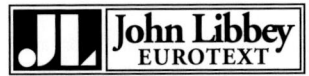

ISSN: 0969-0301
ISBN: 978-2-7420-1488-0

Cover illustration: Dynamic decomposition, Umberto Boccioni, 1913, Civico Gabinetto dei Disegni, Castello Sforzesco, Milan. Copyright: Municipality of Milan, all rights reserved.

Technical and language editor: Oliver Gubbay.

Published by

Éditions John Libbey Eurotext
127, avenue de la République, 92120 Montrouge, France
Tel.: +33 (0)1 46 73 06 60
Fax: +33 (0)1 40 84 09 99
e-mail: contact@jle.com
www.jle.com

© 2017 John Libbey Eurotext. All rights reserved.

Unauthorized duplication contravenes applicable laws.

It is prohibited to reproduce this work or any part of it without authorization of the publisher or of the Centre Français d'Exploitation du Droit de Copie (CFC), 20, rue des Grands Augustins, 75006 Paris, France.

Contents

Foreword	*Antonio V. Delgado-Escueta*	VII
Preface	*The Editors*	IX
Chapter 1	The history of progressive myoclonus epilepsies *Pierre Genton, Pasquale Striano and Berge A. Minassian*	1
Chapter 2	Neurophysiology of myoclonus and progressive myoclonus epilepsies *Giuliano Avanzini, Hiroshi Shibasaki, Guido Rubboli, Laura Canafoglia,* *Ferruccio Panzica, Silvana Franceschetti and Mark Hallett*	11
Chapter 3	Unverricht-Lundborg disease *Arielle Crespel, Edoardo Ferlazzo, Silvana Franceschetti, Pierre Genton,* *Riadh Gouider, Reetta Kälviäinen, Miikka Korja, Maria K. Lehtinen,* *Esa Mervaala, Michele Simonato and Annika Vaarmann*	35
Chapter 4	Lafora disease *Julie Turnbull, Pasquale Striano, Pierre Genton, Stirling Carpenter,* *Cameron A. Ackerley and Berge A. Minassian*	49
Chapter 5	SCARB2/LIMP2 deficiency in action myoclonus-renal failure syndrome *Leanne M. Dibbens, Michael Schwake, Paul Saftig and Guido Rubboli*	79
Chapter 6	Neuronal ceroid lipofuscinoses *Dragos A. Nita, Sara E. Mole and Berge A. Minassian*	93
Chapter 7	Sialidoses *Silvana Franceschetti and Laura Canafoglia*	115
Chapter 8	Myoclonic epilepsy in mitochondrial disorders *Costanza Lamperti and Massimo Zeviani*	121
Chapter 9	Progressive myoclonic epilepsy associated with neuroserpin inclusion bodies (neuroserpinosis) *Benoit D. Roussel, David A. Lomas and Damian C. Crowther*	133

Chapter 10	*GOSR2*: a progressive myoclonus epilepsy gene Leanne M. Dibbens and Guido Rubboli	143
Chapter 11	*KCTD7*-related progressive myoclonic epilepsy Patrick Van Bogaert	149
Chapter 12	Autosomal recessive progressive myoclonus epilepsy due to impaired ceramide synthesis Edoardo Ferlazzo, Pasquale Striano, Domenico Italiano, Tiziana Calarese, Sara Gasparini, Nicola Vanni, Floriana Fruscione, Pierre Genton and Federico Zara	155
Chapter 13	Spinal muscular atrophy associated with progressive myoclonic epilepsy Haluk Topaloglu and Judith Melki	165
Chapter 14	Myoclonus epilepsy and ataxia due to potassium channel mutation (MEAK) is caused by heterozygous *KCNC1* mutations Fábio A. Nascimento and Danielle M. Andrade	173
Chapter 15	Autosomal dominant cortical tremor, myoclonus and epilepsy Pasquale Striano and Federico Zara	179
Chapter 16	Myoclonus and seizures in PMEs: pharmacology and therapeutic trials Roberto Michelucci, Elena Pasini, Patrizia Riguzzi, Eva Andermann, Reetta Kälviäinen and Pierre Genton	187
Chapter 17	Post-modern therapeutic approaches for progressive myoclonus epilepsy Berge A. Minassian	199

Foreword

In his 2015 State of the Union address, US President Barack Hussein Obama launched a National Precision Medicine Initiative and allocated US$215 million to revitalize research into precision medicine across the USA. That announcement makes this volume entitled **'Progressive Myoclonus Epilepsy – State of the Art'** all the more timely and necessary if the 'epilepsy community' is to apply 'high-speed' whole-genome sequencing (WGS) and whole-exome sequencing (WES) to the progressive myoclonic epilepsies (PMEs), to further understand genomic contributions to disease mechanisms and tailor and optimize genome-based diagnosis and treatments.

In line with the work in precision medicine, this volume and its 17 chapters aim to provide a comprehensive account of the genetic/genomic aspects of PMEs, as well as the associated fundamental disease pathways. Chapters 1 and 2 narrate the history of PMEs and their neurophysiological mechanisms. These two chapters provide a platform and framework on which the genotype of PMEs can be expanded and the forms of autosomal recessive inheritance (with the exception of heterozygous *de novo* mutations in *KCNC1*) and disease pathways explored (chapters 3 to 15), leading to translational research into clinical genetic testing and potential treatments (chapters 16 and 17).

Chapter 1 elegantly tracks the origin of the term 'myoclonia' and the notion of seizure, which began some 134 years ago with Prichard and spread through the treatises of Delasiauve (1854), Rabot (1899), and Friedreich (1881). The progressive, severe and distressing course for a subset of families with myoclonias led Lundborg (1903) and Unverricht (1891), and then Lafora (1911), to the concept of separate recognizable PMEs.

Having been abandoned for more than a century, the concept of PMEs would have fossilized with traditional descriptive neuropathology and electrophysiology were it not for the application of biochemical genetics in Batten CLN3 and the use of 'high-tech reverse genetics' and positional cloning in the discovery of cystatin B for Unverricht-Lundborg type PME and laforin/dual specificity phosphatase and malin/ubiquitin ligase 3 for Lafora type PME (chapter 4). There was no need for researchers in molecular biology to wait for high-speed whole-genome or whole-exome sequencing, since causative associations between mutated genes and PMEs were identified by linkage mapping and positional cloning (except for the case of *KCNC1* for which WES was performed).

The discoveries of the various mutations presumed to cause Unverricht-Lundborg type PME, with or without severe cognitive problems, are reconstructed in chapter 3 (cystatin B mutations), chapter 5 (*SCARB2/LIMP2* mutations), chapter 10 (*GOSR2* mutations in North Sea PME), chapter 11 (*KCTD7* mutations), chapter 12 (ceramide synthase 1 and 2 gene mutations), chapter 13 (acid ceramidase or *ASAH1* mutations), and chapter 14 (*KCNC1* mutations). The same approach to biochemical genetics and positional cloning was used to identify protein abnormalities in neuronal ceroid lipofuscinosis (chapter 6), sialidosis (chapter 7), mitochondrial disorders (chapter 8), and neuroserpinoses (chapter 9). Chapter 15 focuses on the as yet unsolved syndrome of autosomal dominant cortical tremor, myoclonus and epilepsy (ADCTME), also referred to as FAME, for familial adult myoclonic epilepsy. Three separate chromosomal loci have been linked to ADCME, namely, chromosome 2p11.1-q12.2, chromosome 5p15.3-p15, and chromosome 3q26.3.

For molecular biologists, 'high-speed' WGS and WES are brought to the laboratory for the primary purpose of identifying disease-associated variants that, in turn, lead to the elucidation of molecular disease mechanisms and cures. For clinicians, the primary purpose is to search for disease-causing genetic variants that can be used to support medical decision-making. Both are necessary if the precision medicine initiative is to show concrete results.

Presently, one year after US President Obama announced his initiative, the main result has been to raise the profile and 'hype' around precision medicine and advertise transformational medical diagnosis and treatment. The true practical use of precision medicine will not be in the recognition of the very rare Mendelian disorders to identify break-through treatment, but rather in the 'grunt work' of understanding molecular disease mechanisms using cell lines and tissue cultures, as well as *Drosophila Melanogaster* fly models and transgenic mice. These are exemplified in the studies on cystatin B and laforin and malin in chapters 3 and 4. The subsequent crucial experiments to rescue/suppress the phenotypes of diseases in transgenic mice are exemplified in Lafora type PME and set out by the editors and authors of this volume of PMEs. The true practical use of precision medicine will also involve the enormous task of vetting putative pathogenic variants of candidate genes for PMEs. This will be achieved through the guidelines established by the US National Human Genome Research Institute (NHGRI) and the American College of Medical Genetics and Genomics/Association for Molecular Pathology (ACMG) for assigning disease causality to sequence variants and distinguishing disease-causing genetic variants from false positive reports of causality. Finally, the editors' aspirations of future treatments are outlined in chapter 17, with the application of small molecules, antisense oligonucleotides, CRISPR/Cas, gene therapy, and protein replacement which can be performed with precision in order to rescue pathogenic variants, their disease mechanisms, and the clinical phenotypes of PME. Results from research laboratories and clinical genome diagnostic centres will justify and heighten the use of WGS and WES in clinical precision medicine, as applied to the PMEs.

In summary, this book highlights the PME syndromes according to the descriptions by clinicians, the studies on pathogenic gene variants/mutations by molecular biologists and biochemical geneticists, as well as the day-to-day work of many scientists along the way in pursuit of cures. This work is, however, more than justified and is inspired by the personal grit and courage of those affected by PME and the gravity of the situation faced by their families and other loved ones. Let us not forget that it is indeed the families affected by PMEs that fuel and inspire our research.

Antonio V. Delgado-Escueta, MD, PhD (Honoris Causa)
David Geffen School of Medicine at UCLA
Veterans Administration Greater Los Angeles Healthcare System

Preface

The progressive myoclonus epilepsies (PMEs) are 'progressive', because they worsen with time and are generally fatal. They are 'myoclonus', because these patients generally have frequent, often constant, myoclonus, which is commonly, though not invariably, cortical. They are 'epilepsies', because in addition to the myoclonus the patients suffer convulsive and other types of seizures, which are soon intractable, and which in many cases precipitate death in status epilepticus. But the PMEs are in most cases more. They are often associated with blindness, because the retina is nervous tissue, and what is wrong with that nervous tissue is what is wrong with the brain itself, namely neurodegeneration. The PMEs are therefore also ataxia, and dementia, and general demise of the brain. The PMEs are yet more. They are children who are born and grow and go to school and love and are loved, before they are struck. They are therefore not static early tragedies that families adjust to from the get-go, but are children with whom the family has grown and who are slipping daily a little bit more into greater pain, towards greater intellectual and emotional separation, and towards death. And yet that death does not come fast in most cases, because these are children generally with otherwise healthy bodies. They and their families therefore suffer for years, sometimes decades before the end.

Yet again the PMEs are something more. Almost all are monogenic diseases. As such, however horrible, they are genetically simple. As such, and because each has an open window of health prior to significant neurodegeneration, they will be among the first brain diseases to be treated by interventions such as gene replacement therapy. Also, because they are genetically simple, they will be understood ahead of genetically complex neurological disorders.

We are therefore dealing with the worst and best of all neurological worlds. This series of chapters reviews the PMEs and provides the most up-to-date knowledge of their basic mechanisms. It concludes with an outlook at upcoming gene knowledge empowered therapies. It is hoped that the next book written on this subject will include real examples of available cures, and a dream shared by all neurologists, that when they see a family with a PME they would be able to say: 'This is what you have. Take this'.

The editors would like to thank Dr. Maria Majno from the Mariani Foundation for her tireless work in helping organize this series, her insights, and her steady gentle prodding to realize this project. At the Mariani Foundation, we would also like to thank Ms. Valeria Basilico for her outstanding productive coordination.

We are very grateful to Pr. Alexis Arzimanoglou at *Epileptic Disorders* for his expert guidance and chief-editing towards ensuring excellent clinical and scientific accessibility of all the manuscripts. The educational missions of both the Mariani Foundation and *Epileptic Disorders* are certainly being fulfilled, and so well.

A word of appreciation is due to all the leaders and teachers in the field of PMEs over the decades. We are certainly forgetting many, but these names include the team from the Montreal Neurological Institute, Drs. Eva and Fred Andermann, Samuel Berkovic now in Australia, previously trained with the Andermanns, and Guy Rouleau; the group in Helsinki led by Anna-Elina Lehesjoki; the Marseille group (the late Dr Joseph Roger and his team: Charlotte Dravet, Pierre Genton and Michelle Bureau); and the Los Angeles group (Antonio Delgado-Escueta and his trainee now a leader in Spain, Jose-Maria Serratosa).

Finally, the greatest thanks go to each and every child we have all seen, who taught us so much about the brain generally, for the sake of countless future patients, and all the families who teach us every day what humanity is at its best.

Berge A. Minassian, Pasquale Striano, Giuliano Avanzini

Chapter 1

The history of progressive myoclonus epilepsies

Pierre Genton[1], Pasquale Striano[2] and Berge A. Minassian[3]

[1] Centre Saint-Paul – Hôpital Henri-Gastaut, 300 Bd De Sainte Marguerite, 13009 Marseille, France
[2] Epilepsy Center, Department of Neurological Sciences, Federico II University, Napoli, and the Unit of Muscular and Neurodegenerative Disease, Institute 'G. Gaslini', Genova, Italy
[3] The Hospital for Sick Children and University of Toronto, 555 University Avenue, Toronto, Ontario, M5G 1X8, Canada
piergen@aol.com
strianop@gmail.com
berge.minassian@sickkids.ca

Summary

The history of the progressive myoclonus epilepsies (PMEs) spans more than a century. However, the recent history of PMEs begins with a consensus statement published in the wake of the Marseille PME workshop in 1989 (Marseille Consensus Group, 1990). This consensus helped define the various types of PME known at the time and set the agenda for a new era of genetic research which soon led to the discovery of many PME genes.

Prior to the Marseille meeting, and before the molecular era, there had been much confusion and controversy. Because investigators had but limited and biased experience with these rare disorders due to the uneven, skewed distribution of PMEs around the world, opinions and nosologies were based on local expertise which did not match well with the experiences of other researchers and clinicians. The three major areas of focus included: (1) the nature and limits of the concept of PME in varying scopes, which was greatly debated; (2) the description of discrete clinical entities by clinicians; and (3) the description of markers (pathological, biological, neurophysiological, *etc.*) which could lead to a precise diagnosis of a given PME type, with, in the best cases, a reliable correlation with clinical findings.

In this chapter, we shall also examine the breakthroughs achieved in the wake of the 1989 Marseille meeting and recent history in the field, following the identification of several PME genes. As in other domains, the molecular and genetic approach has challenged some established concepts and has led to the description of new PME types. However, as may already be noted, this approach has also confirmed the existence of the major, established types of PME, which can now be considered as true diseases.

The concept of progressive myoclonus epilepsy

The relationship between 'myoclonia' and epilepsy was recognized by Prichard in 1822 (quoted by Rabot [1899]). Delasiauve had also noticed the existence of myoclonic jerks in patients with epilepsy and in his 1854 treatise on epilepsy, labelled them *'petit mal moteur'*. The myoclonic jerks, well described by many authors, were found in patients with various conditions, ranging from a comparatively benign, non-progressive type that would later be described as *'impulsive petit mal'* (Janz & Christian, 1957), to many more severe examples.

Following Friedreich's *'paramyoclonus multiplex'* (1881), it was admitted that the jerks probably originated in the spinal cord. No clear disease entity was associated with these jerks (Friedreich, 1881).

The concept of 'progressive myoclonus epilepsy' was introduced by Herman Lundborg (Fig. 1) in 1903 (Lundborg, 1903), on the basis of several Swedish families with a common ancestor and (among other markers of 'degeneration') a particular form of epilepsy associated with progressive myoclonus and varying degrees of severity (Fig. 2). He acknowledged the previous reports from Estonia by Heinrich Unverricht (Unverricht, 1891) (Fig. 3) who had described two families with *'Myoclonie'* (1891) or *'familiäre Myoklonie'* (1895). Both authors had aptly described a fairly 'pure' type of PME which did not include major symptoms other than the myoclonias and epileptic seizures. It took, however, nearly a century for this condition to be rightly recognised as 'Unverricht-Lundborg' disease (ULD). Their contributions were widely read and commented upon, but failed to convince later authors that they had described a recognisable, specific condition. In order to reach a consensus, there were obviously too few cases in the patienthood of major neurologists at the time. When Lafora (Fig. 4) described the pathological inclusion found in the brain of a patient with a 'myoclonic epilepsy', which he also aptly described, he did not believe that his patient was different from those of Unverricht and Lundborg (Lafora, 1911).

Hunt (Fig. 5) contributed to the complexity of the matter by describing patients with signs of Friedreich's ataxia associated with action myoclonus and (in some cases) epilepsy (Hunt, 1921). The 'Ramsay Hunt syndrome' (RHS; not to be confused with the description by the same author of the herpes infection of the geniculate ganglion, with resulting facial paresis and skin eruption) covered many clinical conditions, including ULD (Roger *et al.*, 1968). RHS was finally discarded as a useful entity (Andermann *et al.*, 1989a), however, at that time not for the right reasons, but because it was felt that the recent recognition of mitochondrial diseases with progressive myoclonus and seizures had cleared the way.

There were, however, efforts to try and introduce order to the PMEs. Van Bogaert approached the issue from a mixed neuropathological and clinical point of view, and supported the concept of PME, but failed to establish clear boundaries between the various types (Van Bogaert, 1968). In 1973, Diebold defined a nucleus of 'hereditary myoclonus-epilepsy-dementia nuclear syndromes' (*erbliche myoklonisch-epileptisch-dementielle Kernsyndrome*), which he differentiated from the 'borderline syndromes' occurring in diseases which only fit the PME definition in some cases (Diebold, 1973). Heralding the modern approach, the Montreal group also acknowledged the concept of PME and proposed a classification that was, subjectively, based on the relative frequency of these rare conditions (Berkovic *et al.*, 1986). Before the genetic advances of the past twenty years had really had an impact, the Marseille group (Genton *et al.*, 1990) proposed to divide the PMEs into those with known biochemical mechanisms (*e.g.* MERRF and sialidosis), those with a definite and reliable pathological marker (*e.g.* Lafora's disease, the neuronal ceroid lipofuscinoses [NCLF]), and those without any marker (the 'degenerative' types, with purely clinical diagnosis and exclusion of other aetiologies: *e.g.* ULD and DRPLA).

Chapter 1 The history of progressive myoclonus epilepsies

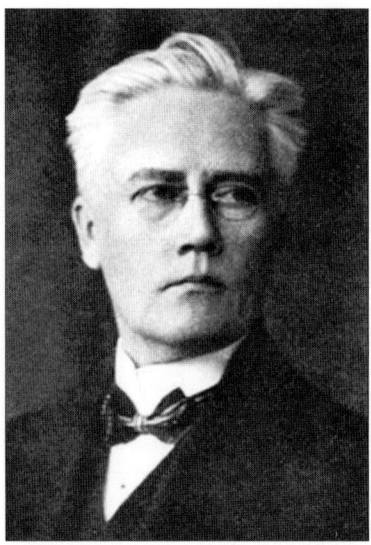

Fig. 1. Herman Lundborg (1868-1943).
Herman Lundborg wrote his dissertation in 1903 at the Karolinska Institutet, in Stockholm, about a family with the condition previously described by Unverricht, which he studied from a clinical point of view but also from a genetic perspective. His interest in genetics led him to found the notorious State Institute of Racial Biology, in Uppsala, in 1922. He came under strong criticism and disrepute due to his adherence to Nazi ideology and his advocacy of eugenics and the sterilisation of 'genetically unworthy' persons.

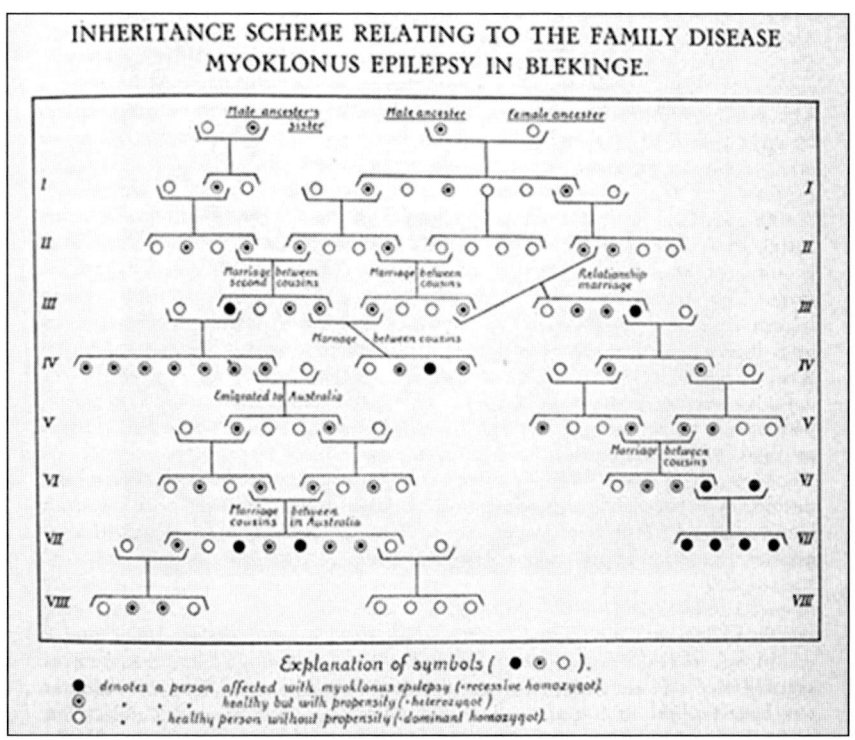

Fig. 2. A pedigree showing recessive transmission in a family with Unverricht-Lundborg disease (from Lundborg & Runnstom [1921]).

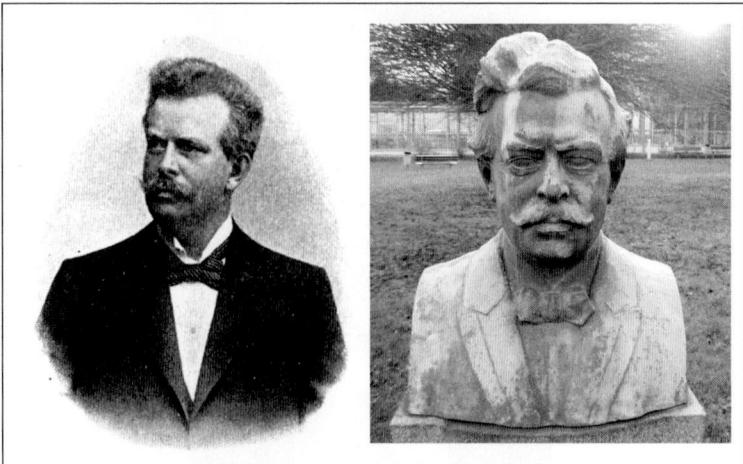

Fig. 3. Heinrich Unverricht (1853-1912).
Bust erected in 1914 at Magdeburg University. During his short tenure at Dorpat (now Tartu, Estonia), which he left because of the Russification policies of the occupying forces, Heinrich Unverricht described a family with 'Myoclonie', i.e. with the condition now named after him, 'Unverricht-Lundborg disease'. He was a prolific internist who also described other conditions (polymyositis and pneumonia). His contribution is regarded as the founding description of progressive myoclonus epilepsy.

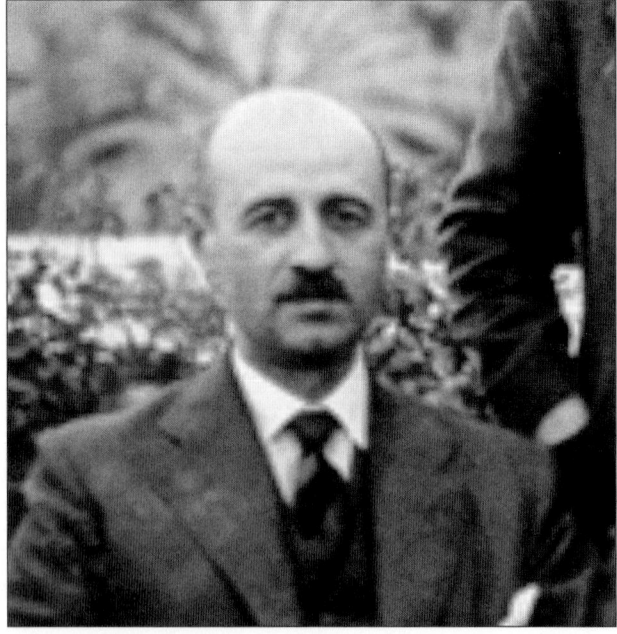

Fig. 4. Gonzalo Rodriguez Lafora (1886-1971).
After studying in Spain (with Santiago Ramón Cajal), France (with Pierre Marie and Joseph Jules Dejerine), Germany (with Alois Alzheimer and Emil Kraepelin) and the USA, Gonzalo Rodriguez Lafora returned to Spain (which he had left for Mexico during the Civil War in 1938; he returned to Madrid in 1947). As a psychiatrist, he introduced the Freudian doctrine to both Spain and Argentina, but mainly dedicated his life to the care of intellectually disabled children. During his tenure as a neuropathologist at the Government Hospital for the Insane in Washington DC, he published his landmark paper on 'myoclonic corpuscles', in German.

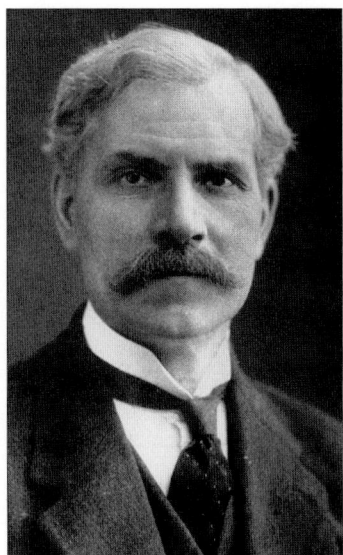

Fig. 5. James Ramsay Hunt (1874-1937).
After studying in Philadelphia, Paris, Berlin and Vienna, James Ramsay Hunt practised and taught neurology in New York City (Cornell University and Columbia University). His name is associated with a small cutaneous zone innervated by the ganglion geniculi. *His contribution to the field of PME from 1914 onward was the source of great confusion; from his area of low prevalence, he selected several unrelated cases with myoclonus (and other symptoms). The term 'Ramsay Hunt Syndrome', when applied to a neurological condition with myoclonus, was used to refer to many disparate entities. The term is no longer in use, following the delimitation of discrete PME types.*

Clinical descriptions and pathological markers

Table 1 summarizes, for the major PMEs, the progression from clinical descriptions to molecular elucidation, which is currently nearly complete. However, it appears that the process was fairly uneven. Some descriptions preceded the molecular characterisation of the condition by more than a hundred years, while in other cases, a 'new' disease was described on the basis of a singular clinical, pathological or genetic feature.

In the classic sequence of events, a clinical description occurred first, followed by a more or less specific biological or neurophysiological marker which helped ascertain the diagnosis. This was the case for the various forms of NCLF. The juvenile type of NCLF was described by Stengel, a general practitioner in 1826, in a geographic isolate of inland Norway (Stengel, 1826), but it took nearly a century to distinguish this and other forms of NCLF from other forms of *'amaurotic idiocy'*, which included non-PME disorders such as Tay-Sachs disease. While Batten had not initially distinguished these conditions from one another (Batten, 1902), in 1903 an ophthalmologist, Alfred Bielschowsky, characterised the ocular findings in the late infantile form of NCLF. The more specific pathological, ultrastructural changes associated with the infantile and juvenile types of NCLF were only described in the 1970s (Zeman *et al.*, 1970). Although it took some time to differentiate NCLF from other types of degenerative childhood diseases, which included mental decline and retinal impairment, they were fairly well distinguished, on clinical grounds, from other types of PMEs. However, another condition with optional ophthalmological symptoms, sialidosis, was only clearly identified in the 1970s (Rapin *et al.*, 1978).

Table 1. Discovery and description of the main classic PME types, showing the timescale, from clinical description to diagnostic marker and genetic localisation and elucidation, in chronological order of initial clinical descriptions. In some cases, such as Lafora's disease, the discovery of a pathological marker preceded the comprehensive clinical description by many years. For a detailed history of the various types of PME, refer to the relevant chapter. NCLF: neuronal ceroidlipofuscinosis.

PME type	First description (year, author)	Pre-genetic diagnostic marker (year)	Locus/gene (year)
Juvenile NCLF	1826 Stengel, Norway 1908 Spielmeyer, Germany 1931 Sjögren, Sweden	Finger print profiles (1963)	1989
Unverricht-Lundborg disease	1891 Unverricht, Estonia 1905 Lundborg, Sweden	None	1991
Lafora's disease	1911 Lafora Spain/USA 1963 Van Heycop Ten Ham, Netherlands	'Myoclonic corpuscles' (1911)	1995
Late-infantile NCLF	1913 Bielschowsky, Germany	Curvilinear profiles (1963)	1997
Adult NCLF	1925 Kufs, Germany	Various	2011
Sialidosis	1978 Rapin, USA	Enzyme defect (1978)	1996
MERRF	1980 Fukuhara, Japan	Ragged red fibres in muscle (1980)	1990
DRPLA	1982 Naito and Oyanagi, Japan	None	1995
Action myoclonus-renal failure syndrome	1986 Andermann, Canada	None	2008

In the case of Lafora's disease, the pathological marker, the presence of amyloid deposits in the brain, was described by Gonzalo Lafora in 1911, together with a fairly precise clinical depiction of the condition named after him. But it took half a century of controversies before a sound and precise clinical description of Lafora's disease (LD) was reached in the Netherlands (Van Heycoptenhamm & De Jager, 1963). From this point onwards, LD was for most, but not all, a clearly identifiable entity. In subsequent years, several refinements were made to the clinical description, focusing on the characteristic EEG presentation and on the occurrence of occipital lobe seizures (Roger et al., 1983; Tinuper et al., 1983).

Diagnosis was much more difficult in the absence of precise markers, when the clinician was left to speculate on patient cases purely on the basis of clinical traits. Some neurophysiological features were shared by several, clearly different conditions. As an example, the spectacular occurrence of runs of polyspikes during REM sleep which was described in several 'myoclonic' and progressive conditions, such as Ramsay-Hunt syndrome (soon to become Unverricht-Lundborg disease [ULD]), was also seen in post-anoxic myoclonus, or MERRF. Indeed, based on their own experience, various authors promoted a regional type of PME, which dominated local experiences. In Finland, close to the original sites of Unverricht's and Lundborg's descriptions, the 'Baltic myoclonus' was the prototype of PMEs (Koskiniemi et al., 1974; Koskiniemi, 1986). Likewise, RHS was repeatedly described in Marseille following Roger et al. (1968) and was, in the light of the Finnish publications, labelled 'Mediterranean myoclonus' and considered to constitute a milder entity than the 'Baltic' type and MERRF (Genton et al., 1990). An explanation had already been given for the difference in severity; in Northern Europe, phenytoin, the most prescribed anticonvulsant for epilepsies with convulsive seizures (including myoclonic seizures), had clearly contributed to an artificial aggravation of the condition (Elridge *et al.*, 1983), in contrast to Mediterranean patients, who were more likely to be treated (or over-treated) with phenobarbital, which lacked this aggravating effect.

In the 1980s, convincing descriptions of new entities emerged, such as mitochondrial encephalopathy with ragged-red fibres (MERRF) (Fukuhara *et al.*, 1980), and dentato-rubro-pallido-luysian atrophy (DRPLA) (Naito & Oyanagi, 1982), and it was tempting to ascribe previously unresolved cases to these new findings, thus rendering the RHS concept obsolete (Berkovic *et al.*, 1986; Andermann *et al.*, 1989a). The time had come to compare the experience of researchers from Europe, America and Japan; an international workshop was organised in Marseille in June 1989, which heralded the modern, genetic and molecular era in PME research (Fig. 6).

The genetic era

Prior to 1989, the year of the Marseille conference, it had only been possible to identify the gene for only one autosomal recessive PME (NEU1; sialidosis), using classic biochemical methods (Rapin *et al.*, 1978). The Marseille conference coincided with momentous developments in the history of genetics. 1989 was the year when the promise of reverse genetics, identifying a disease gene by first mapping its chromosomal location, was first fulfilled with the discovery of the cystic fibrosis gene (*CFTR*) (Rommens *et al.*, 1989). While *CFTR* was mapped using restriction length polymorphisms, that same year the discovery of microsatellite polymorphisms was also first reported (Weber & May, 1989). The microsatellite maps that rapidly followed had just the right density for homozygosity and linkage mapping of autosomal recessive Mendelian diseases, and since the vast majority of PMEs are inherited in this fashion, their genes quickly began to be identified in the years that followed.

PME gene discoveries proceeded in the approximate order in which the diseases themselves had been described, which is likely to be a reflection of the relative frequencies of the various diseases. The *CLN1* (Infantile NCL) and *CLN3* (Batten's disease) genes were identified in 1995 (Vesa *et al.* 1995; The International Batten Disease Consortium, 1995), the ULD gene in 1996 and 1997 (Pennacchio *et al.*, 1996; Lafrenière *et al.*, 1997; Lalioti *et al.*, 1997; Virtaneva *et al.*, 1997), and the LD genes between 1998 and 2003 (Minassian *et al.*, 1998; Serratosa *et al.*, 1999; Chan *et al.*, 2003). The most 'myoclonic' of the NCL genes, *CLN2*, was cloned not through reverse genetics, but by using an elegant biochemical approach, taking advantage of the realisation that most NCL are lysosomal diseases. The authors isolated lysosomal proteins and looked for a missing spot in two-dimensional gels in patients with late-infantile NCL, in order to identify CLN2, a lysosomal dipeptidyl peptidase (Sleat *et al.*, 1997). The remaining childhood NCL genes followed in the first decade of the new millennium, again for the most part through homozygosity and linkage mapping (see Chapter 6).

The gene for Action Myoclonus Renal Failure Syndrome (Andermann *et al.*, 1989b) was one of the first disease genes to be identified using the more abundant polymorphisms established in the 2000s, namely single nucleotide polymorphisms (SNPs), which made it possible to rely on very few patients in order to identify disease genes (Berkovic *et al.*, 2008). Most recently, disease genes, including PME genes, emerged in larger numbers, through combined use of SNP mapping arrays and next-generation (whole-exome and whole-genome) sequencing. Here, identification of disease genes can be based on as few as one patient. The best example of this technical progress relates to Kufs disease (adult-onset NCL). While this disease has been known for 88 years, it was not until advanced mapping and sequencing techniques became routinely used that its genetic cause was uncovered. This turned out not to be a single gene but, to date, at least four different genetic entities (detailed in Chapter 6).

Some PMEs are very rare, caused by private mutations in single families. One example of this is the PME due to mutations in *PRICKLE1* (Bassuk et al., 2008). It is expected that many such PMEs will be identified, as has been the case for other diseases. Mutation for certain genes is limited to allow for viability, but may result in a specific pathology that cannot be replicated by other defects of the same protein. Other PMEs are allelic to previously known PMEs, for example, the most common form of Kufs disease is allelic to the late-infantile variant NCL, CLN6 (Arsov et al., 2011).

As recessively inherited diseases, many PMEs occur fairly frequently in pets and farm animals, due to inbreeding. This includes LD, which is widespread in certain breeds of dog (Lohi et al., 2005), and various forms of NCL in dogs and sheep. In some cases, PME genes were first discovered in animals and then translated to humans, e.g. the severest form of NCL, CLN10, with fatal neonatal disease (Siintola et al., 2006; Steinfeld et al., 2006; Tyynela et al., 2000). PME comparisons between humans and animals has also yielded fascinating insights into genome biology. For example, human ULD is a disease which is not due to the complete absence of the responsible gene (*EPM1*), but to drastic downregulation of the gene's expression caused by expansion of a dodecamer repeat sequence. This repeat is present in the promoter of the human *EPM1* gene but not in the promoter of the orthologous genes in animals. In humans, expansion of this dodecamer leads to significant downregulation but not to the complete absence of *EPM1* mRNA. No patient is reported to have, or probably exists with, a total loss of *EPM1*. Because of the unique genomic particularity within the promoter sequence of the *EPM1* gene, ULD is, therefore, a uniquely human disease and no natural animal model of the disease has been reported. As a second example, the dog genome has a similar dodecamer repeat in the *Epm2b* gene, one of the genes mutated in LD. Recurrent expansion of this repeat in *canine Epm2b* makes LD particularly common in dogs, but this mechanism does not occur in human cases with LD (Lohi et al., 2005).

Conclusions

PMEs comprise a group of rare, heterogeneous genetic (mainly autosomal recessive) disorders, characterised by cortical myoclonus, other types of epileptic seizures, and progressive neurocognitive impairment. PMEs usually present in late childhood or adolescence, which distinguishes them from epileptic encephalopathies that start with polymorphic seizures in early infancy. However, adult-onset PMEs may be due to rare gene defects or to immune or late degenerative disorders. Recent advances in this area have clarified molecular genetic basis, biological basis, and natural history, and have also provided a rational approach to diagnosis. However, PMEs still remain uncommon disorders which are difficult to diagnose in the absence of extensive experience with such conditions, and this severely limits the number of expert groups in the field. Thus, despite the advances in molecular medicine, aetiology remains undetermined in a substantial proportion of patients. In particular, there are still huge areas in medically developing parts of the world, where the diagnosis of PME is probably overlooked. Therefore, the actual prevalence of these conditions is still debatable. The history of PMEs shows that international collaboration and sharing experience is the right way to proceed. The Marseille conference occurred at a perfectly opportune moment, serving to clarify and classify the many PME syndromes known at that time. This was the springboard from which scientists, armed with the genetic and genomic tools that were then being invented, were able to rapidly identify causative defects. It is probably safe to say that we have now identified most PME genes, but it is equally safe to expect that many others remain to be found. Each one, however unique, will fill one of the gaps in the great PME puzzle. This will enable us to better understand this severe brain disease, and to move forward towards grasping some of the mysteries of the human brain. At the same time, the emerging picture and biological insights will allow us to find ways to provide our patients with meaningful treatment.

Conflicts of interest: none.

References

Andermann, F., Berkovic, S., Carpenter, S. & Andermann, E. (1989a): Viewpoints on the Ramsay Hunt syndrome. 2. The Ramsay Hunt syndrome is no longer a useful diagnostic category. *Mov. Disord.* **4**, 13–17.

Andermann, E., Andermann, F., Carpenter, S., *et al.* (1989b): Action myoclonus-renal failure syndrome: a previously unrecognised disorder unmasked by advances in nephrology. In: *Myoclonus. Advances in Neurology Vol. 43*, ed. S. Fahn S. New York: Raven Press, pp. 87–103.

Arsov, T., Smith, K.R., Damiano, J., *et al.* (2011): Kufs disease, the major adult form of neuronal ceroid lipofuscinosis, caused by mutations in CLN6. *Am. J. Hum. Genet.* **88**, 566–573.

Bassuk, A.G., Wallace, R.H., Buhr, A., *et al.* (2008): A homozygous mutation in human *PRICKLE1* causes an autosomal-recessive progressive myoclonus epilepsy-ataxia syndrome. *Am. J. Hum. Genet.* **83**, 572–581.

Batten, F.E. (1902): Cerebral degeneration with symmetrical changes in the maculae in two members of a family. *Transactions of the Ophthalmological Societies of the United Kingdom* **23**, 386–390.

Berkovic, S., Andermann, F., Carpenter, S., Andermann, E. & Wolfe, L.S. (1986): Progressive myoclonus epilepsies: specific causes and diagnosis. *N. Engl. J. Med.* **315**, 296–305.

Berkovic, S.F., Dibbens, L.M., Oshlack, A., *et al.* (2008): Array-based gene discovery with three unrelated subjects shows SCARB2/LIMP-2 deficiency causes myoclonus epilepsy and glomerulosclerosis. *Am. J. Hum. Genet.* **82**, 6.

Chan, E.M., Young, E.J., Ianzano, L., *et al.* (2003): Mutations in *NHLRC1* cause progressive myoclonus epilepsy. *Nature Genet.* **35**, 125–127.

Diebold, K. (1973): Die erblichen myoklonisch-epileptisch-dementiellen Kernsyndrome. Springer: Berlin.

Elridge, R., Iivanainen, M., Stern, R., Koerber, I. & Wilder, B.J. (1983): 'Baltic' myoclonus epilepsy: hereditary disorder of childhood made worse by phenytoin. *Lancet* **2**, 838–842.

Friedreich, N. (1881): Paramyoclonus multiplex. *Virchows Archiv.* 86.

Fukuhara, N., Tokiguchi, S., Shirakawa, K. & Tsubaki, T. (1980): Myoclonus epilepsy asociated with ragged-red fibers (mitochondrial abnormalities). Disease entity or a syndrome? *J. Neurol. Sci.* **47**, 117–133.

Genton, P., Michelucci, R., Tassinari, C.A. & Roger, J. (1990): The Ramsay Hunt syndrome revisited: mediterranean myoclonus versus mitochondrial encephalomyopathy with ragged red fibers and Baltic myoclonus. *Acta Neurol. Scand.* **81**, 8–15.

Hunt, J.R. (1921): Dyssynergia cerebellaris myoclonica -primary atrophy of the dentate system: a contribution to the pathology and symptomatology of the cerebellum. *Brain* **44**, 490–538.

Janz, D. & Christian, W. (1957): Impulsiv petit-mal. *Dtsch. Z. Nervenheilk* **176**, 346–386.

Koskiniemi, M.L. (1986): Baltic myoclonus. In: *Myoclonus. Advances in Neurology, Vol. 43*, eds. S. Fahn, C.D. Marsden & M. Van Woert. New York: Raven Press, pp. 57–64.

Koskiniemi, M., Donner, M., Majuri, H., Haltia, M. & Norio, R. (1974): Progressive myoclonus epilepsy: a clinical and histopathological study. *Acta Neurol. Scand.* **50**, 307–332.

Lafora, G.R. (1911): Über das Vorkommen amyloider Körperchen im Innerender Ganglienzellen. *Virchows Arch. Pathol. Anat.* **205**, 295–303.

Lafrenière, R.G., Rochefort, D.L., Chrétien, N., *et al.* (1997): Unstable insertion of the 5-prime flanking region of the cystatin B gene is the most common mutation in progressive myoclonus epilepsy type 1, EPM1. *Nature Genet.* **15**, 298–302.

Lalioti, M.D., Scott, H.S., Buresi, C., *et al.* (1997): Dodecamer repeat expansion in cystatin B gene in progressive myoclonus epilepsy. *Nature* **386**, 847–851.

Lohi, H., Young, E.J., Fitzmaurice, S.N., et al. (2005): Expanded repeat in canine epilepsy. *Science* **307**, 81.

Lundborg, H. (1903): Die progressive myoclonusepilepsie (Unverrichts myoklonie). Uppsala: Almqvist and Wiskell.

Lundborg, H. & Runnstom, J. (1921): The Swedish nation in word and picture. Stockholm, Swedish Society for Race Hygiene.

Marseille Consensus Group. (1990): Classification of progressive myoclonus epilepsies and related diseases. *Ann. Neurol.* **28**, 113–116.

Minassian, B.A., Lee, J.R., Herbrick, J.-A., et al. (1998): Mutations in a gene encoding a novel protein tyrosine phosphatase cause progressive myoclonus epilepsy. *Nature Genet.* **20**, 171–174.

Naito, H. & Oyanagi, S. (1982): Familial myoclonus epilepsy and choreoathetosis: hereditary dentatorubral- pallidoluysian atrophy. *Neurology* **32**, 798–807.

Pennacchio, L.A., Lehesjoki, A.-E., Stone, N.E., et al. (1996): Mutations in the gene encoding cystatin B in progressive myoclonus epilepsy (EPM1). *Science* **271**, 1731–1733.

Rabot, L. (1899): De la myoclonie épileptique. Medical thesis, Paris.

Rapin, I., Goldfisher, S., Katzman, R., Engel, J. & O'Brien, J.S. (1978): The cherry-red spot myoclonus syndrome. *Ann. Neurol.* **3**, 234–242.

Roger, J., Soulayrol, R. & Hassoun, J. (1968): La dyssynergie cérébelleuse myoclonique (syndrome de Ramsay-Hunt). *Rev. Neurol.* **119**, 85–106.

Roger, J., Pellissier, J.F., Bureau, M., Dravet, C., Revol, M. & Tinuper, P. (1983): Le diagnostic précoce de la maladie de Lafora. Importance des manifestations paroxystiques visuelles et intéret de la biopsie cutané. *Rev. Neurol.* **139**, 115–124.

Rommens, J.M., Iannuzzi, M.C., Kerem, B. et al. (1989): Identification of the cystic fibrosis gene: chromosome walking and jumping. *Science* **245**, 1059–1065.

Serratosa, J.M., Gomez-Garre, P., Gallardo, M.E., et al. (1999): A novel protein tyrosine phosphatase gene is mutated in progressive myoclonus epilepsy of the Lafora type (EPM2). *Hum. Molec. Genet.* **8**, 345–352,

Siintola, E., Partanen, S., Stromme, P., et al. (2006): Cathepsin D deficiency underlies congenital human neuronal ceroid-lipofuscinosis. *Brain* **129**, 1438–1445.

Sleat, D.E., Donnelly, R.J., Lackland, H., et al. (1997): Association of mutations in a lysosomal protein with classical late-infantile neuronal ceroid lipofuscinosis. *Science* **277**, 1802–1805.

Steinfeld, R., Reinhardt, K., Schreiber, K., et al. (2006): Cathepsin D deficiency is associated with a human neurodegenerative disorder. *Am. J. Hum. Genet.* **78**, 988–998.

Stengel, C. (1826): Beretning om et mærkeligt Sygdomstilfelde hos fire Sødskende. *Account of a singular illness among four siblings in the vicinity of Røraas.* Eyr (Christiana) 1, 347–352. English translation, 1982. In: *Ceroid lipofuscinosis (Batten's disease)*, eds. D. Armstrong, N. Koopand & J.A. Rider. Amsterdam, New York, Oxford: Elsevier Biomedical Press, pp. 17–19.

The International Batten Disease Consortium. (1995): Isolation of a novel gene underlying Batten disease, CLN3. *Cell* **82**, 949–957.

Tinuper, P., Aguglia, U., Pellissier, J.F. & Gastaut, H. (1983): Visual ictal phenomena in a case of Lafora disease proven by skin biopsy. *Epilepsia* **24**, 214–218.

Tyynela, J., Sohar, I., Sleat, D.E., et al. (2000): A mutation in the ovine cathepsin D gene causes a congenital lysosomal storage disease with profound neurodegeneration. *EMBO J.* **19**, 2786–2792.

Unverricht, H. (1891): Die Myoclonie. Leipzig, Vienna: Franz Deuticke.

Van Bogaert, L. (1968): L'épilepsie myoclonique progressive d'Unverricht–Lundborg et le probléme des encéphalopathies progressives associant épilepsies et myoclonies. *Rev. Neurol.* **119**, 47–57.

Van Heycoptenhamm, M.W. & De Jager, H. (1963): Progressive myoclonus epilepsy with Lafora bodies. Clinical-pathological features. *Epilepsia* **4**, 95–119.

Vesa, J., Hellsten, E., Verkruyse, L.A., et al. (1995): Mutations in the palmitoyl protein thioesterase gene causing infantile neuronal ceroid lipofuscinosis. *Nature* **376**, 584–587.

Virtaneva, K., D'Amato, E., Miao, J., et al. (1997): Unstable minisatellite expansion causing recessively inherited myoclonus epilepsy, EPM1. *Nat. Genet.* **15**, 393–396.

Weber, J.L. & May, P.E. (1989): Abundant class of human DNA polymorphisms which can be typed using the polymerase chain reaction. *Am. J. Hum. Genet.* **44**, 388–396.

Zeman, W., Donahue, S., Dyken, P. & Green, J. (1970): The neuronal ceroid-lipofuscinoses (Batten-Vogt syndrome). In: *Handbook of Clinical Neurology, vol. 10*, eds. PS Vinken, GW Bruyn. Amsterdam: Elsevier North-Holland, pp. 588–679.

Chapter 2

Neurophysiology of myoclonus and progressive myoclonus epilepsies

Giuliano Avanzini[1], Hiroshi Shibasaki[2], Guido Rubboli[3,4], Laura Canafoglia[1], Ferruccio Panzica[1], Silvana Franceschetti[1] and Mark Hallett[5]

[1] *Fondazione I.R.C.C.S. Istituto Neurologico Carlo Besta, via Celoria 11, 20133 Milan, Italy*
[2] *Department of Brain Pathophysiology, Faculty of Medicine, Kyoto, Japan*
[3] *IRCCS Institute of Neurological Sciences, Bellaria Hospital, Bologna, Italy*
[4] *Danish Epilepsy Center, Epilepsihospital, Dianalund, Denmark*
[5] *National Institute of Neurological Disorders and Stroke, NIH, Bethesda, MD, USA*
avanzini@istituto-besta.it

Summary

The precise temporal resolution of neurophysiological recordings makes them particularly suited to establishing an accurate description of a time course of rapid events, such as myoclonus, and measurement of their temporal relationship with other related activities. In progressive myoclonus epilepsies (PMEs), polygraphy with simultaneous EMG-EEG recordings is a crucial tool for defining the characteristics of myoclonic jerks; their time course, the topography of the different muscles involved (namely antagonists), and the relationship with muscle activation and stimulation. Moreover, on polygraphic recordings it is possible to detect EEG activities associated with myoclonic jerks and define their temporalrelationship with myoclonus, thus differentiating cortical types of myoclonus from those that are subcortically generated. As a result of the back-averaging technique, non-obvious time-locked EEG potentials can be detected on polygraphy. Furthermore, for stimulus-sensitive myoclonus, the analysis can include the potential evoked by the somatosensory stimulus (SEP). The polygraphic recording also provides information on muscle activity suppression occurring after a jerk or as pure negative myoclonus. Besides the time domain analysis, techniques based on frequency analysis have been developed to evaluate EEG-EMG coherence.

The neurophysiological techniques provide investigators and clinicians with invaluable information with which to define the type of myoclonus and its generating circuitry, thus substantially contributing to the diagnosis and management of PMEs.

Neurophysiological features associated with myoclonusin progressive myoclonus epilepsies

Neurophysiological recordings may be conducted over a relatively long period of time,making them particularly suited to establishing an accurate description of the time course of the shock-likemuscle contractions which characterize myoclonus. Moreover, the combination ofelectroencephalographic (EEG) and electromyographic (EMG) recordings allows detection ofany EEG correlates of myoclonus and high precision measurement of their temporalrelationshipto muscle jerks. For these reasons, neurophysiological analysis is a first-line approach to myoclonicsyndromes, both in terms of clinical characterization and pathophysiologicalinvestigation.

The first section of this chapter deals with the neurophysiological techniques suitable for characterizingdifferent types of myoclonus, while the second section addresses the value of neurophysiologyin defining the clinical presentation of some progressive myoclonus epilepsies(PMEs).

Neurophysiological analysis of myoclonus

The correlation between EEG and EMG activities associated with myoclonus is the basis for investigating the pathophysiology of myoclonus as well as the clinical diagnosis of PMEs. Several signal analysis techniques relating to time and frequency domains, which are currently employed to detect EEG correlated with myoclonus and used to investigate its pathophysiology, will be highlighted in this first section.

Polygraphic recordings and EEG-EMG correlations in progressive myoclonus epilepsy

In epileptic disorders, polygraphy with simultaneous recording of EEG-EMG activity can provide relevant information for defining the characteristics of a motor manifestation and the relationship with concomitant EEG activity. Moreover, it can be useful to identify subtle and apparently subclinical manifestations, and is necessary for precise investigation of the temporal relationship between EEG and EMG phenomena (Tassinari & Rubboli, 2008).

In PMEs, polygraphic recording can be a crucial tool for the investigation and definition of the characteristics of myoclonic phenomena, which represent one of the cardinal features of this vast group of diseases. EMG is usually recorded using surface electrodes placed on the skin overlying the muscles involved in myoclonic activity, which should be clearly identified by clinical examination (Fig. 1). The cortical correlates of myoclonus have also been analyzed using magneto-encephalography (MEG), which can complement the EEG information in terms of the cortical generators of myoclonus (Mima *et al.*, 1998).

Myoclonus is an essential and defining feature of PMEs. It can occur spontaneously or be induced or exacerbated by a variety of stimuli (such as light, sound, touch and emotional strain) and active movement or posture maintenance. At rest, in PMEs, myoclonus is commonly fragmentary and multifocal, and is particularly apparent in the musculature of the face and distal limbs (Fig. 2; left panel). Action myoclonus, in which movement (as an attempt or intention to move) initiates jerking, is a common feature in almost all the conditions underlying PMEs, and can be extremely disabling.

At rest, the EMG expression of myoclonus is a burst of myoclonic potentials of brief (100 ± 50 ms) duration, typically occurring synchronously in agonist and antagonist muscles. If myoclonus occurs in a contracting muscle, then after the myoclonus there is a brief (50-100 ms) suppression of muscle activity.

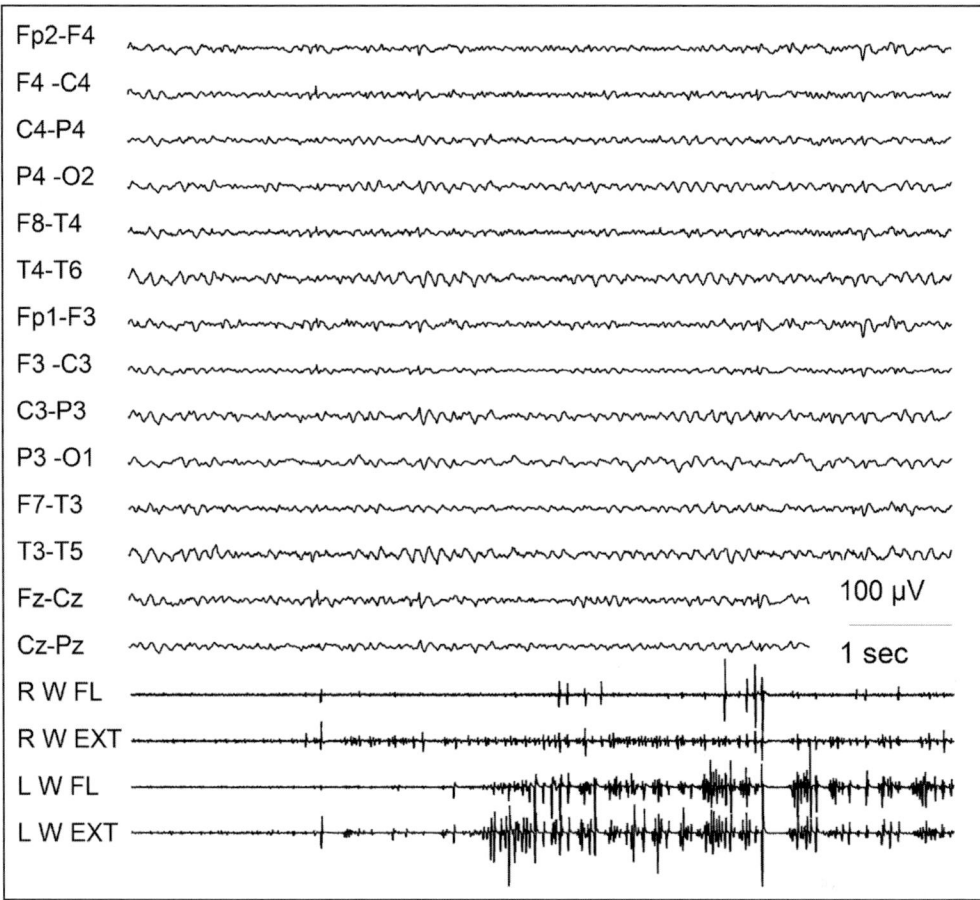

Fig. 1. Patient with Unverricht-Lundborg disease. Polygraphic recording with the patient at rest showing fragmentary multifocal myoclonus without overt EEG correlate (EMG artefacts due to myoclonic jerks involving the face are superimposed onto the EEG trace).

A period of suppression of muscle activity without a preceding myoclonus can also produce a negative jerk, due to a sudden interruption and resumption of ongoing muscular activity. This latter phenomenon is referred to as 'negative myoclonus' and is related to a mechanism of supraspinal inhibition lasting from 100 to 500 ms. In PMEs, a mixture of positive and negative myoclonus is common in the same patient. The EMG correlate of a single action myoclonus is an EMG potential of short duration (20 to 30 ms), which appears synchronously in agonist and antagonist muscles (Fig. 3). It is usually followed by an EMG-silent period lasting 40 to 120 ms (in rare cases up to 300 ms). The myoclonic bursts and silent periods are seldom related to EEG spike and waves or polyspike and waves (Tassinari et al., 1974). More often, the EEG correlate is small in transient amplitude, merging with spontaneous EEG activity. The cortical nature of the myoclonic event can be assumed when a time-locked spike or other EEG paroxysmal event is detected on EEG-EMG polygraphic recordings either by visual inspection (see Fig. 1) or by the back-averaging techniques that will be described in detail below. Cortical myoclonus, regardless of whether it is positive or negative, is attributed to a pathologically enhanced excitability of the primary sensorimotor cortex (Obeso et al., 1985), although negative

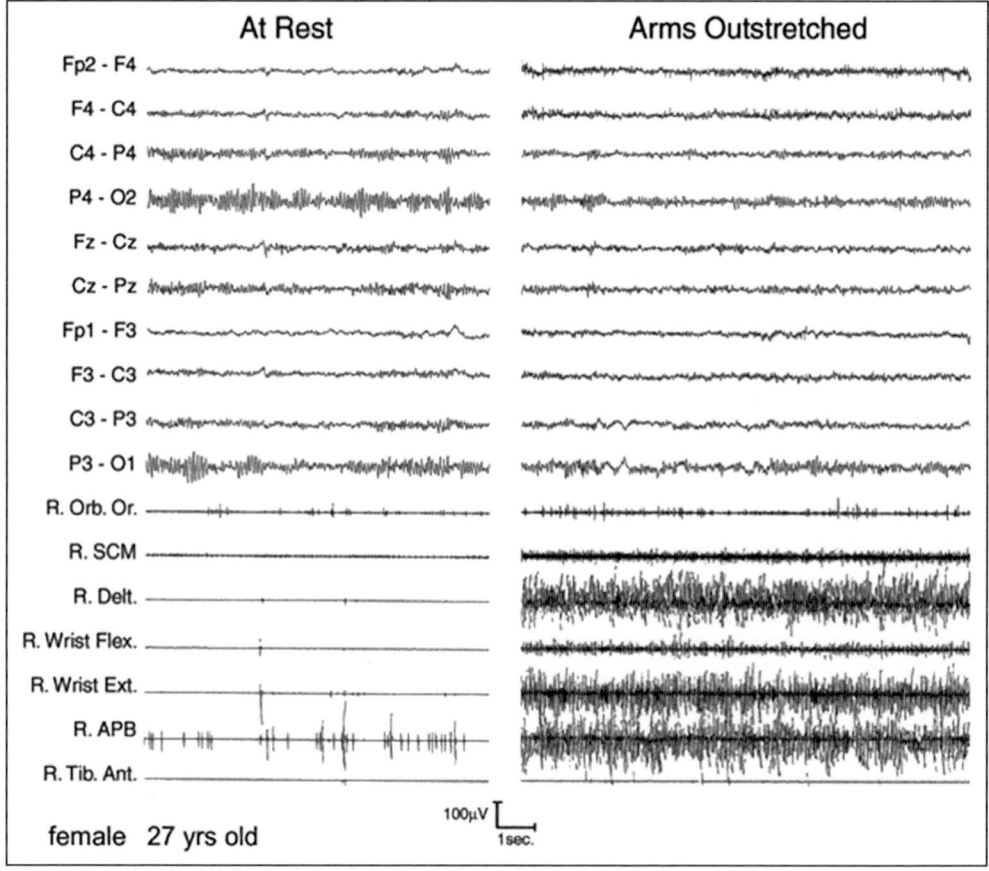

Fig. 2. Patient with PME associated with SCARB2 mutation, at disease onset. Left panel: the patient is at rest; EEG shows preserved background activity without epileptiform abnormalities; on the EMG channels, erratic multifocal myoclonic jerks without EEG correlate are evident. Right panel: the patient keeps her arms outstretched; the EMG channels show continuous rhythmic cortical myoclonic activity at a frequency around 12-20 Hz.

myoclonus may also originate from the pre-motor or supplementary motor area (Rubboli *et al.*, 2006). Additionally, increased excitability of subcortical circuits is considered to be the causative mechanism of subcortical myoclonus which may coexist with cortical myoclonus in PMEs. Additional findings that support the cortical or subcortical origin of myoclonus and their pathophysiological implications will be discussed in detail below.

Polygraphic recordings of PMEs can be complemented with stimulation procedures aimed at revealing their stimulus sensitivity. Photic stimulation should always be applied due to the high frequency of photic reflex myoclonus and/or EEG photosensitivity. Intermittent photic stimulation (IPS) may induce bursts of polyspike-wave discharges associated with massive myoclonic jerks. If the triggering stimulus is prolonged, the clinical response may progress to a generalized convulsion. The mechanism of photic reflex myoclonus involves both occipital and motor cortices, with bilateral spread, presumably mediated by transcallosal connections and propagation down the spinal cord via fast-conducting cortico-spinal pathways (Rubboli *et al.*, 1999).

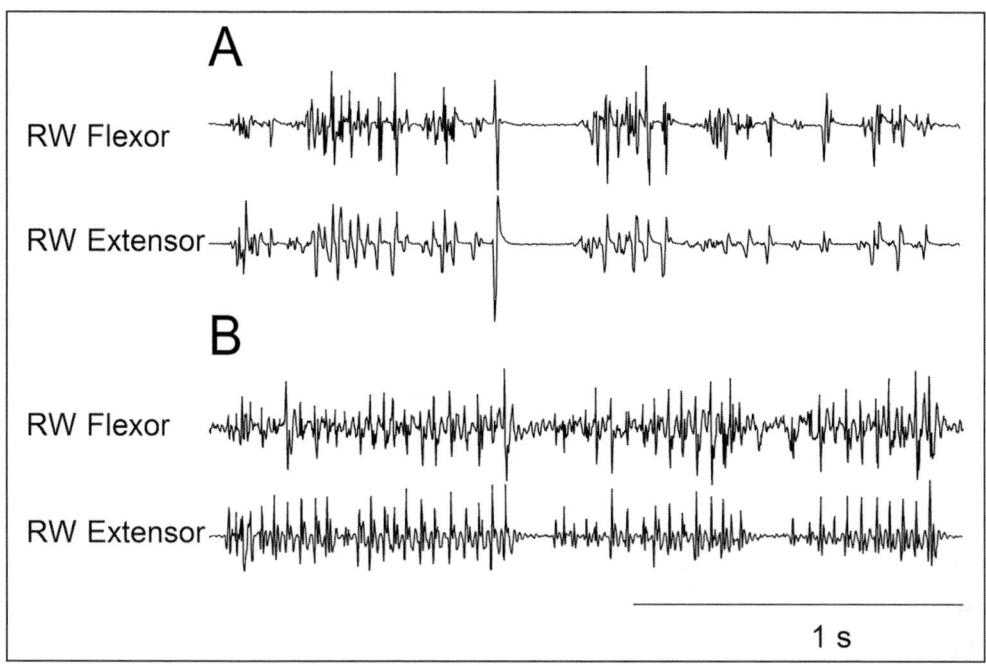

Fig. 3. EMG recording from two antagonist muscles of the right wrist (RW) showing the presence of synchronous EMG bursts with an irregular (A) and quasi-rhythmic (B) course.

Although cortical positive myoclonus usually occurs irregularly, it may appear fairly rhythmical, and may even resemble a tremor (hence the term 'cortical tremor') in some cases of PME (Toro et al., 1993). Brown & Marsden (1996) reported repetitive myoclonus, both spontaneous and stimulus-evoked, at short intervals of around 20 ms in patients with cortical reflex myoclonus. This was associated with repetitive EEG discharges of the same frequency. Enhanced motor cortex hyperexcitability, as the result of loss of intracortical inhibition, possibly due to abnormal GABA-B mediated inhibitory circuits, has been postulated to underlie the susceptibility to generate rhythmic myoclonic activity (Valzania et al., 1999). Rhythmic cortical myoclonus, at a frequency of around 12-20 Hz has also been reported in the recently described PME associated with *SCARB2* mutations (Berkovic et al., 2008; Rubboli et al., 2011) (Fig. 2, right panel). This rhythmic myoclonus, reminiscent of postural tremor, can be evident at disease onset. Its cortical origin has been demonstrated mainly by coherence and phase analysis of EEG-EMG signals, indicating a significant EEG-EMG coupling and a direct corticospinal transfer (Rubboli et al., 2011). Rhythmic jerks in the beta band have also been described in some PMEs associated with rare storage diseases (Brown et al., 1999; Panzica et al., 2003; Canafoglia et al., 2006).

Additional information can be drawn from sleep recordings which should be performed in the PME work-up whenever possible. The results of sleep studies in different PMEs will be discussed in the second section of this chapter.

Coherence study of EEG-EMG relationship in progressive myoclonus epilepsies

Since synchronization between muscles and cortical activities was demonstrated in the 1990s (McLachlan & Leung, 1991; Farmer *et al.*, 1993), methods of analysis relating to the frequency domain have become an important tool for investigating the human motor system, particularly in terms of studying whether specific patterns of neuronal synchrony may be of diagnostic value (Brown *et al.*, 1999; Grosse *et al.*, 2003).

In the last decade, spectral analysis, namely coherence and phase analysis, has been increasingly applied to investigations of the relationship between rhythmic or quasi-rhythmic myoclonic events and EEG oscillations. Indeed, the relationship between EEG or MEG activity and voluntary or involuntary muscle contraction can be studied by calculating the linear cross-correlation over certain frequency bands (coherence) during sustained muscle contraction (corticomuscular coherence) (Conway *et al.*, 1995; Salenius *et al.*, 1997; Halliday *et al.*, 1998; Mima & Hallett, 1999).

Spectral analysis appears to be a powerful method for detecting EEG-EMG coherence (Mima & Hallett, 1999) and MEG-EMG (Salenius *et al.*, 1997; Silen *et al.*, 2000) or EMG-EMG relationships in cortical myoclonus, and has several advantages over the more commonly used jerk-locked back-averaging technique (see below) for a number of reasons. High-frequency myoclonic discharges do not prevent the analysis, no arbitrary trigger level has to be chosen, results can be evaluated from a statistical point of view, and the technique can be automated, such that long sections of signal traces can be analyzed over a short epoch. However, the estimation of EEG-EMG coherence requires relatively artefact-free EEG/MEG epochs, and the recording itself, particularly in children with myoclonus or involuntary jerks, may be difficult and time-consuming.

Brown and colleagues (1999) demonstrated cortical activity related to myoclonic jerking through frequency analysis in five patients in whom jerk-locked back-averaging failed to show any clear EEG transient associated with myoclonic jerks. To estimate coherence and phase spectra, couples of channels are usually investigated by means of cross-spectral analysis based on traditional Fast Fourier Transform (FFT). Selected data are usually divided into consecutive non-overlapping segments, transformed in the frequency domain and then averaged. A trade-off should be considered in the FFT approach between frequency resolution and spectral variance. As window length decreases, variance also decreases, but spectral resolution becomes poorer.

An alternative approach is based on parametric autoregressive (AR) models. The main advantages of spectral AR estimates over FFT-based methods are that they significantly improve frequency resolution since parametric spectra can be evaluated numerically at any number of frequencies and do not require any averaging to obtain a smoothed spectrum (Gath *et al.*, 1992; Pardey *et al.*, 1996; Spyers-Ashby *et al.*, 1998). Conversely, the FFT-based spectra can be evaluated only on the number of samples (N) with harmonically related frequencies. This advantage is particularly important for the analysis of short sequence lengths or epochs characterized by rapid dynamic changes. Moreover, AR spectra can be obtained without windowing the data since no assumptions about samples outside the data sequence are needed. In addition, the inclusion of a noise term in the AR model means that the estimated spectrum is smooth, since its shape depends only on the values of the coefficients used to model the signal. In contrast, in the FFT-based analysis, random fluctuations due to noise can be reduced only by the averaging procedure. The improvement is related to the number of degrees of freedom of the AR model, which is given by N/p where N is the number of samples and p is the model order (Gath *et al.*, 1992). Using the AR model, the number of AR parameters needed to model a time series is typically much lower than the total number of data points composing the signal, and this therefore gives a statistically desirable compact representation of the signal. For FFT methods, by comparison, it is necessary to determine as many coefficients as there are points in a particular data segment. In itself, this is statistically undesirable and this is the reason why one needs to average over a large number of data segments in order to obtain an appropriate spectrum. As a result, it is commonly claimed that AR spectral estimates tend to be more robust than FFT estimates when working with a small data set. These characteristics make it possible to estimate the myoclonic bursts that need to be isolated from periods of normal muscle contractions (as is the case with Unverricht-Lundborg patients), or from the spontaneous 'epileptic' myoclonus associated with diffuse spike-wave discharges (as is the case with Lafora patients) (Panzica *et al.*, 2003). The main problem with AR models is the choice of model order. It is important to stress that the model order determines the number of frequency components contained in the spectra (in a univariate model, the maximum number of peaks in the power spectrum is half of that of the model order and thus determines the 'frequency resolution of the spectrum' (Schlogl & Supp, 2006). The main advantage of the FFT over AR spectral estimation is its computational efficiency.

Using a parametric approach, multivariate AR models can be used to provide a multivariate representation of the signals, from which appropriate measures of coupling can be estimated. In 1991, Kaminski and Blinowska proposed the Directed Transfer Function (DTF) (Kaminski & Blinowska, 1991), a multichannel estimator of the intensity and direction of activity flow, based on a multichannel autoregressive model between couples of channels as a function of the frequency (Mima *et al.*, 2001; Cassidy & Brown, 2003).

In 2001, Baccalá and Sameshima proposed a different multichannel approach, the partial directed coherence (PDC), which allows the direction of information flow between any of the two channels to be estimated by subtracting the interactions and possible common influences due to other remaining simultaneously observed time series (Baccalá & Sameshima, 2001; Meng *et al.*, 2008). By applying this approach, Panzica and collaborators (2014) were recently able to demonstrate, in patients with cortical myoclonus, a significant increase in cortical outflow towards activated muscles, in comparison to healthy controls. Moreover, they showed a more robust EMG outflow toward ipsi and contralateral cortical areas which could maintain jerk recurrence.

In addition, non-stationary or time-varying multivariate AR models have recently been developed and can be applied to study dynamical changes associated with cortico-muscular coupling in patients with myoclonus, when the statistical properties of the signals change substantially over time. Panzica and collaborators (2010) studied myoclonus-related EEG changes in patients with two forms of progressive myoclonus (Unverricht-Lundborg disease and sialidosis) using bivariate time-varying autoregressive models (TVAR). The results indicated that it was possible to detect the presence of prominent peaks of EEG-EMG coherence between the EMG and contralateral frontocentral EEG derivation by TVAR analysis in all patients and, most importantly, differences were disclosed relating to time-frequency spectral profiles correlated with the severity of myoclonus (Fig. 4).

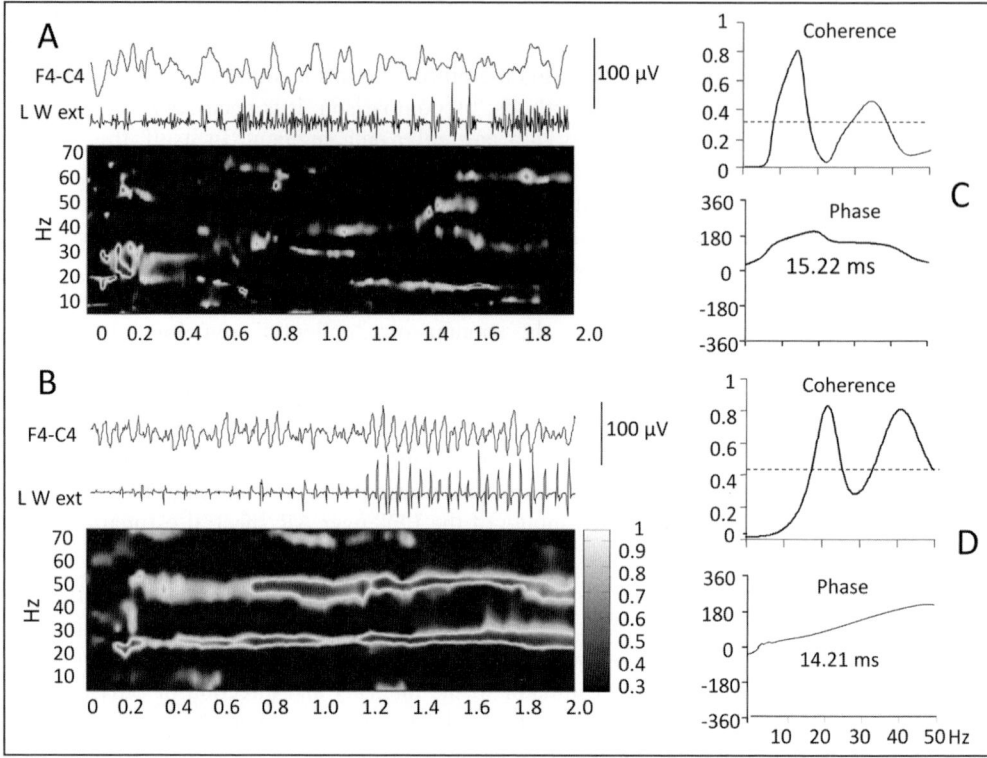

Fig. 4. TVAR analysis of a movement-activated myoclonus in a patient with Unverricht-Lundborg disease (A) and sialidosis (B). Note in the coherence spectrum (B), the presence of significant EEG-EMG coherence in the beta and gamma bands remaining consistent throughout the movement, in contrast with the intermittent course in the ULD patient. (C and D) Mean coherence (the dotted line indicates the 95 per cent confidence limit) and phase spectra obtained from TVAR analysis. The estimated time lag was fitted with a cortico-spinal time transfer.

In patients with cortical myoclonus, regardless of aetiology, frequency analysis showed the presence of an exaggerated coherence peak in the beta band (mainly at 15-20 Hz) between sensorimotor cortex activity and EMG activity that is normally rectified, recorded from muscles co-activated by myoclonic jerks. In this frequency range, often the cortical activity precedes EMG by a time period which is appropriate for conduction in the fast conduction pyramidal pathway (Brown & Marsden, 1996; Brown et al., 1999; Valzania et al., 1999; Silen et al., 2000; Grosse et al., 2003; Panzica et al., 2003). Sometimes, however, the phase difference indicates a time lag that is lower than expected for the fastest conducting pathway (Brown et al., 1998; Ohara et al., 2000). This phenomenon may be due to the presence of multidirectional activities which contribute to the cortico-muscular coherence between muscle and cortex (efferent control from the primary motor cortex to muscle and afferent feedback from the periphery) (Panzica et al., 2012). These findings support the idea that myoclonus may be due to an exaggeration of the cortical drive to muscle observed during voluntary contractions in healthy subjects (Brown et al., 1999).

Unlike coherent beta activity, a coherent gamma peak is not a consistent feature. In healthy subjects, a similarly inconsistent presence of coherent gamma activity has been hypothetically attributed to the variable cortical activation associated with attention or differences in functional cortical-muscular coupling depending on the strength of the muscle contraction (Brown *et al.*, 1998; Mima & Hallett, 1999). Panzica *et al.* (2003), based on a study of patients with different types of PMEs, found constant coherent gamma coherence only in the patients with sialidosis (Fig. 4). In these patients, myoclonic jerks entirely replaced the physiological muscle contractions, which occurred at the onset of movement and throughout posture maintenance, with a rather rhythmic and protracted course, reminiscent of the rhythmical nature of a tremor.

Brown (2007) suggested that prominent and extensive synchronization in the beta band might limit the ability of sensorimotor neurons to code information in time and space, since these neurons preferentially fire at a frequency locked to the beta rhythm. These synchronized discharges of pyramidal neurons are transferred through the pyramidal tract to the peripheral motor system, resulting in synchronous motor unit discharges that may lead to myoclonic jerks, rather than the sustained muscle contractions or movements normally resulting from the relatively asynchronous activation of motor units.

Neurophysiological investigation of brain circuitry sub-serving myoclonus

In this section, we review some neurophysiological techniques in the time domain that may complement the frequency analysis of EEG-EMG polygraphic recordings to investigate whether muscle jerk is associated with any EEG activity and to define their reciprocal time relationship. The first important point concerns the existence of myoclonus-associated scalp electrographical events that precede the myoclonic jerk, thus supporting a cortical origin of myoclonus.

Jerk-locked back-averaging

The potential of this technique to detect non-obvious EEG correlates of myoclonus was first reported by Shibasaki and Kuroiwa (1975) and has been widely employed since then to study involuntary movements.

The principle upon which it is based is that of averaging the EEG (or MEG) recording preceding the muscle jerk such that all activities which are not consistently time related to the jerk are subtracted from one other, while the time-locked EEG potentials preceding myoclonus will summate, resulting in easily recognizable transients which are well-suited to morphological analysis and time relationship calculation (Fig. 5).

According to Kornhuber and Deecke (1965) in their original study of movement-related EEG activities, the backward analysis could be performed by playing back a magnetic tape where polygraphic the EEG-EMG recording has been stored or by introducing a delay-line analogue circuit into the EEG recording system (Franceschetti *et al.*, 1980). With the increased availability of digitized recordings, analysis of the EEG preceding the myoclonic jerk can be easily obtained by setting the analysis window at 200 ms before and 200 ms after the myoclonus onset. The trigger pulse is generated by the myoclonus-related EMG potential either in its original or rectified shape. The definition of the true onset of the EMG potential is crucial to ensure reliable results. The method can also be applied to the study of the negative myoclonus of cortical origin, in which the onset of the EMG silent period is used as a trigger for back-averaging EEG (Ugawa *et al.*, 1989).

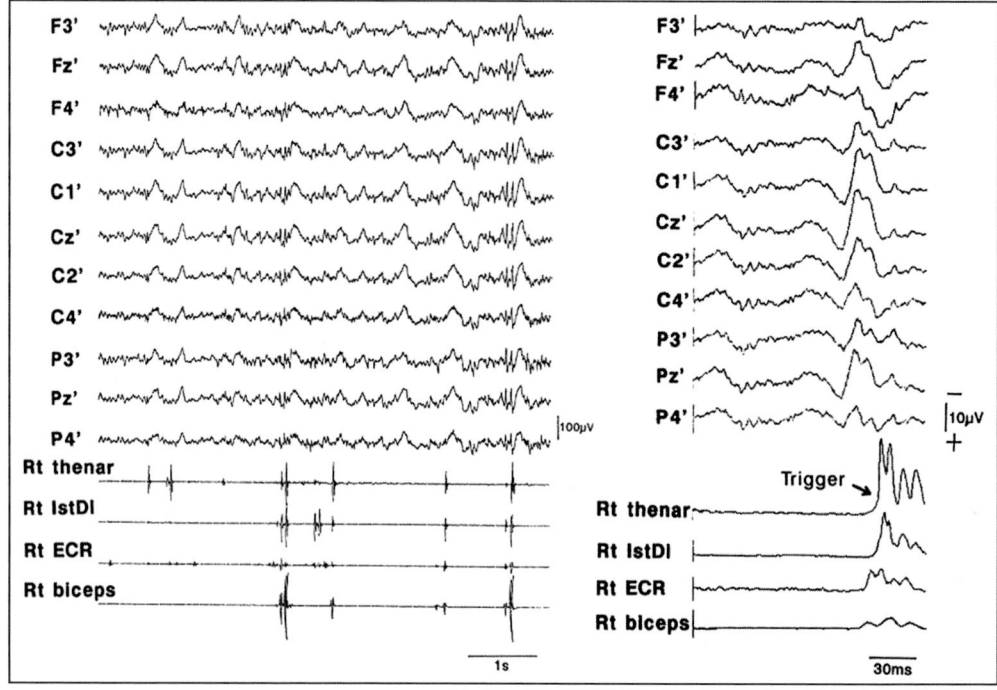

Fig. 5. Left panel: EEG-EMG polygraphic recording in a patient with PME manifesting positive myoclonus in the hands at rest. Note that most myoclonic jerks were associated with a spike-and-wave complex on EEG, and the upward negativity recorded from the ipsilateral earlobe electrode. ECR: extensor carpi radialis muscle; 1stDI: first dorsal interosseous muscle; Rt: right. Right panel: recordings of jerk-locked back-averaging obtained from the same patient. The onset of the EMG discharge from the right thenar muscle was used as a trigger pulse to back-average multichannel EEGs. EEG was recorded from the ipsilateral earlobe electrode. A positive-negative, biphasic EEG spike is observed maximally near the midline vertex, slightly shifted to the left (C1-Cz), and widespread over the scalp. Note that the myoclonic EMG discharge, which was also averaged with respect to the same fiducial point, spreads rapidly from the proximal muscles to the distal ones (modified from Shibasaki & Hallett [2005]).

An EEG potential preceding the muscle jerk by 15-20 ms may express a cortical discharge responsible for the myoclonus and is therefore considered to be compatible with its cortical origin. Shorter intervals or an inverted time relationship with the jerk preceding the EEG potential would rather support a cortical response evoked by the muscle jerk originating in some subcortical structure.

Electrophysiological study of reflex myoclonus

In 1939, Adrian and Moruzzi showed that the stimulus-evoked myoclonus observed in cats anaesthetised with chloralose was due to a discharge travelling in the pyramidal tract and time-locked to a cortical wave (Adrian & Moruzzi, 1939). This 'cortical reflex myoclonus' did not fully account for the muscle jerk observed in the anaesthetised animals, as decortication did not eradicate it completely. The origin of the residual component was found to be in the reticular formation. The observation of stimulus-sensitive myoclonus in different human diseases made it possible to characterize cortical versus reticular reflex myoclonus in several pathological disorders, including PMEs. Their main features are summarized here, in line with the work by Shibasaki and Hallett (2005) and Shibasaki (2012).

Cortical reflex myoclonus

Cortical reflex myoclonus, evoked by electrical shocks delivered to the median nerve at the wrist, is associated with a giant somatosensory evoked potential (SEP), first reported by Dawson in 1947 (Dawson, 1947), with an extreme enlargement of P25 and subsequent components (up to 10 times as large as the normal value), whereas the initial components N20 and P20 are normal or only slightly enhanced (Fig. 6).

However, the studies of somatosensory evoked magnetic fields (Karhu et al., 1994; Mima et al., 1998) shows that M20 is also slightly enhanced in some cases, suggesting hyperactivity of the sensorimotor thalamo-cortical loop. Moreover, these studies demonstrate that the hyperactivity involves the primary somatosensory cortex but not the second somatosensory area, which is not hyperexcitable.

Giant potentials can also be evoked by flash stimulation in photosensitive myoclonus, which is also considered a type of cortical reflex myoclonus (Shibasaki & Neshige, 1987). The areas of enhanced excitability include the occipital and frontal cortices, in which hyperexcitability is considered to account for photo-induced muscle jerks.

The somatosensory stimulus-induced cortical reflex myoclonus is readily evoked in the thenar muscle by stimulating the median nerve at the wrist with a latency of 45 ms, which corresponds to that of the long-loop reflex known as the C reflex (C for 'cortical'), as reported by Sutton and Mayer (1974). The P25 peak of giant SEP and cortical potential preceding the muscle jerk, as revealed by jerk-locked back-averaging, show a similar topography and time interval relationship to myoclonus and are considered to be related to the same pathophysiological mechanisms, *i.e.* cortical hyperexcitability (Shibasaki et al., 1978). Analysis of the latencies of the cortical reflex myoclonus recorded from different muscles shows a rostro-caudal order of activation, compatible with a cortical origin of the myoclonus, generating a signal which travels down the brainstem (Hallett et al., 1979).

Reticular reflex myoclonus

Reticular reflex myoclonus differs from cortical reflex myoclonus in terms of SEP, which is not enhanced, and order of activation of muscles; bulbar muscles are activated first and rostral cranial (*i.e.* facial muscles) muscles and caudal muscles (*i.e.* limb muscles) are involved only subsequently (Hallett et al., 1977).

Cortical and reticular reflex myoclonus can coexist in the same patients with PME. The coexistence of subcortical and cortical myoclonus has been demonstrated on the basis of the discrepancies between the latency of reflex myoclonus and the sum of afferent and efferent times to and from the cortex, as evidenced by TMS studies (Cantello et al., 1997).

Neurophysiological findings in different progressive myoclonus epilepsy forms

PMEs share common neurological signs that include progressively worsening cortical myoclonus and epileptic seizures, with classic onset in late childhood and adolescence. Other neurological symptoms, namely dementia and ataxia, are typically associated with myoclonus-epilepsy syndromes, and occasionally further signs and symptoms are due to the specific impairment of nervous or other systems (Marseille Consensus Group, 1990).

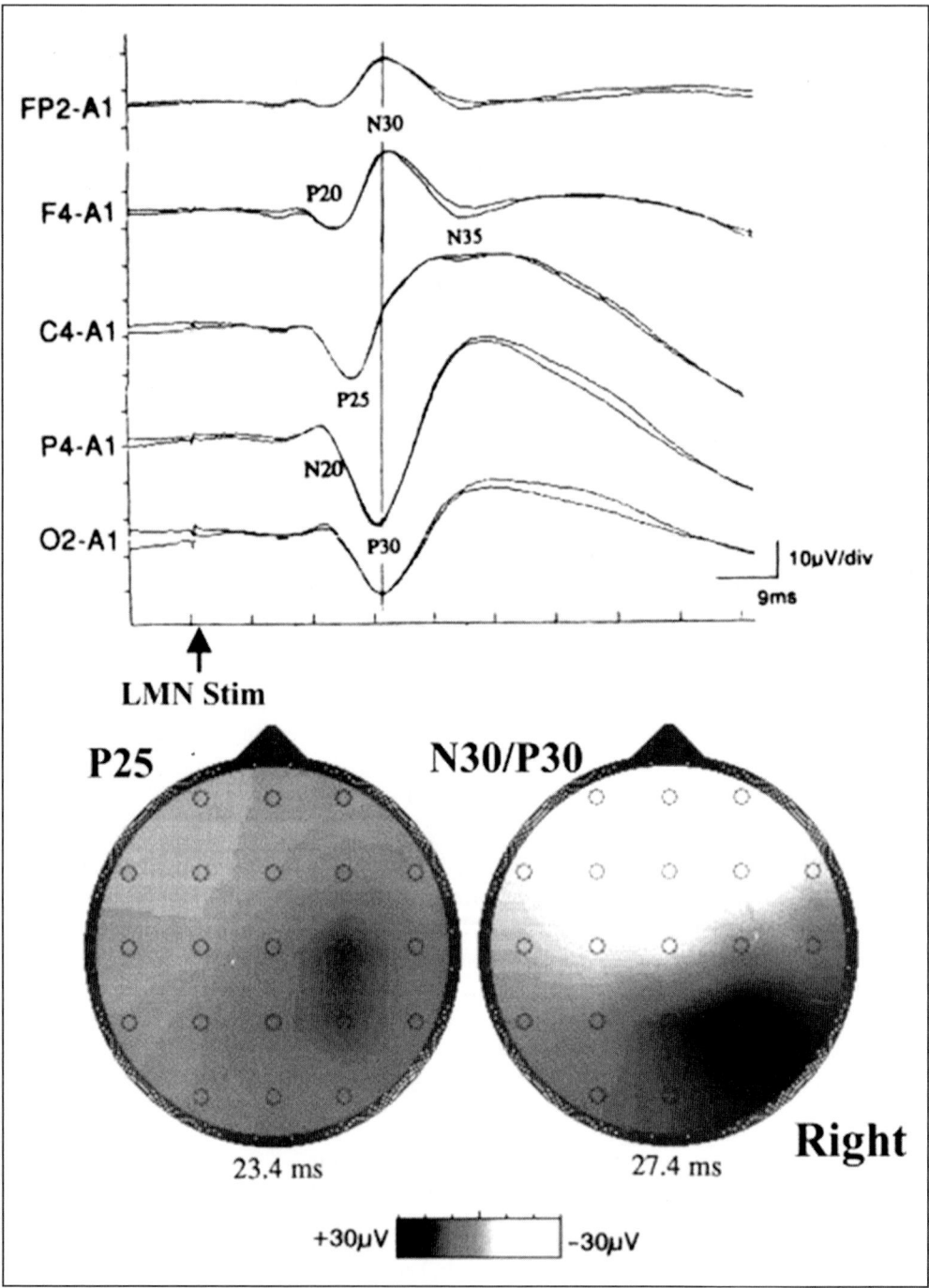

Fig. 6. Somatosensory evoked potential (SEP) waveforms following electrical stimulation of the left median nerve (LMN Stim) of the wrist in a patient with Lafora disease presenting with PME (upper panel), with scalp topography consisting of two peaks (lower panel). Four peaks are clearly distinguishable: N20/P20, P25, N30/P30, and N35. N30/P30 shows a similar distribution to N20/P20 (not shown here), although with opposite polarity. A1: left earlobe electrode. Note the upward negativity. (From Ikeda et al., 1995.)

The PME phenotype includes a 'core' symptom: multi-focal reflex (action-induced) myoclonus. This type of myoclonus is assumed to be cortically generated, since it is typically associated with 'subtle' central EEG changes that can be studied using EEG-EMG relationship analysis (including jerk-locked back-averaging and other techniques). Moreover, cortical myoclonus is coupled with neurophysiological features reflecting neocortical hyperexcitability, such as 'giant' evoked potentials and enhanced long-loop reflexes (Shibasaki, 1988; Shibasaki & Thompson, 2011).

PMEs are derived from heterogeneous genetic disorders (Serratosa *et al.*, 1999; Ramachandran *et al.*, 2009; de Siqueira, 2010), probably with distinct pathological mechanisms, including neural degeneration (Unverricht-Lundborg and dentatorubral-pallidoluysian atrophy), storage disorders (Lafora disease, neural-ceroid-lipofuscinoses, sialidoses, Gaucher III, Niemann Pick type C, and action myoclonus-renal failure syndrome), mitochondrial disorders (myoclonic epilepsy associated with ragged-red fibres), and ion channel dysfunction (Azizieh *et al.*, 2011). Advances in biomolecular research continuously enrich our knowledge of the genetic background of PMEs and their pathogenesis.

Since the causes of PMEs are heterogeneous, they can be expected to affect cortical and subcortical brain structures in varying ways and probably by different mechanisms.

Due to different pathogenetic/neuropathological mechanisms, PME syndromes may present partially different neurophysiological features, which can reflect the prominent dysfunction of distinct cerebral areas or the occurrence of associated symptoms (for instance, the involvement of the peripheral nervous system). Specific neurophysiological findings may be important for diagnostic assessment and phenotypic classification (Kasai *et al.*, 1999; Panzica *et al.*, 2003; Canafoglia *et al.*, 2004; Canafoglia *et al.*, 2010) and may help quantify the severity of the clinical disorder (Garvey *et al.*, 2001) at diagnosis and during follow-up. Indeed, changes in neurophysiological findings relating to the disease course may reflect spontaneous evolution or relate to therapeutic interventions (Kobayashi *et al.*, 2011).

In this section, we address the differences between neurophysiological findings in the main PME forms, Unverricht-Lundborg (EPM1) and Lafora body disease (EPM2), and in some rarer diseases: sialidoses and neuronal-ceroid-lipofuscinoses (NCL) in adults (Kufs disease). With this aim, we report on the EEG-EMG features and neurophysiological findings obtained using somatosensory evoked potentials (SSEPs), long-loop reflexes (LLR) and transcranial magnetic stimulation in these diseases and their changes over time.

EEG-EMG findings may be useful to differentiate between different PMEs

EEG-EMG polygraphy

EPM1

The EEG-EMG features of EPM1, originally described in patients with Baltic myoclonus from a restricted geographical area (Koskiniemi *et al.,* 1974; Norio & Koskiniemi, 1979), include diffuse EEG background slowing with recurrent paroxysms of spike and polyspike and waves, focal spikes in the central region, and marked photosensitivity. A different disease course, probably resulting from more effective treatment (usually including valproate), emerged in more recent observations of large case series. Indeed, EPM1 patients observed in recent years have generally demonstrated normal to slightly slow EEG background and brief and rare epileptic paroxysms of spikes or polyspikes, occasionally associated with spontaneous isolated myoclonic jerks (Canafoglia *et al.*, 2004; Ferlazzo *et al.*, 2007). Segmental myoclonic jerks occurring with voluntary or passive movements (action myoclonus), unrelated to obvious EEG 'epileptic' paroxysms, remain the prominent symptom. Epileptic paroxysms and photosensitivity tend to disappear over the years, together with a relatively stationary phase of the disease (Magaudda et al., 2006; Kälviäinen et al., 2008; Genton, 2010), while some observations indicate progressive impairment of the physiological EEG sleep pattern (Ferlazzo et al., 2007).

EPM2

The EEG-EMG picture observed in EPM2 patients is strikingly different from that of Unverricht-Lundborg, at least in the intermediate and advanced stages. As described by Tassinari et al. (1978), in the first disease period, EEG features may resemble those of primary generalized epilepsy due to preserved background activity and the occurrence of fast spikes, polyspikes, waves and photosensitivity. However, shortly after onset, despite advanced pharmacological treatments, the EEG background markedly slows and posterior or diffuse paroxysms of multiple spikes, associated with atypical (myoclonic-atonic) seizures or absences, sometimes resulting in a non-convulsive status (Fernández-Torre et al., 2012), recur with a high frequency.

Moreover, myoclonus in EPM2 patients shows rather peculiar features, including prominent negative EMG phenomena (Shibasaki, 1995). Voluntary motor activity consistently enhances the occurrence of myoclonic jerks on the activated segment, but it is often difficult to distinguish action myoclonus from the almost incessant spontaneous myoclonus (Canafoglia et al., 2004).

Sialidoses

EEG background activity is substantially preserved, although it may include a moderate amount of theta activity. Brief paroxysms of bilateral spikes and polyspikes and waves, with maximum amplitude on the central EEG regions, may be present, combined with rare spontaneous bilateral myoclonic jerks. Photosensitivity is mild or absent. Myoclonus mainly occurs during motor activity and typically takes a pseudo- rhythmic course (Rapin et al., 1978; Canafoglia et al., 2011).

Rhythmic EEG fast activities are sometimes visible on central and vertex regions, occasionally associated with spikes. The movement-activated central fast rhythm (Kelly et al., 1978), sometimes intermingled with spikes, constitutes a rather typical correlate of the rythmic myoclonus observed during motor activation.

NCL

Clinical and electrophysiological features of adult-onset NCL (Kufs disease) were critically revised by Berkovic et al. (1988). Recently, *CLN6* gene mutations have been found in PME patients with Kufs disease (Arsov et al., 2011). The EEG shows paroxysms of spike-and-slow-wave complexes (Berkovic et al., 1988) or multiple generalized spikes without any slow component (Binelli et al., 2000). Multiple spike discharges may be synchronized with myoclonus and the slow waves with brief EMG, silent in limb muscles (Berkovic et al., 1988). The photoparoxysmal and myoclonic response to photic stimuation is particularly strong both at slow and high (1 to 100 Hz) stimulus frequencies, and low-frequency photoparoxysmal response might be an early clue for diagnosis (Guellerin et al., 2012). Table 1 summarizes the information on EEG-EMG features.

Table 1. EEG-EMG features (in treated patients)

	Background	Epileptic paroxysms		PPR	Spontaneous myoclonus	Action myoclonus
		type	Occurrence		Occurrence	
EPM1	alpha-theta	Diffuse SW/PSW	+	+	+	+++
EPM2	theta-delta	Diffuse SW/PSW and occipital SW	+++	++	+++	++
Sialidoses	alpha-theta	Diffuse SW/PSW	+	+/-	+	+++
Kufs	alpha-theta	Diffuse SW/PSW	++	+++	++	+++

Evolution of EEG-EMG findings during sleep

In Unverricht-Lundborg disease, sleep studies demonstrate: (1) a lack of activation of generalized paroxysmal discharges; and (2) the appearance of focal multiple fast spikes occurring in repetitive bursts, localized over the midline and centroparietal regions, more frequently during REM sleep, particularly when eye movements are abundant. These fast spikes can be time-locked to myoclonic jerks, particularly in muscles which show a striking action myoclonus during wakefulness. In Lafora disease, sleep organization is radically altered, with the barely recognizable different stages. Paroxysmal activity does not appear to increase during sleep; diffuse multiple fast spikes show variable amplitude and topography and can be intermixed with fast activity, while posterior spikes persist during slow sleep and can appear enhanced during REM sleep.

Somatosensory evoked potentials

Giant potentials

In PME patients, early SEP components are typically enlarged, with major emphasis of the P25-N33 waves, which are thought to be connected to the occurrence of reflex myoclonus (Kakigi & Shibasaki, 1987). In a study performed in EPM1 and EPM2 patients (Canafoglia *et al.*, 2004), the peak-to-peak amplitude of N20-P25 was abnormally enlarged in both groups, but N33 was often poorly defined in EPM2 patients, merging in a broad negative wave (N3, peaking between 43.8 to 66.6 ms). Moreover, the P25-N60 and N60 amplitudes were significantly larger in EPM2 patients in comparison to both controls and EPM1 patients (Fig. 7).

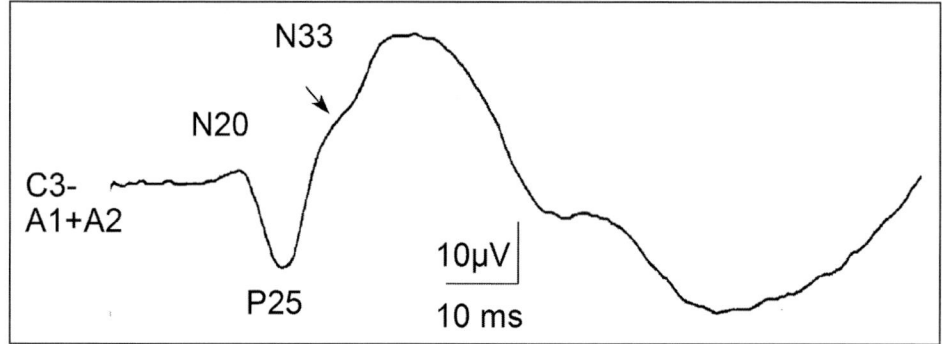

Fig. 7. Giant SEP recorded in a patient with Lafora body disease showing an enlarged N20-P25 component and extremely enhanced P25-N33, merged into a very large middle-latency wave.

Increased SSEP amplitudes may also occur less consistently in patients with sialidoses and Kufs disease, however, they are unlikely to be useful in the differential diagnosis (Berkovic *et al.*, 1988; Canafoglia *et al.*, 2011).

The amplitude of the SSEP components may change over the course of the disease. A recent study (Kobayashi *et al.*, 2011) suggested that in EPM1 patients, the reduction or disappearance of a middle-latency cortical component (labeled N40) is associated with a decrease in epileptiform discharges at the plateau stage of the disease. Conversely, in EPM2 patients, early and middle-latency SSEP components may increase during the disease, alongside the worsening course of the myoclonus and seizures.

SEP latencies

Various studies indicate that the latencies of the early cortical SSEP components increase (Mervaala *et al.*, 1984; Canafoglia *et al.*, 2004) due to a delay in the central conduction pathway from the thalamus to the somatosensory cortex, while in EPM2 patients, the conduction studies gave normal results (Canafoglia *et al.,* 2004) (Fig. 8A).

In patients with sialidosis, the possible co-occurrence of polyneuropathy is typically associated with prolonged latencies (Canafoglia *et al.*, 2011).

Long latency reflex (LLR)

LLR is the neurophysiological correlate of reflex myoclonus. A comparative study has suggested that facilitated LLRs are more common in EPM1 than EPM2 patients, probably reflecting the prominence of reflex myoclonus in this disorder. LLR latencies were briefer in EPM1 than in EPM2 patients (Canafoglia *et al.*, 2004) (Fig. 8B).

In sialidoses patients, the shape of LLR often includes multiple waves, probably reflecting the rhythmic occurrence of the jerks (Franceschetti *et al.*, 1980; Tobimatsu *et al.*, 1985; Canafoglia *et al.*, 2011).

Cortical relay time (CRT)

According to a comparative study (Canafoglia *et al.*, 2004) the CRT was significantly briefer in both EPM1 and EPM2 patients, in comparison to that of healthy controls. The CRT was particularly brief in EPM1 patients, due to their delayed N20 latency, together with short LLR latency (Fig. 8C).

Transcranial magnetic stimulation

Resting motor threshold is typically high in most PME patients, a finding that can be probably explained by the AED treatment (Reutens *et al.*, 1993; Manganotti *et al.*, 2001; Canafoglia *et al.*, 2004; Danner *et al.*, 2009, 2013). The high threshold means that, in some patients, MEPs cannot be produced. In EPM1 and EPM2 patients, MEP latencies may be either normal or slightly prolonged (Canafoglia *et al.*, 2004; Danner *et al.*, 2009), while for sialidoses they are typically prolonged due to delays in both peripheral and central conduction (Canafoglia *et al.*, 2011). The silent period (SP) tested in EPM1 patients is abnormally prolonged (Danner *et al.*, 2009). In patients with sialidosis type I, the SP was, conversely, reduced (Huang *et al.*, 2008).

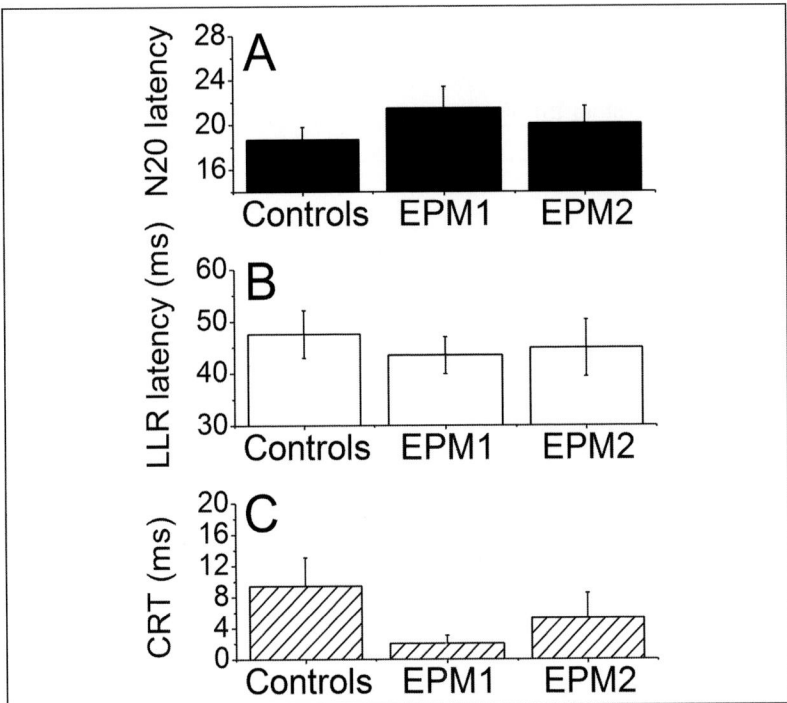

Fig. 8. Graphic representation of N20 latency (A), LLR latency (B) and cortical relay time (C), comparing healthy controls with patients with Unverricht-Lundborg disease (EPM1) or Lafora body disease (EPM2).

Modulation of the motor evoked potentials (MEPs) by afferent somatosensory stimuli

The evaluation of MEP modulation by means of multimodal stimulation protocols suggests some clues about cortical excitability in different PMEs.

Both healthy subjects and PME patients had larger MEP amplitudes after conditioning stimuli (R2) to peripheral mixed nerves, in comparison to basal (non-conditioned) MEP amplitudes (R1); this finding was more evident at inter-stimulus intervals (ISIs), ranging from 30 to 80 ms (Reutens et al., 1993; Cantello et al., 1997; Canafoglia et al., 2004). Digital stimulation markedly facilitated conditioned motor evoked potentials at ISIs ranging from 25 to 40 ms in all patients. This pattern was significantly different from the inhibition observed in controls at the same ISIs (Manganotti et al., 2001).

A comparative analysis of the results obtained in EPM1 and EPM2 patients (Canafoglia et al., 2004) indicated that the degree and time course of MEP facilitation was different for EPM1 compared to EPM2. Indeed, EPM2 patients maintained a significantly higher MEP facilitation at ISIs of between 40 and 60 ms, whereas EPM1 patients had a higher facilitation only at an ISI of between 20 and 40 ms (Fig. 9).

Intracortical inhibition and facilitation tested with paired magnetic pulses

In patients with cortical myoclonus, short interval intracortical inhibition (SICI) is generally reduced (Brown et al., 1996; Manganotti et al., 2001; Hanajima et al., 2008). A comparative study in patients with EPM1 and EPM2 (Canafoglia et al., 2010) indicated that both the EPM1 and EPM2 patients showed significantly less inhibition than the healthy subjects, with no difference between the two patient groups, with the exception of an ISI of 6 ms; at this ISI there was a significant enhanced inhibition in EPM2 with respect to EPM1 patients. Intracortical facilitation (ICF) was normal in EPM1 patients, while there was a significantly reduced facilitation in EPM2 patients at an ISI of 10 ms.

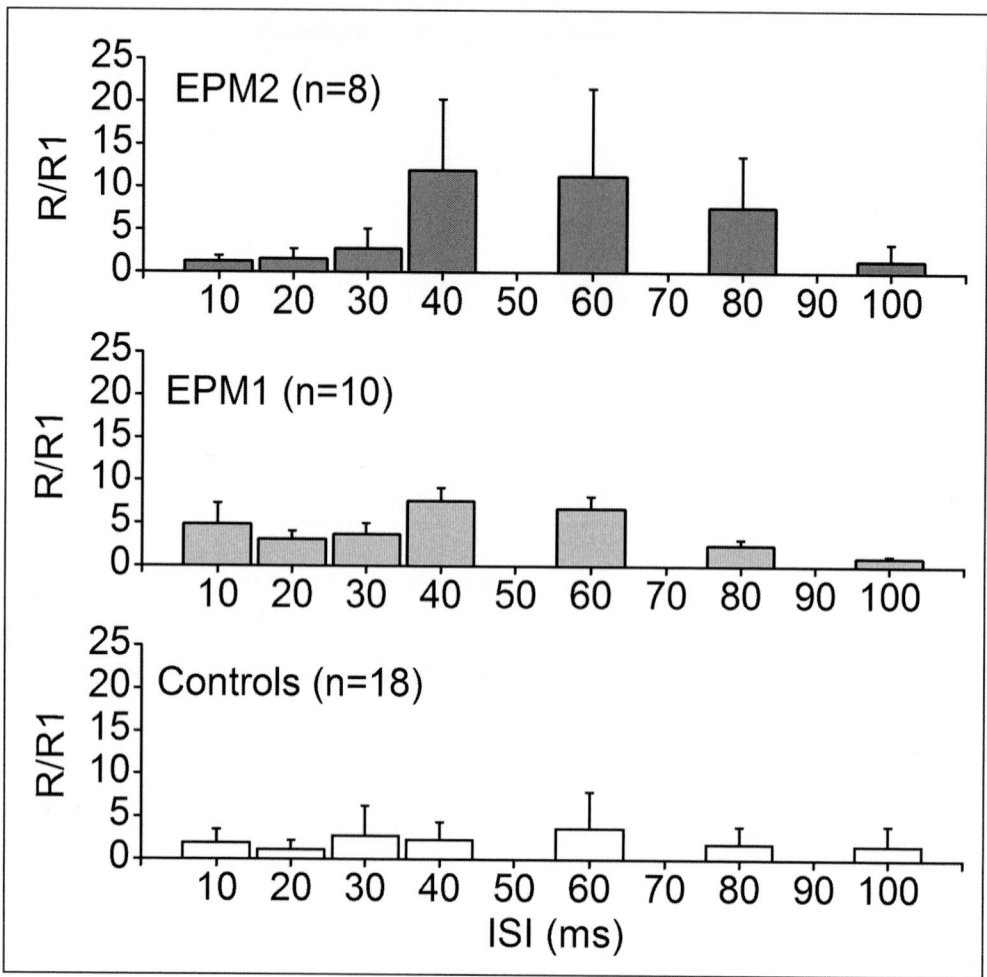

Fig. 9. *Graphic representation of interaction between peripheral somatosensory stimuli and transcranial magnetic stimulation (TMS). Note the different profiles between controls and both PME groups indicating the amplification of the effect of sensory stimulus on motor cortex excitability. Moreover, Lafora patients show a larger and long-lasting excitatory interaction.*

Data obtained in sporadic patients with sialidosis (Brown et al., 1996; Manganotti et al., 2001) and in a homogeneous series of patients with sialidosis type I (Huang et al., 2008) indicated a reduced SICI. In those patients, ICF was normal.

Long interval intracortical inhibition (LICI) was generally impaired in patients with cortical myoclonus (Valzania et al., 1999). However, a comparative study in patients (Canafoglia et al., 2010) with EPM1 and EPM2 revealed significantly less inhibition in EPM2 patients with afferent stimuli (ISIs: 20 and 40 ms; ISIs: 30-80 ms).

Table 2. Neurophysiological parameters in different PMEs

	SSEP	LLR	SP	CRT	MEP facilitation	SICI	ICF	LICI
EPM1	Enlarged N20-P25	++	Prolonged	Reduced	+++	Reduced	Normal	Normal
EPM2	N20-P25 and N3 giant	+	ND	Reduced	+++	Reduced	Reduced	Reduced
Sialidoses	Normal or giant	++	Reduced	Reduced	ND	ND	Normal	ND
Kufs	Normal or giant	ND	ND	ND	ND	ND	ND	ND

Cortical plasticity

Cortical plasticity may be tested by means of repetitive TMS protocols. A study performed using a paired associative stimulation protocol indicated altered plasticity of the sensorimotor cortex in EPM1 patients. These patients exhibited an average decrease of 15 per cent in motor-evoked potential amplitudes, 30 minutes after paired associative stimulation, while in the control subjects, there was a significant increase (Danner *et al.*, 2011). Again, AEDs may have an important influence upon these results.

Conclusions

The neurophysiological evaluation of patients with different PMEs demonstrates the presence of peculiar features that, although not strictly distinctive, suggest different mechanisms underlying the generation of myoclonus. Most patients who were included in the study protocols were treated with multiple drugs, mainly AEDs, which may have influenced some results. However, since the treatment was relatively similar in the various PME syndromes, the differences observed actually suggest different dysfunctions affecting the circuitries sustaining myoclonic jerks.

In EPM1 patients, myoclonus was regularly induced by action and was associated with exaggerated LLRs and early facilitation of the motor cortex by afferent stimuli. These findings, associated with the increased P25-N33 SSEP component, completely fit the definition of cortical reflex myoclonus (Shibasaki & Thompson, 2011). The finding of a short cortical relay time suggests the possibility of an alternative transcortical loop generating reflex myoclonus, passing through the thalamus directly to the motor cortex (Canafoglia *et al.*, 2004). This hypothesis also agrees with the finding in EPM1 patients, of an early facilitation of the motor cortex by conditioning stimuli (possibly following premature invasion of the motor cortex by somatosensory afferent volleys).

The findings obtained with paired TMS stimulation clearly indicated a defective inhibition, probably due to defective GABA circuitry (Canafoglia *et al.*, 2010), in line with the observation made in the CSTB mouse model, suggesting a prominent reduction in GABA-dependent inhibitory function in both the hippocampus and neocortex (Franceschetti *et al.*, 2007; Buzzi *et al.*, 2012).

The finding of abnormal cortical plasticity indicating defective sensorimotor integration may be associated with the previously reported structural and physiological abnormalities of the primary motor cortex in EPM1 patients (Danner et al., 2011).

In EPM2 patients, neurophysiological findings differ from those found in EPM1 patients, suggesting a more complex circuitry sustaining the severe myoclonic presentation. LLRs are more often within the normal range, corresponding to a less significant reflex myoclonus. Conversely, the prolonged late facilitation of motor cortex found by applying sensory stimuli followed by magnetic stimuli, and the enhanced middle latency SSEP components can, conversely, match a more complex circuitry, generating the high propensity of these patients to show spontaneous epileptic myoclonus. The profile of cortical excitability revealed by paired pulse with TMS, showing multiple abnormalities, not limited to short-time interaction or even late interaction, revealed by ICF and LICI, may support this interpretation, suggesting a more complex, hyperexcitable network and a more extensive defect of the inhibitory mechanisms, possibly related to GABA-B mediation (Ziemann, 2004).

Polyglucosan accumulation in dendrites typically occurring in this disorder (Chan et al., 2004) may directly cause an imbalance between GABAergic and glutamatergic post-synaptic inputs to the dendrite tree or changes in the dendrite electrotonic properties capable of modifying the transfer of inputs to the neuronal soma.

In sialidoses, neurophysiological findings mainly overlap those observed in EPM1, since myoclonus prominently presents as a reflex phenomenon and as action-activated. The most characteristic feature is the rhythmic time course of action myoclonus, which substantially replaces the normal muscle contraction throughout the movement. In accordance with this finding, LLR mostly features repetitive components, probably reflecting pathological loops involving the motor cortex, leading to a reverberating circuitry and recurrence of jerks.

Although sialidoses are lysosomal disorders leading to neuron storage which may in turn lead to cell death, only mild spongiosis and lipofuscin granules have been found in the neocortical structures of patients with sialidosis (Allegranza et al., 1989). Thus, the hyperexcitability sustaining myoclonus in this disorder probably arises from subtle circuitry rearrangements rather than from massive cell loss. The circuitry rearrangement resulting from sialidoses may lead to extreme synchronization of the neuronal pools sustaining action-activated jerks.

In conclusion, although PME presentations always include findings reflecting neocortical hyperexcitability, the recognition of subtle differences in diverse genetic disorders may help in designing the diagnostic work-up. Moreover, these differences suggest peculiar dysfunctions in the neuronal network responsible for myoclonus. At present, we can only hypothesize that different modulating mechanisms derived from extra cortical regions (possibly subcortical nuclei and cerebellum) or due to complex cortico-cortical interaction, potentially lead to these different presentations.

In this chapter, we report evidence obtained in the two more common PME forms (EPM1 and EPM2) and for sialidoses, in which different neurophysiological features reflect the different clinical presentation and severity of stimulus reflex vs. spontaneous myoclonus. However, this certainly also occurs for other, rarer PMEs, which are often reported in single cases or minimal case series, preventing an analysis of the comparability of the results obtained by the applied examination protocols. The opportunity to share similar examination procedures could significantly promote better recognition of the specific phenotypes and could better address significant hypotheses to explain genotype-phenotype relationships.

Conflicts of interest: none.

References

Adrian, B.E. & Moruzzi G. (1939): Impulses in the pyramidal tract. *J. Physiol.* **97**, 153–199.

Allegranza, A., Tredici, G., Marmiroli, P., Di Donato, S., Franceschetti, S. & Mariani, C. (1989): Sialidosis type I: pathological study in an adult. *Clin. Neuropathol.* **8**, 266–271.

Arsov, T., Smith, K.R., Damiano, J., et al. (2011): Kufs disease, the major adult form of neuronal ceroid lipofuscinosis, caused by mutations in CLN6. *Am. J. Hum. Genet.* **88**, 566–573.

Azizieh, R., Orduz, D., Van Bogaert, P., et al. (2011): Progressive myoclonic epilepsy-associated gene *KCTD7* is a regulator of potassium conductance in neurons. *Mol. Neurobiol.* **44**, 111–121.

Baccalà, L.A. & Sameshima, K. (2001): Partial directed coherence: a new concept in neural structure determination. *Biol. Cybern.* **84**, 463–474.

Berkovic, S.F., Carpenter, S., Andermann, F., Andermann, E. & Wolfe, L.S. (1988): Kufs' disease: a critical reappraisal. *Brain* **111**, 27–62.

Berkovic, S.F., Dibbens, L.M., Oshlack, A., et al. (2008): Array-based gene discovery with three unrelated subjects shows SCARB2/LIMP-2 deficiency causes myoclonus epilepsy and glomerulosclerosis. *Am. J. Hum. Genet.* **82**, 673–684.

Binelli, S., Canafoglia, L., Panzica, F., Pozzi, A. & Franceschetti, S. (2000): Electroencephalographic features in a series of patients with neuronal ceroid lipofuscinoses. *Neurol. Sci.* **21**, S83–S87.

Brown, P. (2007): Abnormal oscillatory synchronisation in the motor system leads to impaired movement. *Curr. Opin. Neurobiol.* **17**, 656–664.

Brown, P. & Marsden, C.D. (1996): Rhythmic cortical and muscle discharge in cortical myoclonus. *Brain* **119**, 1307–1316.

Brown, P., Ridding, M.C., Werhahn, K.J., Rothwell, J.C. & Marsden, C.D. (1996): Abnormalities of the balance between inhibition and excitation in the motor cortex of patients with cortical myoclonus. *Brain* **119**, 309–317.

Brown, P., Salenius, S., Rothwell, J.C. & Hari, R. (1998): The cortical correlate of the Piper rhythm in man. *J. Neurophysiol.* **80**, 2911–2917.

Brown, P., Farmer, S.F., Halliday, D.M., Marsden, J. & Rosenberg, J.R. (1999): Coherent cortical and muscle discharge in cortical myoclonus. *Brain* **122**, 461–472.

Buzzi, A., Chikladze, M., Falcicchia, C., et al. (2012): Loss of cortical GABA terminals in Unverricht-Lundborg disease. *Neurobiol. Dis.* **47**, 216–224.

Canafoglia, L., Ciano, C., Panzica, F., et al. (2004): Sensorimotor cortex excitability in Unverricht-Lundborg disease and Lafora body disease. *Neurology* **63**, 2309–2315.

Canafoglia. L., Bugiani, M., Uziel, G., et al. (2006): Rhythmic cortical myoclonus in Niemann-Pick disease type C. *Mov. Disord.* **21**, 1453–1456.

Canafoglia, L., Ciano, C., Visani, E., et al. (2010): Short and long interval cortical inhibition in patients with Unverricht-Lundborg and Lafora body disease. *Epilepsy Res.* **89**, 232–237.

Canafoglia, L., Franceschetti, S., Uziel, G., et al. (2011): Characterization of severe action myoclonus in sialidoses. *Epilepsy Res.* **94**, 86–93.

Cantello, R., Gianelli, M., Civardi, C. & Mutani, R. (1997): Focal subcortical reflex myoclonus. A clinical and neurophysiological study. *Arch. Neurol.* **54**, 187–196.

Cassidy, M.J. & Brown, P. (2003): Spectral phase estimates in the setting of multidirectional coupling. *J. Neurosci. Meth.* **127**, 95–103.

Chan, E.M., Ackerley, C.A., Lohi, H., et al. (2004): Laforin preferentially binds the neurotoxic starch-like polyglucosans, which form in its absence in progressive myoclonus epilepsy. *Hum. Mol. Genet.* **13**, 1117–1129.

Conway, B.A., Halliday, D.M., Farmer, S.F., et al. (1995): Synchronization between motor cortex and spinal motoneuronal pool during the performance of a maintained motor task in man. *J. Physiol. (Lond)* **489**, 917–924.

Danner, N., Julkunen, P., Khyuppenen, J., et al. (2009): Altered cortical inhibition in Unverricht-Lundborg type progressive myoclonus epilepsy (EPM1). *Epilepsy Res.* **85**, 81–88.

Danner, N., Säisänen, L., Määttä, S., et al. (2011): Motor cortical plasticity is impaired in Unverricht-Lundborg disease. *Mov. Disord.* **26**, 2095–2100.

Danner, N., Julkunen, P., Hypponen, J., et al. (2013): Alterations of motor cortical excitability and anatomy in Unverricht-Lundborg disease. *Mov. Disorder* **28**, 1860–1867.

Dawson, G.D. (1947): Investigations on a patient subject to myoclonic seizures after sensory stimulation. *J. Neurol. Neurosurg. Psychiatry* **10**, 141–162.

de Siqueira, L.F. (2010): Progressive myoclonic epilepsies: review of clinical, molecular and therapeutic aspects. *J. Neurol.* **257**, 1612–1619.

Farmer, S.F., Bremner, F.D., Halliday, D.M., Rosenberg, J.R. & Stephens, J.A. (1993): The frequency content of common synaptic inputs to motoneurones studied during voluntary isometric contraction in man. *J. Physiol.* **470**, 127–155.

Ferlazzo, E., Magaudda, A., Striano, P., Vi-Hong, N., Serra, S. & Genton, P. (2007): Long-term evolution of EEG in Unverricht-Lundborg disease. *Epilepsy Res.* **73**, 219–227.

Fernández-Torre, J.L., Kaplan, P.W., Rebollo, M., Gutiérrez, A., Hernández-Hernández, M.A. & Vázquez-Higuera, J.L. (2012): Ambulatory non-convulsive status epilepticus evolving into a malignant form. *Epileptic Disord.* **14**, 41–50.

Franceschetti, S., Uziel, G., Di Donato, S., Caimi, L. & Avanzini, G. (1980): Cherry-red spot myoclonus syndrome and alpha-neuraminidase deficiency: neurophysiological, pharmacological and biochemical study in an adult. *J. Neurol. Neurosurg. Psychiatry* **43**, 934–940.

Franceschetti, S., Sancini, G., Buzzi, A., et al. (2007): A pathogenetic hypothesis of Unverricht-Lundborg disease onset and progression. *Neurobiol. Dis.* **25**, 675–685.

Garvey, M.A., Toro, C., Goldstein, S., et al. (2001): Somatosensory evoked potentials as a marker of disease burden in type 3 Gaucher disease. *Neurology* **56**, 391–394.

Gath, I., Feuerstein, C., Tuan Pham, D. & Rondouin, G. (1992): On the tracking of rapid dynamic changes in seizure EEG. *IEEE Trans. Biomed. Eng.* **39**, 952–958.

Genton, P. (2010): Unverricht-Lundborg disease (EPM1). *Epilepsia* **51**, 37–39.

Grosse, P., Guerrini, R., Parmeggiani, L., Bonani, P., Pogosyan, A. & Brown, P. (2003): Abnormal corticomuscular and intermuscular coupling in high-frequency rhythmic myoclonus. *Brain* **126**, 326–342.

Guellerin, J., Hamelin, S., Sabourdy, C. & Vercueil, L. (2012): Low-frequency photoparoxysmal response in adults: an early clue to diagnosis. *J. Clin. Neurophysiol.* **29**, 160–164.

Hallet, M., Chadwick, D., Adam, J. & Marsden, C.D. (1977): Reticular reflex myoclonus: a physiological type of human post-hypoxic myoclonus. *J. Neurol. Neurosurg. Psychiatry* **40**, 253–264.

Hallett, M., Chadwick, D. & Marsden, C.D. (1979): Cortical reflex myoclonus. *Neurology* **29**, 1107–1125.

Halliday, D.M., Conway, B.A., Farmer, S.F. & Rosenberg, J.R. (1998): Using electroencephalography to study functional coupling between cortical activity and electromyograms during voluntary contractions in humans. *Neuroscience Letters* **241**, 5–8.

Hanajima, R., Okabe, S., Terao, Y., et al. (2008): Difference in intracortical inhibition of the motor cortex between cortical myoclonus and focal hand dystonia. *Clin. Neurophysiol.* **119**, 1400–1407.

Huang, Y.Z., Lai, S.C., Lu, C.S., Weng, Y.H., Chuang, W.L. & Chen, RS. (2008): Abnormal cortical excitability with preserved brainstem and spinal reflexes in sialidosis type I. *Clin. Neurophysiol.* **119**, 1042–1050.

Ikeda, A., Shibasaki, H., Nagamine, T., et al. (1995): Peri-rolandic and fronto-parietal components of scalp-recorded giant SEPs in cortical myoclonus. *Electroencephalogr. Clin. Neurophysiol.* **96**, 300–309. Erratum in: *Electroencephalogr. Clin. Neurophysiol.* (1995) **96**, 484.

Kakigi, R. & Shibasaki, H. (1987): Generator mechanisms of giant somatosensory evoked potentials in cortical reflex myoclonus. *Brain* **110**, 1359–1373.

Kälviäinen, R., Khyuppenen, J., Koskenkorva, P., Eriksson, K., Vanninen, R. & Mervaala, E. (2008): Clinical picture of EPM1-Unverricht-Lundborg disease. *Epilepsia* **49**, 549–556.

Kaminski, M.J. & Blinowska, K.J. (1991): A new method of the description of the information flow in the brain structures. *Biol. Cybern.* **65**, 203–210.

Karhu, J., Hari, R., Paetau, R., Kajola, M. & Mervaala, E. (1994): Cortical reactivity in progressive myoclonus epilepsy. *Electroencephalogr. Clin. Neurophysiol.* **90**, 93–102.

Kasai, J., Onuma, T., Kato, M., et al. (1999): Differences in evoked potential characteristics between DRPLA patients and patients with progressive myoclonic epilepsy: preliminary findings indicating usefulness for differential diagnosis. *Epilepsy Res.* **37**, 3–11.

Kelly, J.J.Jr., Sharbrough, F.W. & Westmoreland, B.F. (1978): Movement-activated central fast rhythms: an EEG finding in action myoclonus. *Neurology* **28**, 1037–1040.

Kobayashi, K., Matsumoto, R., Kondo, T., et al. (2011): Decreased cortical excitability in Unverricht-Lundborg disease in the long-term follow-up: a consecutive SEP study. *Clin. Neurophysiol.* **122**, 1617–1621.

Kornhuber, H.H. & Deecke, L. (1965): Changes in the brain potential involuntary movements and passive movements in man: readiness potential and reafferent potentials. *Pflugers. Arch. Gesamte. Physiol. Menschen. Tiere.* **284**, 1–17.

Koskiniemi, M., Donner, M., Majuri, H., Haltia, M. & Norio, R. (1974): Progressive myoclonus epilepsy. A clinical and histopathological study. *Acta Neurol. Scandinav.* **50**, 307–332.

Magaudda, A., Ferlazzo, E., Nguyen, V.H. & Genton, P. (2006): Unverricht-Lundborg disease, a condition with self-limited progression: long-term follow-up of 20 patients. *Epilepsia* **47**, 860–866.

Manganotti, P., Tamburin, S., Zanette, G. & Fiaschi, A. (2001): Hyperexcitable cortical responses in progressive myoclonic epilepsy. *Neurology* **57**, 1793–1799.

Marseille Consensus Group. Classification of progressive myoclonus epilepsies and related disorders. (1990): Classification of progressive myoclonus epilepsies and related disorders. *Ann. Neurol.* **28**, 113–116.

McLachlan, R.S. & Leung, L.W. (1991): A movement-associated fast rolandic rhythm. *Can. J. Neurol. Sci.* **18**, 333–336.

Meng, F., Tong, K., Chan, S., et al. (2008): Study on connectivity between coherent central rhythm and electromyographic activities. *J. Neural. Eng.* **5**, 324–332.

Mervaala, E., Partanen, J.V., Keränen, T., Penttilä, M. & Riekkinen, P. (1984): Prolonged cortical somatosensory evoked potential latencies in progressive myoclonus epilepsy. *J. Neurol. Sci.* **6**, 131–135.

Mima, T. & Hallett, M. (1999): Corticomuscular coherence: a review. *J. Clin. Neurophysiol.* **6**, 501–511.

Mima, T., Nagamine, T., Ikeda, A., Yazawa, S., Kimura, J. & Shibasaki, H. (1998): Pathogenesis of cortical myoclonus studied by magnetoencephalography. *Ann. Neurol.* **43**, 598–607.

Mima, T., Matsuoka, T. & Hallett, M. (2001): Information?ow from the sensorimotor cortex to muscle in humans. *Clin. Neurophysiol.* **112**, 122–126.

Norio, R. & Koskiniemi, M. (1979): Progressive myoclonus epilepsy: genetic and nosological aspects with special reference to 107 Finnish patients. *Clin. Genet.* **15**, 382–398.

Obeso, J.A., Rothwell, J.C. & Marsden, C.D. (1985): The spectrum of cortical myoclonus. From focal reflex jerks to spontaneous motor epilepsy. *Brain* **108**, 193–224.

Ohara, S., Nagamine, T., Ikeda, A., et al. (2000): Electrocorticogram-electromyogram coherence during isometric contraction of hand muscle in human. *Clin. Neurophysiol.* **111**, 2014–2024.

Panzica, F., Canafoglia, L., Franceschetti, S., et al. (2003): Movement-activated myoclonus in genetically defined progressive myoclonic epilepsies: EEG-EMG relationship estimated using autoregressive models. *Clin. Neurophysiol.* **114**, 1041–1052.

Panzica, F., Varotto, G., Canafoglia, L., Rossi-Sebastiano, D., Visani, E. & Franceschetti, S. (2010): EEG-EMG coherence estimated using time-varying autoregressive models in movement-activated myoclonus in patients with progressive myoclonic epilepsies. *Annual Conf. Proc. IEEE Eng. Med. Biol. Soc.* **2010**, 1642–1645.

Panzica, F., Varotto, G., Canafoglia, L. & Franceschetti, S. (2012): EEG-EMG information flow in movement-activated myoclonus in patients with progressive myoclonic epilepsies. *IJBEM* **14**, 167–171.

Panzica, F., Canafoglia, L. & Franceschetti, S. (2014): EEG-EMG information flow in movement-activated myoclonus in patients with Unverricht-Lundborg disease. *Clin Neurophysiol.* **125**, 1803–1808.

Pardey, J., Roberts, S. & Tarassenko, L. (1996): A review of parametric modeling techniques for EEG analysis. *Med. Eng. Phys.* **18**, 2–11.

Ramachandran, N., Girard, J.M., Turnbull. J. & Minassian, B.A. (2009): The autosomal recessively inherited progressive myoclonus epilepsies and their genes. *Epilepsia* **50**, 29–36.

Rapin, I., Goldfischer. S., Katzman, R., Engel, J.Jr. & O'Brien, J.S. (1978): The cherry-red spot myoclonus syndrome. *Ann. Neurol.* **3**, 234–242.

Reutens, D.C., Berkovic, S., Macdonell, R.A. & Blandin, P.F. (1993): Magnetic stimulation of the brain in generalized epilepsy: reversal of cortical excitability by anticonvulsants. *Ann. Neurol.* **34**, 351–355.

Rubboli, G., Meletti, S., Gardella, E., et al. (1999): Photic reflex myoclonus: a neurophysiological study in progressive myoclonus epilepsies. *Epilepsia* **40**, 50–58.

Rubboli, G., Mai, R., Meletti, S., et al. (2006): Negative myoclonus induced by cortical electrical stimulation in epileptic patients. *Brain* **129**, 65–81.

Rubboli, G., Franceschetti, S., Berkovic, S.F., et al. (2011): Clinical and neurophysiologic features of progressive myoclonus epilepsy without renal failure caused by SCARB2 mutations. *Epilepsia* **52**, 2356–2363.

Salenius, S., Portin, K., Kajola, M., Salmelin, R. & Hari, R. (1997): Cortical control of human motoneuron firing during isometric contraction. *J. Neurophysiol.* **77**, 3401–3405.

Schlogl, A. & Supp, G. (2006): Analyzing event-related EEG data with multivariate autoregressive parameters. In: *Progress in Brain Research*, eds. C. Neuper & W. Klimesch. Amsterdam: Elsevier B.V., vol. 159, pp. 135–157.

Serratosa, J.M., Gardiner, R.M., Lehesjoki, A.E., Pennacchio, L.A. & Myers, R.M. (1999): The molecular genetic bases of the progressive myoclonus epilepsies. *Adv. Neurol.* **79**, 383–398.

Shibasaki, H. (1988): AAEE Minimograph #30: electrophysiologic studies of myoclonus. *Muscle Nerve* **11**, 899–907.

Shibasaki, H. (1995): Pathophysiology of negative myoclonus and asterixis. In: *Adv. Neurol. Negative motor phenomena,* eds. S. Fahn, M. Hallett, H.O. Lüders & CD Marsden. Philadelphia: Lippincott-Raven Publishers, vol. 67, pp. 199–209.

Shibasaki, H. (2012): Cortical activities associated with voluntary movements and involuntary movements. *Clin. Neurophysiol.* **123,** 229–243.

Shibasaki, H. & Kuroiwa, Y. (1975): Electroencephalographic correlates of myoclonus. *Electroenceph. Clin. Neurophysiol.* **39,** 455–463.

Shibasaki, H. & Neshige, R. (1987): Photic cortical reflex myoclonus. *Ann. Neurol.* **22,** 252–257.

Shibasaki, H. & Hallett, M. (2005): Electrophysiological studies of myoclonus. *Muscle Nerve* **31,** 157–174.

Shibasaki, H. & Thompson, P.D. (2011): Milestones in myoclonus. *Mov. Disord.* **26,** 1142–1148.

Shibasaki, H., Yamashita, Y. & Kuroiwa, Y. (1978): Electroencaphalographyc studies of myoclonus. Myoclonus-related cortical spikes and high amplitude somatosensory evoked potentials. *Brain* **101,** 447–460.

Silen, T., Forss, N., Jensen, O. & Hari, R. (2000): Abnormal reactivity of the approximately 20-Hz motor cortex rhythm in Unverricht Lundborg type progressive myoclonus epilepsy. *Neuroimage* **12,** 707–712.

Spyers-Ashby, J.M., Bain, P.G. & Roberts, S.J. (1998): A comparison of fast Fourier transform (FFT) and autoregressive (AR) spectral estimation techniques for the analysis of tremor data. *J. Neurosci. Methods* **83,** 35–43

Sutton, G.G. & Mayer, R.F. (1974): Focal reflex myoclonus. *J. Neurol. Neurosurg. Psychiatry* **37,** 207–217.

Tassinari, C.A. & Rubboli, G. (2008): Polygraphic recordings. In: *Epilepsy. A comprehensive textbook,* eds. J.Jr. Engel, & T.A. Pedley. Philadelphia: Walters Kluwer-Lippincott Williams & Wilkins, pp. 873–894.

Tassinari, C.A., Bureau-Paillas, M., Grasso, E. & Roger, J. (1974): Etude electroencephalographique de la dyssynergie cerebelleuse myoclonique avec epilepsie (syndrome de Ramsay-Hunt). *Rev. EEG Neurophysiol.* **4,** 407–428.

Tassinari, C.A., Bureau-Paillas, M., Dalla Bernardina, B., *et al.* (1978): La maladie de Lafora. *Rev. EEG Neurophysiol. Clin.* **8,** 107–122.

Tobimatsu, S., Fukui, R., Shibasaki, H., Kato, M. & Kuroiwa, Y. (1985): Electrophysiological studies of myoclonus in sialidosis type 2. *Electroencephalogr. Clin. Neurophysiol.* **60,** 16–22.

Toro, C., Pascual-Leone, A., Deuschl, G., Tate, E., Pranzatelli, M.R. & Hallett, M. (1993): Cortical tremor. A common manifestation of cortical myoclonus. *Neurology* **43,** 2346–2353.

Ugawa, Y., Shimpo, T. & Mannen, T. (1989): Physiological analysis of asterixis: silent period locked averaging. *J. Neurol. Neurosurg. Psychiatry* **52,** 89–92.

Valzania, F., Strafella, A.P., Tropeani, A., Rubboli, G., Nassetti, S.A. & Tassinari, C.A. (1999): Facilitation of rhythmic events in progressive myoclonus epilepsy: a transcranial magnetic stimulation study. *Clin. Neurophysiol.* **110,** 152–157.

Ziemann, U. (2004): TMS and drugs. *Clin. Neurophysiol.* **115,** 1717–1729.

Chapter 3

Unverricht-Lundborg disease

Arielle Crespel[1], Edoardo Ferlazzo[2], Silvana Franceschetti[3], Pierre Genton[4], Riadh Gouider[5], Reetta Kälviäinen[6], Miikka Korja[7], Maria K. Lehtinen[8], Esa Mervaala[9], Michele Simonato[10] and Annika Vaarmann[11]

[1] *Epilepsy Unit, Hôpital Gui-de-Chauliac, Montpellier, France;*
Research Unit 'Movement Disorders' (URMA), Department of Neurobiology,
Institute of Functional Genomics, Montpellier, France
[2] *Magna Graecia University of Catanzaro, Department of Medical and Surgical Sciences, Italy*
[3] *Neurophysiopathology and Epilepsy, Fondazione I.R.C.C.S. Istituto Neurologico Carlo Besta, via Celoria 11,*
20133 Milan, Italy
[4] *Hôpital Henri-Gastaut, Marseille, France*
[5] *Razi Hospital, University of Medicine of Tunis, Tunisia*
[6] *University of Eastern Finland, Kuopio, Finland*
[7] *Department of Neurosurgery, University of Helsinki and Helsinki University Hospital, Finland*
[8] *Department of Pathology, Boston Children's Hospital, Harvard Medical School, Boston, USA*
[9] *University of Eastern Finland, Kuopio, Finland*
[10] *San Raffaele Hospital, Milan, Italy*
[11] *Department of Pharmacology, University of Tartu, Tartu, Estonia*
Maria.Lehtinen@childrens.harvard.edu

Summary

We first review the clinical presentation and current therapeutic approaches available for treating Unverricht-Lundborg disease (ULD), a progressive myoclonus epilepsy. Next, we describe the identification of disease-causing mutations in the gene encoding cystatin B (*CSTB*). A *CSTB*-deficient mouse model, which recapitulates the key features of ULD including myoclonic seizures, ataxia, and neuronal loss, was generated to shed light on the mechanisms contributing to disease pathophysiology. Studies with this model have elucidated the diverse biological roles for Cstb from functioning as a protease inhibitor, to regulating glial activation, oxidative stress, serotonergic neurotransmission, and hyperexcitability. These findings set the stage for future studies that may open avenues to improved therapeutic approaches.

Introduction

Unverricht-Lundborg disease (ULD) (EPM1) is the 'purest' type of progressive myoclonus epilepsy (PME), with only minor symptoms associated with epileptic seizures and myoclonus. H. Unverricht and H. Lundborg described the condition in 1891 (in Estonia) and 1904 (in Sweden), respectively. The recognition of ULD is still lacking in areas of low prevalence, moreover, the distribution of ULD around the world is highly variable which is due to several factors: i) unequal distribution of the genetic defect between different populations; ii) an autosomal recessive mode of inheritance, which implies higher prevalence in areas and cultures with high consanguinity or a founder effect; and iii) variable availability of modern diagnostic procedures, including molecular biological techniques. Although ULD remains uncommon, it has been increasingly diagnosed among patients with drug-resistant myoclonic epilepsy, as shown, for instance, in Holland (de Haan *et al.*, 2004). However, whereas the most common mutation in ULD affects the cystatin B gene (*CSTB*), no evidence for a role of this gene was found in sporadic or familial cases of juvenile myoclonic epilepsy (JME) (Mumoli *et al.*, 2015). The availability of molecular genetic diagnostic techniques in developed countries has certainly helped.

ULD is still considered a severe and disabling condition, however, recent years have witnessed a shift for ULD, from a very severe, even lethal entity, towards a comparatively bearable disability with little impact, for instance, on life expectancy. Aggravation by phenytoin (PHT) (Elridge *et al.*, 1983) has contributed to poor prognosis of ULD in countries where PHT is heavily used and titrated to high doses for resistant seizures. The aim of this chapter is to review the clinical features, prognosis, management, and pathogenesis of ULD.

Clinical characteristics

Onset occurs in late childhood and early adolescence, peaking at around age 12-13. Sex distribution is equal.

Generalized tonic-clonic seizures (GTCSs) are usually grounds for an initial referral. They occur typically at awakening or during sleep. At onset, GTCS cannot be easily differentiated from those observed in JME, and may occur without prior myoclonic jerks. However, with disease progression, they may evolve into *cascade seizures* (Kyllerman *et al.*, 1991), characterized by a build-up of increasingly intense and violent myoclonic jerks, culminating into a short GTCS; some patients do not report clear consciousness and more or less retain normal contact during this type of seizure. Often, patients experience GTCS or major seizures after a period of progressive increase in myoclonus and subsequently experience less myoclonus, with a decreased risk of major seizures for a period that can last days to weeks; this periodicity has already been described by Unverricht and reported for other PMEs (Ferlazzo *et al.*, 2009; Vanni *et al.*, 2014). Besides awakening, there are no clear triggering factors for GTCSs. Of course, modern drug therapy has contributed to the control of these major seizures, which also seem to decrease spontaneously with advancing age (see below).

Myoclonus is already present in the very early stages, with diffuse myoclonic jerks that predominate at awakening. Over a relatively short period (months to a few years), and in spite of antiepileptic treatment, myoclonus becomes movement-related and increases with stress. It also becomes physically challenging for patients, *e.g.* patients may fear using stairs or physical strain, and bilateral, violent myoclonus becomes less apparent (unless the patient is challenged or stressed), and partial, erratic myoclonus predominates. Reflex myoclonus, triggered by sensory stimulation (touch, light, *etc.*), initiation of movement, and surprise, is a prominent feature in some patients. Remarkably, myoclonus is less severe or even absent at rest or during sleep. In the early stage of ULD and in patients who are insufficiently treated, myoclonus may fluctuate within the same day (with maximal myoclonus in the morning and in the latter part of the day, when patients are tired) or with an interval of a number of days, sometimes with marked periodicity. These features, however, become less prominent over the subsequent years and with effective drug therapy. Contrary to major seizures, myoclonus does not spontaneously abate in the long term, but may even slowly increase in some adult or middle-aged patients.

In the more severely affected patients, myoclonus causes major disability; a wheelchair may have to be used and feeding becomes problematic and slow, especially with the intake of liquids (using a straw may be helpful).

Absence, simple motor, or complex focal seizures may occur, but few video-EEG reports of these seizure types have been documented (Kälviäinen *et al.*, 2008).

Photosensitivity, detected in the EEG laboratory for nearly all patients in the early years of the disease, does not pose major problems in daily life, and tends to abate after 5 to 10 years of disease (Ferlazzo *et al.*, 2007).

Associated neurological symptoms are few. Ataxia, impaired walking, and instability upon standing up are associated with the severity of myoclonus. In our experience, patients cease to be ataxic when myoclonus is fully controlled.

Cognitive impairment may be absent or vary from mild to moderate. Many of our patients reached university level and are qualified professionals. However, whenever possible, ULD patients should avoid professions that involve significant physical activity or fine and precise handling of small objects. Neuropsychological impairment may slightly progress over the years. Early evidence points to a 10-point loss of IQ over ten years (Koskiniemi, 1974), and the presence of short-term memory, attention, and executive function impairment is particularly apparent, based on recent studies (Ferlazzo *et al.*, 2009; Giovagnoli *et al.*, 2009).

Psychiatric comorbidities are frequent in ULD but have not been systematically studied. Suicidal behaviour, with loss of interest in life and neglect of therapy, is a common behaviour, however, only one in 60 of our patients committed suicide. Depression is common and was found in six of eight patients by Chew *et al.* (2008).

Prognosis

The long-term evolution is characterized by limited progression after the first five to ten years (Magaudda *et al.*, 2006), with a varying but fairly stable level of disability thereafter; the outcome in adults ranges from independent active life with minimal impairment to severe disability and wheelchair-bound or even bedridden patients. Early death has a comparatively low incidence and may be due to suicide or accidents, but also to SUDEP, the latter mostly in 'undertreated' patients, in relation to persisting convulsive seizures (Khiari *et al.*, 2009).

Management: diagnosis and genetic counselling

Given the absence of specific clinical or pathological markers, a confirmation of diagnosis of ULD based on genotyping is necessary. Diagnosis used to rely on a combination of positive signs and on the absence of the more specific symptoms and markers of other PMEs, but nowadays can be considered to depend entirely on molecular biological techniques. It is our opinion that this procedure, which remains costly, should be justified by solid evidence, and should not be performed, together with a variety of tests, to screen all possible genetic aetiologies in poorly assessed subjects with epilepsy and myoclonus.

The diagnosis of ULD is based on three levels of evidence:

1. Clinical evidence: a combination of history-taking (age at onset, familial and ethnic background, circumstances, and aspects and progression of seizures and myoclonus), examination (including cognitive assessment showing the absence of major and progressive cognitive impairment, and exclusion of associated manifestations such as sensory deficits), and video documentation of myoclonus.

2. Complementary evidence: based on a thorough evaluation of the EEG, polygraphic EEG, and video-EEG recordings (with assessment of changes over time); neurophysiological studies may also help distinguish ULD from other adolescent-onset PMEs, *e.g.* Lafora disease (in which EEG changes are much more spectacular) or juvenile ceroid-lipofuscinosis (with prominent single-flash responses on EEG). A lack of any of the signs and symptoms associated with other PMEs is likely to indicate a diagnosis of ULD, however, other less common PMEs that were recently identified among genetically negative 'ULD' patients may complicate the diagnosis (Franceschetti *et al.*, 2014; Muona *et al.*, 2015)

3. Confirmation of diagnosis: provided nowadays by the demonstration of a pathogenic mutation in both alleles of the *EPM1* gene.

The diagnosis of ULD can be made, or suspected, in various clinical settings. In particular, the most common clinical situation is when idiopathic generalized epilepsy (IGE) or JME has been diagnosed, with a re-assessment of the patient's situation because of an unusual evolution or apparent drug resistance; the clinical work-up should help exclude the possibility of aggravation of IGE by inappropriate AEDs, which may result in a pseudo-PME phenotype.

In some patients with a very likely diagnosis of ULD, the genetic testing of *EPM1* remains negative. Such patients should be discussed with PME specialists; if the clinical work-up has been thorough, there is usually no need to screen the genes associated with the very typical PMEs which manifest within the same age group (LD, juvenile or adult neuronal ceroid lipofuscinosis, MERRF, DRPLA; *etc*), although recently described genetic defects in *SCARB2/LIMP2*, *KCNC1* or *PRICKLE* might be considered. When the molecular defect remains elusive, and the general condition is very much compatible with ULD, the patient should be diagnosed with ULD (or 'ULD-like PME') and managed as other patients with ULD, with reassessment of the case at two- to five-year intervals by specialized teams.

The diagnosis of ULD should not be given to the family before a final and definitive confirmation, because of the multiple psychological problems that surround the diagnosis of this genetic disease. However, it should be given to the patient and caregivers when confirmed, together with as much information as possible about the condition and its prognosis. Patient organizations can be contacted, and quality information is available on the web. The patients should be encouraged to learn more about the condition and to follow the scientific progress on ULD.

The consequences of a diagnosis of ULD for the family of the proband should not be underestimated. Regarding the prospects, time should be devoted to the change in the patient's and family's lives (see below), but also to counselling on the following topics:

The understandable, expected feelings of guilt and resentment associated with the diagnosis of a genetically transmitted condition should be alleviated, with the use of a few simple statements: inheritance is bilateral (*i.e.* the disease is not transmitted specifically from either the father or mother, but potentially from both), the disease results from a very uncommon co-occurrence of abnormal genes (even in consanguineous marriages), and subjects with a single abnormal gene will not have the disease.

One major concern is the possible occurrence of ULD in other family members. The risk can be practically excluded in older, fully asymptomatic siblings, but cannot be excluded in *younger* asymptomatic siblings, *a fortiori* in yet unborn siblings, if the parents are young enough to have other children. Whether siblings, especially younger ones, should be referred for molecular screening is still debatable. For *pre*symptomatic ULD cases, there is no reliable, recommended prophylactic treatment to prevent or delay the appearance and progression of symptoms, but this may change in the near future. Having provided all the relevant information, the physician should come to an agreement with the family and obtain their informed consent for all the possible procedures performed for non-affected family members. Concerning future pregnancies for the parents of a patient with ULD, the risks are easy to explain (the risk of ULD is 25 per cent).

The risk of carrying an abnormal gene and transmitting the condition to other generations is also a major concern in families with ULD. Several of our ULD patients have children but none are affected; following medical advice, they had married 'outside the family', an unusual option in some ethnic contexts. Their siblings, or parents (when wanting children with another spouse), as well as other collaterals, may benefit from molecular screening in order to assess the presence or absence of the pathogenic gene found in the proband.

An important aspect of diagnosis and genetic counselling is financial and the conditions of insurance and reimbursement (or, more basically, the availability of procedures, tests, and medications) differ greatly between countries and social systems. The families should always be informed about the costs involved; the search for a mutation is expensive, but simple screening for a known mutation is less costly. Similarly, the regulations covering genetic diagnosis, screening, and counselling may differ between countries, and clinicians should always conform to local laws. Obtaining informed consent for the successive steps of diagnostic and screening procedures is a minimum.

Management: medical treatment

This type of PME is characterized by two important features:

– The severity of the condition varies greatly between subjects, even within sibships, and a significant proportion of patients will be able to create a family and lead normal, productive lives with normal or adapted employment, while a significant minority will be severely disabled and dependent upon their family or have an institutionalized life. In a previously published series of 20 ULD patients followed for more than 20 years (Magaudda *et al.*, 2006), eight lived autonomously, six had a family with children, six were normally employed, and seven were dependent on others, including two who were wheelchair-bound. In the largest cross-sectional series (77 subjects) evaluated using modern methodology in Finland, one third of the patients had mild myoclonus, one third had moderate myoclonus, and one third were wheelchair-bound due to severe myoclonus (Koskenkorva *et al.*, 2009).

– The disease has limited progression. Over several (up to 10) years following clinical onset, major seizures and photosensitivity disappear in most patients, while myoclonus stabilizes or progresses only minimally (Magaudda *et al.*, 2006). Thus, a reasonably accurate prognosis can be made fairly early during the course of the condition, 5 to 10 years after onset.

AEDs and piracetam (PIR), a more specific antimyoclonic agent, alleviate the burden of seizures and myoclonus, and their effect is felt throughout the course of the disease; unfortunately, this effect is partial in some cases, as medication does not influence the natural course of the disease.

Patients will usually receive an AED after the first GTCS, typically valproic acid (VPA). VPA is normally effective in suppressing, for some time, most GTCS, photosensitivity, and some of the myoclonus. Other AEDs can be used at this stage (Genton et al., 2012); lamotrigine (LTG) is not very advisable in the context of a myoclonic epilepsy, and has been shown to aggravate myoclonus in patients with ULD (Genton et al., 2006); phenobarbital (PB) and primidone are effective, but produce cognitive side effects on top of the complications attributed to the condition; levetiracetam (LEV) is increasingly used early on in adolescents with IGE, hence in ULD cases, even before confirmation of the diagnosis. Other useful drugs include topiramate (TPM) and zonisamide (ZNS), both with marked antimyoclonic effects. Additional relief can be obtained, often transiently, with benzodiazepines (BZD). The latter (usually clobazam, clonazepam, or diazepam) should be used with care because of a marked initial effect followed by rapid tolerance.

For ULD, the paradoxical aggravating effect of some AEDs may be difficult to assess. There is no evidence that carbamazepine (CBZ), oxcarbazepine (OXC), phenytoin (PHT), eslicarbazepine, gabapentin, pregabalin, vigabatrin or lacosamide are of any benefit. Often, withdrawal of one of these AEDs (especially CBZ or OXC) will bring some relief.

For established ULD, AED treatment leads to polytherapy with a combination of several of the drugs quoted above (with the exclusion of LTG); the commonly used combinations are VPA+LEV or TPM or ZNS, with an additional BZD (a three- to five-drug combination is quite usual); one can switch between different BZDs in the event of tolerance. In case of transient worsening, with intense myoclonus and serial seizures, there should be no abrupt change in the usual regimen (except for the interruption of a potentially aggravating AED), and IV BZD as well as IV PHT could be used.

In practice, some patients will fare reasonably well with a limited drug regimen, while others will remain severely disabled, especially with intractable myoclonus, and will have a much heavier pharmacological load. In such patients, specific therapeutic approaches can be discussed:

– vagal nerve stimulation has been tried with success in some individuals (Smith et al., 2000), including three in our personal experience, but the benefit is limited;
– deep brain stimulation has also been used in PME cases, including some patients with ULD; combined subthalamic and thalamic high-frequency stimulation has brought some relief, especially in the least severely affected cases (Wille et al., 2011). Our personal experience with three patients with a severe form of ULD, who received bipallidal stimulation (as used for dystonia and myoclonic dystonia), was disappointing (Crespel, personal communication).

Management: social support

For ULD, a lifelong condition, social support is at least as important as medical treatment. Psychological support can be provided by patient organizations; one such organization exists in France specifically devoted to ULD, but epilepsy organizations in other countries may offer support. The individual patient should also receive professional psychological support whenever necessary throughout the course of ULD. Physical therapy aims at maintaining a good overall muscular condition and at preserving the ability to walk for the more severely affected patients.

Small amounts of alcohol may temporarily relieve myoclonus (Genton and Guerrini, 1990), but patients should be warned about tolerance, and chronic abuse of alcohol clearly worsens the condition. Photosensitivity, with increased myoclonic jerks, usually abates after several years and is seldom a problem in daily life (patients may watch television or use a computer). Most patients experience increased myoclonus (and an increased risk of major seizures) in the morning, especially after abrupt/sudden awakening, during the active phase of the condition, and should be advised to take their time before getting up. The effect of sleep deprivation has not been well documented, but anecdotal evidence shows that it may increase myoclonus and seizures, and should be avoided.

At the onset of seizures, the patient is typically in primary or secondary school and experiencing some difficulties with academic requirements, however, it is usually possible to maintain normal schooling. It is useful to discuss with the parents future professional orientation, in light of the possible disability associated with ULD. In most families, the patient will remain at home, but the environment may need to be adapted, *e.g.* avoidance of the use of stairs or ensuring the proximity of a bathroom. Specialized institutions are used for the most severely disabled patients, or for periods to promote education about the condition.

Re-evaluation at a specialized neurological department can be organized at 6- or 12-month intervals, with acute admissions in case of complications, often due to intercurrent diseases (*e.g.* febrile infections). There should be a link between the reference specialized epilepsy team and the local caregiving structure in case of intercurrent health problems, ranging from dental care to surgical procedures. Long-term psychological support is not always necessary, and additional medication (*e.g.* antidepressants) should be discussed with the reference neurologist. Pregnancies have occurred without major complications in less (or moderately) severe women with ULD.

Adult ULD patients usually reach a level of disability and dependency that will remain fairly stable. As stated above, possibilities range from a fully normal life with minimal impairment and monotherapy (usually with VPA) to institutionalized care.

Pathogenesis of ULD: the role of oxidative stress

Oxidative stress is associated with many neurological conditions, including epilepsies (Chong *et al.*, 2005; Kunz, 2002). Several case reports have suggested that antioxidant therapies, including N-acetylcysteine, may alleviate ULD symptoms (Ben-Menachem *et al.*, 2000; Edwards *et al.*, 2002; Hurd *et al.*, 1996; Selwa, 1999). Consistent with the model in which redox homeostasis may be disrupted in ULD, redox analyses in the *Cstb* knockout mouse have revealed that oxidative damage in the cerebellum contributes to the pathogenesis of murine ULD (Lehtinen *et al.*, 2009). Deregulation of antioxidants, including superoxide dismutase (SOD) and the antioxidant glutathione (GSH), are disrupted in the cerebella of ULD mice. The ratio of oxidized to reduced glutathione (GSSG:GSH), a hallmark of oxidative damage, is also increased in ULD mice. Detailed analyses have uncovered progressive lipid peroxidation in the cerebella of ULD mice. Lipid peroxidation accelerates with age, beginning at baseline in young adult mice (two months of age) and increasing nearly five-fold in six-month-old mice, compared to controls. Evidence for cellular adaptation to accumulating lipid peroxidation was also observed as the activity of glutathione peroxidase, an enzyme that reduces lipid hydroperoxides, increases in ULD mice, compared to controls (Lehtinen *et al.*, 2009).

A hallmark of the ULD mouse model is a progressive loss of cerebellar granule neurons (Pennacchio *et al.*, 1998). Cerebellar granule neurons can be isolated, cultured, and genetically manipulated *in vitro* (Lehtinen *et al.*, 2006), thus providing a powerful experimental tool for investigating the cellular role of Cstb. In these types of *in vitro* studies, healthy neurons upregulate *Cstb* transcription when challenged by peroxide-induced oxidative stress (Lehtinen *et al.*, 2009). Most patients with classic autosomal recessive ULD harbour an unstable dodecamer repeat expansion (5'-CCC-CGC-CCC-GCG-3') in at least one allele in the *Cstb* promoter region (Pennacchio *et al.*, 1996; Joensuu *et al.*, 2008; Lafreniere *et al.*, 1997; Lalioti *et al.*, 1997). Introducing a similar expansion into neurons prevents *Cstb* upregulation during oxidative stress, suggesting that the inability to upregulate *Cstb* expression impairs normal neuronal responses to oxidative stress. Consistent with this model, reducing *Cstb* expression by RNA interference (RNAi) or genetic deletion in knockout mice sensitizes neurons to oxidative stress-induced death (Lehtinen *et al.*, 2009).

As part of its downstream signalling, Cstb inhibits the lysosomal protease cathepsin B (Turk and Bode, 1991). Cathepsin B over-expression promotes neuronal death, and cathepsin B activity is upregulated in both *Cstb*-deficient cells, as well as in ULD patients with *CSTB* mutations (Rinne *et al.*, 2002). Importantly, the neuronal cell death that occurs upon *Cstb* loss can be inhibited by a concomitant decrease in cathepsin B both *in vitro* (Lehtinen *et al.*, 2009) and *in vivo* (Houseweart *et al.*, 2003), supporting the model that homeostasis related to Cstb-cathepsin B signalling regulates neuronal survival in the mouse model of ULD.

The identification of a role for Cstb in oxidative stress responses in neurons, together with reports that antioxidant therapies alleviate some symptoms of ULD (Ben-Menachem *et al.*, 2000; Edwards *et al.*, 2002; Hurd *et al.*, 1996; Selwa, 1999), provide us with a better understanding of ULD disease pathophysiology. However, whether oxidative damage is a primary cause of disease onset and progression remains to be elucidated. It will be important in future studies to further investigate Cstb-cathepsin B signalling, as well as the downstream consequences of selective oxidative damage to cerebellar lipids. These types of studies may shed light on new approaches to selectively tailor therapies for ULD.

Pathogenesis of ULD: disruption in serotonin metabolism

5-hydroxytryptamine (5HT) metabolism may contribute to ULD pathogenesis. Indeed, an early report identified decreased availability of L-tryptophan (TRP) and its metabolites in cerebrospinal fluid and blood of ULD patients (Pranzatelli *et al.*, 1995). These observations supported the hypothesis that insufficient serotonergic neurotransmission contributes to ULD. Studies using *Cstb*-deficient mice failed to identify changes in serum TRP concentrations. However, serum levels of 5HT and 5-hydroxyindole acetic acid (5HIAA), an intermediate metabolite of 5HT, tend to be reduced (Vaarmann *et al.*, 2006). These data suggest that the observed disruption in 5HT metabolism in ULD patients may be causally related to *Cstb* deficiency, rather than being affected by systemic TRP availability or drug therapy. In contrast to TRP concentrations in serum, the brains of *Cstb* knockout mice have increased levels of TRP and its metabolites (Vaarmann *et al.*, 2006). Kynurenine, the first metabolic intermediate in the TRP kynurenine pathway, is also elevated in the *Cstb* knockout cerebellum. The myoclonus in ULD is believed to arise from impaired intracortical inhibition leading to secondary hyperexcitability of the motor cortex (Franceschetti *et al.*, 2007). Interestingly, *Cstb*-deficient mice exhibit significantly higher levels of 5HT and 5HIAA in the cerebral cortex and cerebellum (Vaarmann *et al.*, 2006), the structures where the greatest cellular atrophy and glial appearance have been described (Pennacchio *et al.*, 1998; Shannon *et al.*, 2002). The enhanced serotonergic neurotransmission may result from the loss of GABAergic interneurons, which play a critical role in controlling the serotonergic network in these regions, and are damaged in the *Cstb* knockout cortex (Buzzi et al., 2012; Franceschetti et al., 2007). While a direct relationship between altered serotonergic neurotransmission and ULD remains to be elucidated, these data suggest that disrupted serotonergic transmission is associated with the disease.

Pathogenesis of ULD: loss of *Cstb* contributes to defective inhibitory neurotransmission

In addition to its role in redox homeostasis and 5HT metabolism, *Cstb* protects a cell from endogenous proteases that have the potential to damage neuronal circuitry. *Cstb* deficiency leads to hyperexcitability and impaired neuronal function of cortical neuronal networks in both ULD patients and in *Cstb* knockout mice. Several studies have investigated the molecular mechanisms underlying neuronal hyperexcitability by pairing analyses of neurodegeneration with network changes occurring in the hippocampus following kainate treatment, a proconvulsant that triggers excitotoxicity and epileptic events (Arundine et al., 2003). Early *in vitro* hippocampal slice experiments suggested that during kainate perfusion, afferent synaptic activation evokes multiple population spikes in both *Cstb*-deficient and wild-type control mice (Franceschetti et al., 2007). The appearance of such hyperexcitable responses coincides with a rapid decline in the amplitude of the evoked field potentials in slices from *Cstb*-deficient mice. Spontaneous epileptic discharges (SEDs) occur in a subset of slices prepared from wild-type controls, with a delay of about 15 minutes following the onset of kainite perfusion, and persisting until the end of the kainate exposure. In contrast, in *Cstb*-deficient mice, SEDs begin within minutes of kainate perfusion, and progressively decrease in amplitude, ultimately disappearing along with the field responses evoked by electrical stimulation (Franceschetti et al., 2007). To test if increased susceptibility to pro-convulsant agents can be recapitulated *in vivo*, *Cstb*-deficient and control mice received intraperitoneal injections of kainate (30 mg/kg), and their behaviour was recorded for two hours thereafter. Consistent with *in vitro* findings, in this paradigm, *Cstb*-deficient mice display an increased susceptibility to kainite-induced seizures, such that the latency to generalized seizure onset is reduced and the behavioural seizure scores (cumulative seizure score and seizure index) are increased (Franceschetti et al., 2007). To investigate the extent of seizure-induced damage, brain damage was evaluated in *Cstb*-deficient mice and controls one day following kainate administration using several markers of neurodegeneration, including Fluoro-Jade B (Schmued and Hopkins, 2000). The degree of degeneration correlates with the severity of the seizures, and is higher in *Cstb*-deficient mice than in control mice (Franceschetti et al., 2007). In addition, *Cstb*-deficient mice display more neurodegeneration compared to controls with identical seizure scores, suggesting that seizure-induced brain damage is more pronounced in animals lacking *Cstb*. Analyses using immunohistological markers reveal a loss of GABAergic hippocampal neurons, suggesting that the observed hyperexcitability may depend, at least in part, on defective GABAergic inhibition (Franceschetti et al., 2007). To test if ULD is accompanied by a progressive loss of cerebral cortical GABAergic inhibition, cortical GABAergic neurotransmission was analyzed in *Cstb* knockout mice at various ages by histologically visualizing GABAergic nerve terminals, by examining GABA release from isolated nerve terminals, and electrophysiologically evaluating cortical GABAergic tone. While the overall cell numbers are reduced in the *Cstb* knockout cortex, the loss of GABAergic interneurons is more pronounced compared to the general loss of neurons, indicating that GABA interneurons are selectively more vulnerable to kainate-induced damage compared to other neuronal subtypes (Buzzi et al., 2012). A progressive reduction in the density of GABAergic nerve terminals (marked by VGAT staining) is also observed in the sensorimotor cortex of 4-, 8-, and 12-month-old *Cstb* knockout mice. One post-mortem ULD patient sample has shown a reduction in cortical thickness and a striking loss of VGAT-labelled GABAergic nerve terminals (Buzzi *et al.*, 2012). Experiments performed in mouse sensorimotor cortex using the paired-pulse paradigm, which is a stimulus protocol to test depression of the conditioned stimulus resulting primarily from GABAergic inhibition, show decreased inhibition in *Cstb* knockout mice at inter-pulse intervals in cortical layers II-III and V, compared to controls (Buzzi *et al.*, 2012). Perfusion with low concentrations of the GABAA antagonist bicuculline, at 0.5 µM, a concentration suitable for slightly reducing GABAergic-neurotransmission, results in an amplification of the field responses in cortical layers II-III and V of *Cstb* knockout brain slices (Buzzi *et al.*, 2012). Bicuculline leads to a pronounced decrease in depression profile in the paired-pulse protocol in *Cstb* knockout mice, while only minimally affecting control mice (Buzzi *et al.*, 2012). These effects result from the reduction of early GABAergic inhibition occurring simultaneously with the postsynaptic excitatory potential. Taken together, these data support the model that *Cstb* deficiency increases the susceptibility to seizures and to seizure-induced cell death. *In vitro*, hippocampal slices from *Cstb* knockout mice are hyperexcitable, and when perfused with kainate, display precocious and pronounced epileptic-like responses that couple with an early impairment in cellular function. *In vivo*, *Cstb* knockout mice display increased susceptibility to kainate-induced seizures and develop enhanced seizure-induced cell damage with higher degrees of neurodegeneration. The observation of decreased hippocampal GABAergic interneurons suggests that these neuronal subtypes are especially prone to cell damage resulting from *Cstb* loss. The reduction in GABAergic synaptic transmission observed in the sensorimotor cortex implicates a reduction in GABAergic synaptic transmission in ULD. Together, these findings support the model that one key factor contributing to the pathophysiology of ULD is the progressive loss of cortical GABAergic signalling which, with time, leads to hyperexcitability, myoclonus, and seizures.

ULD pathogenesis: precocious microglial activation

Glial activation, and particularly microglial activation, contributes to the mechanisms underlying brain pathologies including neuronal ceroid lipofuscinoses which also display PME (Cooper, 2010). In an early study using aged mice (16-20 months old), GFAP-positive astrocytes were reported to be more abundant in *Cstb* knockout mice than in controls, especially in the hippocampus (Shannon *et al.*, 2002). A recent study including both pre-symptomatic (P14) and symptomatic mice (one month old), suggests that precocious glial activation is a key mechanism contributing to the pathogenesis of ULD (Tegelberg *et al.*, 2012; Okuneva *et al.*, 2015). Systematic histological analyses using an unbiased stereological approach revealed early and localized glial activation in the brain, as well as in the thalamocortical system. Microglial activation entailed the expression of p-p38 MAPK, a marker of inflammation. While the proportion of pro-inflammatory M1 and anti-inflammatory M2 microglia favours the M2 type earlier in development, the ratio shifts in favour of the M1 type by P30 (Joensuu *et al.*, 2014; Okuneva *et al.*, 2015). The observed microglial activation precedes the onset of myoclonus, and is followed by gliosis and neuronal loss. Interestingly, active microglia undergo morphological changes during ULD disease progression, from that of phagocytic brain macrophages in young animals, to thickened branch processes in older animals (Tegelberg *et al.*, 2012). Consistent with a requirement for microglial activation during disease progression, neuronal loss was not observed in brain regions lacking glial activation (*e.g.* thalamic relay nuclei). These findings are consistent with previous studies suggesting that ULD is a neurodegenerative disease (Pennacchio *et al.*, 1998; Shannon *et al.*, 2002). Indeed, recent approaches using magnetic resonance imaging and diffusion tensor imaging have uncovered white matter degeneration in *Cstb*-deficient mice (Manninen *et al.*, 2014), as well as in patients (Manninen *et al.*, 2015). Taken together, these findings reveal the timing and progression of pathological events in the *Cstb*-deficient mouse brain, highlighting the potential role of glial activation during the initial stages of ULD.

Conclusion

Although nowadays ULD can be treated effectively (albeit only symptomatically) which has led to reduced severity, patients may experience significant disability. A precise molecular diagnostic technique is available. Major progress can be expected in the near future, as elucidation of the mechanisms causing seizures, myoclonus, and associated symptoms (which are mild and mainly cognitive) are likely to bring about pathogenetically-oriented treatment for ULD.

Genetic deletion of *Cstb* in the mouse has provided a powerful tool for modelling ULD in the laboratory. These mice display the triad of symptoms associated with ULD, including myoclonus, ataxia, and neuronal loss. Because *Cstb* is ubiquitously expressed and functions in healthy cells as an inhibitor of the cathepsin family of proteases, it is not surprising that loss of *Cstb* affects a broad range of cellular biological functions, including neuronal death, redox homeostasis, hyperexcitability, and glial activation. The studies reviewed in this chapter suggest that glial activation may be one of the earliest events contributing to *Cstb*-deficient brain pathology and is accompanied by oxidative stress, neuronal death, aberrant serotonin regulation, and hyperexcitability. Because *Cstb* is ubiquitously expressed, systemic knockout of *Cstb* results in the loss of *Cstb* in all cells of the body. Therefore, a limitation of the present ULD mouse model is the inability to reveal whether the observed phenotypes arise from primary defects in a specific cell type (*i.e.* neurons *vs.* glial cells). It is possible that some observed phenotypes are secondary to defects originating in neighbouring cells.

Collectively, these findings lay the foundation for future studies, which, by harnessing the potential of the ULD mouse model, should improve our understanding of the pathophysiology of ULD and open avenues for tailoring new therapeutic approaches.

Conflicts of interest: none.

References

Arundine, M., Chopra, G.K., Wrong, A., *et al.* (2003): Enhanced vulnerability to NMDA toxicity in sublethal traumatic neuronal injury in vitro. *J. Neurotrauma.* **20**, 1377–1395.

Ben-Menachem, E., Kyllerman, M. & Marklund, S. (2000): Superoxide dismutase and glutathione peroxidase function in progressive myoclonus epilepsies. *Epilepsy Res.* **40**, 33–39.

Berkovic, S., Andermann, F., Carpenter, S., Andermann, E. & Wolfe, L.S. (1986): Progressive myoclonus epilepsies: specific causes and diagnosis. *N. Engl. J. Med.* **315**, 296–305.

Buzzi, A., Chikhladze, M., Falcicchia, C., *et al.* (2012): Loss of cortical GABA terminals in Unverricht-Lundborg disease. *Neurobiol. Dis.* **47**, 216–224.

Chew, N.K., Mir, P., Edwards, M.J., *et al.* (2008): The natural history of Unverricht-Lundborg disease: a report of eight genetically proven cases. *Mov. Disord.* **23**, 107–113.

Chong, Z., Li, F. & Maiese, K. (2005): Oxidative stress in the brain: novel cellular targets that govern survival during neurodegenerative disease. *Prog. Neurobiol.* **75**, 207–246.

Cooper, J.D. (2010): The neuronal ceroid lipofuscinoses: the same, but different? *Biochem. Soc. Trans.* **38**, 1448–1452.

de Haan, G.J., Halley, D.J., Doelman, J.C., *et al.* (2004): Unverricht-Lundborg disease: underdiagnosed in the Netherlands. *Epilepsia* **45**, 1061–1063.

Edwards, M.J., Hargreaves, I.P., Heales, S.J., *et al.* (2002): N-acetylcysteine and Unverricht-Lundborg disease: variable response and possible side effects. *Neurology* **59**, 1447–1449.

Eldridge, R., Iivanainen, M., Stern, R., Koerber, T. & Wilder, B.J. (1983): 'Baltic' myoclonus epilepsy: hereditary disorder of childhood made worse by phenytoin. *Lancet* **2**, 838–842.

Ferlazzo, E., Magaudda, A., Striano, P., *et al.* (2007): Long-term evolution of EEG in Unverricht-Lundborg disease. *Epilepsy Res.* **73**, 219–227.

Ferlazzo, E., Gagliano, A., Calarese, T., *et al.* (2009): Neuropsychological findings in patients with Unverricht-Lundborg disease. *Epilepsy Behav.* **14**, 545–549.

Ferlazzo, E., Italiano, D., An, I., *et al.* (2009): Description of a family with a novel progressive myoclonus epilepsy and cognitive impairment. *Mov. Disord.* **24**, 1016–1022.

Franceschetti, S., Sancini, G., Buzzi, A., *et al.* (2007): A pathogenetic hypothesis of Unverricht-Lundborg disease onset and progression. *Neurobiol. Dis.* **25**, 675–685.

Franceschetti, S., Michelucci, R., Canafoglia, L., *et al.* (2014): Progressive myoclonic epilepsies: definitive and still undetermined causes. *Neurology* **82**, 405–411.

Genton, P. & Guerrini, R. (1990): Antimyoclonic effects of alcohol in progressive myoclonus epilepsy. *Neurology* **40**, 1412–1416.

Genton, P., Gélisse, P. & Crespel, A. (2006): Lack of efficacy and potential aggravation of myoclonus with lamotrigine in Unverricht-Lundborg disease. *Epilepsia* **47**, 2083–2085.

Genton, P., Delgado Escueta, A., Serratosa, J.M., Michelucci, R. & Bureau, M. (2012): Progressive myoclonus epilepsies. In: *Epileptic Syndromes in Infancy, Childhood and Adolescence (5th ed).* M. Bureau, P. Genton, A. Delgado Escueta, Ch. Dravet, C.A. Tassinari, P. Thomas, P. Wolf, eds. John Libbey Eurotext Ltd., pp 575–606.

Genton, P., Michelucci, R., Tassinari, C.A. & Roger, J. (1990): The Ramsay Hunt Syndrome revisited: Mediterranean Myoclonus versus mitochondrial encephalomyopathy with ragged red fibers and Baltic Myoclonus. *Acta. Neurol. Scand.* **81**, 8–15.

Genton, P., Malafosse, A., Moulard, B., *et al.* (2005): Progressive myoclonus epilepsies. In: *Epileptic Syndromes in Infancy, Childhood and Adolescence (4th ed).* J. Roger, M. Bureau, C. Dravet, P. Genton, C.A. Tassinari, P. Wolf, éd. John Libbey Eurotext, Paris, 441–465.

Giovagnoli, A.R., Canafoglia, L., Reati, F., *et al.* (2009): The neuropsychological pattern of Unverricht-Lundborg disease. *Epilepsy Res.* **84**, 217–223.

Heyes, M.P., Saito, K., Devinsky, O. & Nadi, N.S. (1994): Kynurenine pathway metabolites in cerebrospinal fluid and serum in complex partial seizures. *Epilepsia* **35**, 251–257.

Houseweart, M.K., Pennacchio, L.A., Vilaythong, A., Peters, C., Noebels, J.L. & Myers, R.M. (2003): Cathepsin B but not cathepsins L or S contributes to the pathogenesis of Unverricht-Lundborg progressive myoclonus epilepsy (EPM1). *J. Neurobiol.* **56**, 315–327.

Hurd, R.W., Wilder, B.J., Helveston, W.R. & Uthman, B.M. (1996): Treatment of four siblings with progressive myoclonus epilepsy of the Unverricht-Lundborg type with Nacetylcysteine. *Neurology* **47**, 1264–1268.

Joensuu, T., Lehesjoki, A.E. & Kopra, O. (2008): Molecular background of EPM1- Unverricht-Lundborg disease. *Epilepsia* **49**, 557–563.

Joensuu, T., Tegelberg, S., Reinmaa, E., *et al.* (2014): Gene expression alterations in the cerebellum and granule neurons of Cstb(-/-) mouse are associated with early synaptic changes and inflammation. *PLoS One* 9, e89321.

Kälviäinen, R., Khyuppenen, J., Koskenkorva, P., Eriksson, K., Vanninen, R. & Mervaala, E. (2008): Clinical picture of EPM1-Unverricht-Lundborg disease. *Epilepsia* **49**, 549–556.

Khiari, H.M., Franceschetti, S., Jovic, N., Mrabet, A. & Genton, P. (2009): Death in Unverricht-Lundborg disease. *Neurol. Sci.* **30**, 315–318.

Koskenkorva, P., Khyuppenen, J., Niskanen, E., *et al.* (2009): Motor cortex and thalamic atrophy in Unverricht-Lundborg disease: Voxel-based morphometric study. *Neurology* **73**, 606–611.

Koskiniemi, M., Toivakka, E. & Donner, M. (1974): Progressive myoclonus epilepsy. Electroencephalographical findings. *Acta. Neurol. Scand.* **50**, 333–359.

Koskiniemi, M.L. Baltic myoclonus. (1986): In: Fahn S, Marsden CD, Van Woert M (eds) *Myoclonus, vol. 43.* New York: Raven Press, Advances in neurology 57–64.

Kunz, W.S. (2002):The role of mitochondria in epileptogenesis. *Curr. Opin. Neurol.* **15**, 179–184.

Kyllerman, M., Sommerfelt, K., Hedström, A., Wennergren, G. & Holmgren, D. (1991): Clinical and neurophysiological development of Unverricht-Lundborg disease in four Swedish siblings. *Epilepsia* **32**, 900–909.

Lafreniere, R.G., Rochefort, D.L., Chretien N., et al. (1997): Unstable insertion in the 5' flanking region of the cystatin B gene is the most common mutation in progressive myoclonus epilepsy type 1, EPM1. *Nat. Genet.* **15**, 298–302.

Lalioti, M.D., Scott, H.S., Buresi, C., et al. (1997): Dodecamer repeat expansion in cystatin B gene in progressive myoclonus epilepsy. *Nature* **386**, 847–851.

Lehesjoki, A.E. & Koskiniemi, M. (1999): Progressive myoclonus epilepsy of Unverricht-Lundborg type. *Epilepsia* **40**, 23–28.

Lehtinen, M.K., Yuan, Z., Boag, P.R., et al. (2006): A conserved MST-FOXO signaling pathway mediates oxidative-stress responses and extends life span. *Cell* **125**, 987–1001.

Lehtinen, M.K., Tegelberg, S. & Schipper, H. (2009): Cystatin B deficiency sensitizes neurons to oxidative stress in progressive myoclonus epilepsy, EPM1. *J. Neurosci.* **29**, 5910–5915.

Lehesjoki, A.E., Koskiniemi, M. & Sistonen, P., et al. (1991): Localization of a gene for progressive myoclonus epilepsy to chromosome 21q22. *Proc. Natl. Acad. Sci. USA* **88**, 3606–3699.

Lundborg, H. (1903): Die progressive Myoclonusepilepsie (Unverricht's Myoklonie). Uppsala: Almqvist and Wiskell.

Magaudda, A., Ferlazzo, E., Nguyen, V.H. & Genton, P. (2006):Unverricht-Lundborg disease, a condition with self-limited progression: long-term follow-up of 20 patients. *Epilepsia* **47**, 860–866.

Manninen, O., Laitinen, T., Lehtimäki, K.K., et al. (2014): Progressive volume loss and white matter degeneration in cstb-deficient mice: a diffusion tensor and longitudinal volumetry MRI study. *PLoS One* 9, e90709.

Manninen, O., Koskenkorva, P., Lehtimäki, K.K., et al. (2015): White matter degeneration with Unverricht-Lundborg progressive myoclonus epilepsy: a translational diffusion-tensor imaging study in patients and cystatin B-deficient mice. *Radiology* **269**, 232–239.

Marseille Consensus Group. (1990): Classification of progressive myoclonus epilepsies and related disorders. Marseille Consensus Group. *Ann. Neurol.* **28**, 113–116.

Muona, M., Berkovic, S.F., Dibbens, L.M., et al. (2015): A recurrent de novo mutation in KCNC1 causes progressive myoclonus epilepsy. *Nat. Genet.* **47**, 39–46.

Mumoli, L., Tarantino, P., Michelucci, R., et al. (2015): No evidence of a role for cystatin B gene in juvenile myoclonic epilepsy. *Epilepsia* **56**, e40–43.

Okuneva, O., Körber, I., Li, Z., et al. (2015): Abnormal microglial activation in the Cstb(-/-) mouse, a model for progressive myoclonus epilepsy, EPM1. *Glia* **63**, 400–411.

Pennacchio, L.A., Lehesjoki, A.E., Stone, N.E., et al. (1996): Mutations in the gene encoding cystatin B in progressive myoclonus epilepsy (EPM1). *Science* **271**, 1731–1734.

Pennacchio, L.A., Bouley, D.M., Higgins, K.M., Scott, M.P., Noebels, J.L. & Myers, R.M. (1998): Progressive ataxia, myoclonic epilepsy and cerebellar apoptosis in cystatin B-deficient mice. *Nat. Genet.* **20**, 251–258.

Pranzatelli, M.R., Tate, E., Huang, Y., et al. (1995): Neuropharmacology of progressive myoclonus epilepsy: response to 5-hydroxy-Ltryptophan. *Epilepsia* **36**, 783–791.

Rinne, R., Saukko, P., Jarvinen, M. & Lehesjoki, A.E. (2002): Reduced cystatin B activity correlates with enhanced cathepsin activity in progressive myoclonus epilepsy. *Ann. Med.* **34**, 380–385.

Schmued, L.C. & Hopkins, K.J. (2000): Fluoro-Jade B: a high affinity fluorescent marker for the localization of neuronal degeneration. *Brain Res.* **874**, 123–130.

Selwa, L.M. (1999): N-acetylcysteine therapy for Unverricht-Lundborg disease. *Neurology* **52**, 426–427.

Shannon, P., Pennacchio, L.A., Houseweart, M.K., Minassian, B.A. & Myers, R.M. (2002): Neuropathological changes in a mouse model of progressive myoclonus epilepsy: cystatin B deficiency and Unverricht-Lundborg disease. *J. Neuropathol. Exp. Neurol.* **61**, 1085–1091.

Smith, B., Shatz, R., Elisevich, K., Bespalova, I.N. & Burmeister, M. (2000): Effects of vagus nerve stimulation on progressive myoclonus epilepsy of Unverricht-Lundborg type. *Epilepsia* **41**, 1046–1048.

Tegelberg, S., Kopra, O., Joensuu, T., Cooper, J.D. & Lehesjoki, A.E. (2012): Early microglial activation precedes neuronal loss in the brain of the Cstb-/- mouse model of progressive myoclonus epilepsy, EPM1. *J. Neuropathol. Exp. Neurol.* **71**, 40–53.

Unverricht, H. (1891): Die Myoclonie. Leipzig, Wien: Franz Deuticke.

Vaarmann, A., Kaasik, A. & Zharkovsky, A. (2006): Altered tryptophan metabolism in the brain of cystatin B-deficient mice: a model system for progressive myoclonus epilepsy. *Epilepsia* **47**, 1650–1654.

Vanni, N., Fruscione, F., Ferlazzo, E., et al. (2014): Impairment of ceramide synthesis causes a novel progressive myoclonus epilepsy. *Ann. Neurol.* **76**, 206–212.

Wille, C., Steinhoff, B.J., Altenmüller, D.M., et al. (2011): Chronic high-frequency deep-brain stimulation in progressive myoclonic epilepsy in adulthood-report of five cases. *Epilepsia* **52**, 489–496.

Chapter 4

Lafora disease

Julie Turnbull[1], Pasquale Striano[2], Pierre Genton[3], Stirling Carpenter[4], Cameron A. Ackerley[5] and Berge A. Minassian[1]

[1] *Program in Genetics and Genome Biology and Division of Neurology, Department of Paediatrics, The Hospital for Sick Children and the University of Toronto, Canada*
[2] *Paediatric Neurology and Muscular Diseases Unit, Department of Neurosciences, Rehabilitation, Ophthalmology, Genetics, Maternal and Child Health, University of Genoa, 'G. Gaslini' Institute, Genova, Italy*
[3] *Centre Saint-Paul, Hôpital Henri-Gastaut, 300 Bd De Sainte Marguerite, 13009 Marseille, France*
[4] *Department of Anatomic Pathology, Hospital Sao Joao, Porto, Portugal*
[5] *Division of Pathology, Department of Pathology and Laboratory Medicine, The Hospital for Sick Children and the University of Toronto, Canada*
berge.minassian@sickkids.ca

Summary

Lafora disease (LD) is an autosomal recessive progressive myoclonus epilepsy due to mutations in the *EPM2A* (laforin) and *EPM2B* (malin) genes, with no substantial genotype-phenotype differences between the two. Founder effects and recurrent mutations are common, and mostly isolated to specific ethnic groups and/or geographical locations. Pathologically, LD is characterized by distinctive polyglucosans, which are formations of abnormal glycogen. Polyglucosans, or Lafora bodies (LB) are typically found in the brain, periportal hepatocytes of the liver, skeletal and cardiac myocytes, and in the eccrine duct and apocrine myoepithelial cells of sweat glands. Mouse models of the disease and other naturally occurring animal models have similar pathology and phenotype. Hypotheses of LB formation remain controversial, with compelling evidence and caveats for each hypothesis. However, it is clear that the laforin and malin functions regulating glycogen structure are determinant.

Introduction

Lafora disease (LD, OMIM# 254780) is an autosomal recessive progressive myoclonus epilepsy (PME), first described in 1911. It is particularly frequent in Mediterranean countries (Spain, Italy, France), Northern Africa, the Middle East, and in some regions of Southern India where a high rate of consanguinity is present (Minassian *et al.*, 2001; Striano *et al.*, 2008). It can, nevertheless, be found in any population (Traore *et al.*, 2009), and particularly, as expected, with consanguinity.

LD classically starts in adolescence in otherwise neurologically normal individuals, usually with action and stimulus-sensitive myoclonus, as well as tonic-clonic, absence, atonic, and visual seizures. Neuropsychiatric symptoms, such as behavioural changes, depression and apathy, are also often present. Initial symptoms are followed by rapidly progressing dementia, refractory status epilepticus, psychosis, cerebellar ataxia, dysarthria, mutism, and respiratory failure which lead to death within about a decade (Minassian et al., 2001; Striano et al., 2008). LD is caused by mutations in the EPM2A or EPM2B (NHLRC1) genes, encoding the laforin dual specificity phosphatase and the malin ubiquitin E3 ligase, respectively, both involved in a complex and yet very incompletely understood pathway regulating glycogen metabolism (Minassian et al., 1998; Chan et al., 2003a, 2003b). To date, an additional gene, PRDM8, the mutation of which causes a variant of early childhood-onset phenotype in a single family, has been reported (Turnbull et al., 2012).

A distinctive pathology characterizes LD. Cells of various types exhibit dense accumulations of malformed and insoluble glycogen molecules, known as polyglucosans, which differ from normal glycogen due to the fact that they lack the symmetric branching that allows glycogen to be soluble. These polyglucosan accumulations are called Lafora bodies (LBs) and are profuse in all brain regions and in the majority of neurons, specifically in their cell bodies and dendrites (Minassian et al., 2001; Striano et al., 2008). Neuronal LBs localize in perikarya and dendrites but not in axons, possibly explaining the cortical hyperexcitability seen in LD. The neuropathology of LD patients and LD animal models is described in greater detail below.

Lafora disease: clinical features and diagnosis

The first symptoms of LD appear during late childhood or adolescence (range: 8-19 years; peak: 14-16 years). Characteristically, focal visual seizures are early manifestations and present as transient blindness, or simple or complex visual hallucinations. However, generalized seizure types, e.g. tonic-clonic, absence, or drop attacks, as well as myoclonus, occur soon after. The latter typically occurs at rest and increases with emotion, action, or photic stimulation. In many cases, the disease shows an insidious near-simultaneous, or closely consecutive, appearance of headaches, difficulties at school, myoclonic jerks, generalized seizures, and visual hallucinations (Minassian et al., 2001; Franceschetti et al., 2006; Striano et al., 2008). It is notable that not all visual hallucinations are epileptic in Lafora patients, as some respond initially to antipsychotic, rather than antiepileptic, medications (Andrade et al., 2005).

EEG abnormalities often precede clinical symptoms and initially consist of almost normal or slowed background (Fig. 1A) and generalized or focal paroxysmal activity (Fig. 1B), typically not accentuated by sleep. In particular, the occipital discharges on EEG, arising from a slowed posterior dominant rhythm are, in the proper clinical context, highly suggestive of the disease. Within a few years, a slowing of background activity becomes evident with frequent, superimposed bursts of diffuse epileptic discharges (Fig. 1C). In addition, positive or negative myoclonus (Fig. 1D) and marked photosensitivity (Fig. 1E) are prominent features.

Brain MRI is usually unremarkable at onset. In two reported cases (Jennesson et al., 2010), [18]fluorodeoxyglucose positron emission tomography (FDG-PET) revealed posterior hypometabolism early during the evolution of the disease. Electrophysiological investigations (to examine jerk-locked averaging, somatosensory evoked potentials, C-reflex, and visual evoked potentials) can reveal aberrant integration of somatosensory stimuli and cortical hyperexcitability (i.e. giant evoked potentials). Visual evoked potentials may show increased latencies or absence of response. Other findings obtained by transcranial magnetic stimulation indicate a complex circuitry dysfunction, possibly involving both excitatory and inhibitory systems (Canafoglia *et al.*, 2010). A skin biopsy shows the presence of the characteristic periodic acid-Schiff (PAS)-positive glycogen-like intracellular inclusion bodies in the myoepithelial cells of the secretory acini of the apocrine sweat glands and in the eccrine and apocrine sweat duct cells (Andrade *et al.*, 2003; Lohi *et al.*, 2007). Electron microscopy confirms the presence of fibrillary accumulations, typical of polyglucosans. This diagnostic approach offers limited invasiveness and high sensitivity. Interpretation of the biopsy, however, requires expertise in distinguishing LB from normal polysaccharide contents of apocrine sweat glands, without which false-positive diagnosis is common. Genetic testing is crucial to confirm the diagnosis as it reveals mutations in the *EPM2A* or *EPM2B* gene in more than 95 per cent of patients (Minassian *et al.*, 2001; Ganesh *et al.*, 2006; Striano *et al.*, 2008).

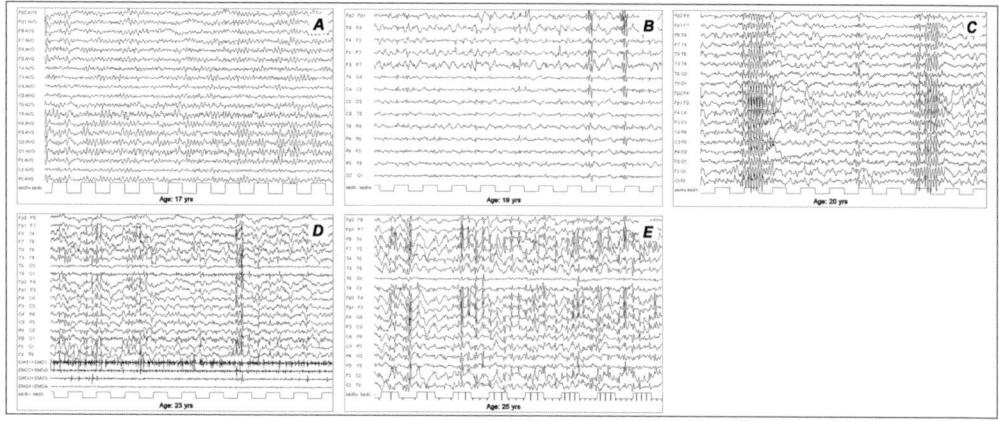

*Fig. 1. Progression of electroencephalographic (EEG) changes in a patient with Lafora disease. (**A**) At the time of disease onset (age 17 years); normal to slightly slowed background activity. (**B**) Two years later (age 19 years) EEG demonstrates asymmetric generalized spikes and polyspikes, maximum over the anterior regions on a slowed background. (**C**) At age 20 years, the occurrence of fast (4-6 cycles per second) spike-waves was concomitant with head drops. During the final stages of the disease, EEG recordings show long bursts of diffuse spike-waves and fast polyspikes associated with major volleys or massive myoclonic jerks (**D**), dramatically enhanced by photic stimulation at low frequency (**E**). Modified from Striano* et al.*, 2008.*

In the years following onset, symptoms of LD progress towards intractable action-sensitive and stimulus-sensitive myoclonus, refractory seizures, psychosis, ataxia, and dysarthria. As the disease progresses, the myoclonus remains asymmetric and segmental but becomes almost constant, and massive myoclonic jerks appear. At this stage, brain MRI may reveal mild cerebellar or cortical atrophy. Moreover, brain ^{1}H MR spectroscopy shows metabolic changes of the cerebellum, basal ganglia, and frontal cerebral cortex (Villanueva *et al.*, 2006; Pichiecchio *et al.*, 2008). Subsequently, a rapidly progressive dementia with apraxia and visual loss soon appears. Speech becomes extremely difficult, and ataxia makes walking impossible. For many years, the patient struggles to maintain normal contact, with communication interrupted by extremely frequent myoclonic absence seizures (Minassian *et al.*, 2001; Striano *et al.*, 2008). Patients finally become totally disabled and bed-bound. Death usually occurs within 10 years from the onset, often during status epilepticus with aspiration pneumonia.

Differential diagnosis

At onset, LD may present with a clinical picture resembling an idiopathic generalized epilepsy, such as juvenile myoclonic epilepsy (Janz syndrome). In the early stages, drug resistance and a slow background with early disrupted sleep patterns should lead to a suspicion of LD. In some patients, the diagnosis is reached only after substantial follow-up of the patient. However, the main differential diagnosis concerns four other forms of PME: Unverricht-Lundborg disease (EPM1), the neuronal ceroid lipofuscinoses, myoclonic epilepsy with ragged red fibers (MERRF), and sialidosis (Berkovic et al., 1986; Minassian et al., 2001; Striano et al., 2008) (Table 1). PMEs are a group of inherited neurodegenerative disorders characterized by progressively worsening myoclonus and epilepsy, variable neurological dysfunction (ataxia, dementia), and possible associated signs and symptoms. LD is one of the main teenage-onset PMEs. Age at onset, presenting symptoms, occurrence of occipital seizures, and the progressive

Table 1. Distinguishing features of some of the more common inherited progressive myoclonic epilepsies

Progressive myoclonic epilepsy	Inheritance	Onset (years)	Suggestive clinical signs	Pathologic features	Gene(s)
Unverricht-Lundborg disease (EPM1)	AR	6-15	Slow progression; mild and late cerebellar impairment; late or absent dementia	None	CSTB
Lafora disease (EPM2)	AR	6-19	Visual symptoms	Polyglucosan inclusions (Lafora bodies)	EPM2A EPM2B
Myoclonic epilepsy with red ragged fibres (MERRF)	Maternal	Any age	Lactic acidosis	Ragged red fibres	MTTK (tRNALys)
Neuronal Ceroid lipofuscinoses (NCLs)	AR, AD	Variable	Macular degeneration and visual impairment (except adult form)	Lipopigment deposits; granular osmiophilic, curvilinear or fingerprints inclusions	CLN1–CLN9
Sialidoses	AR	8–15	Gradual cerebellar impairment; cherry-red spot maculopathy	Urinary oligosaccharides, fibroblast neuraminidase deficit	NEU PPGB

AD: autosomal dominant; AR: autosomal recessive. Modified from Striano et al. (2008).

and rapid course, together with the EEG features, are suggestive of LD, but the diagnosis is definitively confirmed by skin biopsy or genetic analysis. Unverricht-Lundborg disease (EPM1), caused by mutations of the cystatin B gene, is the closest differential. The age at onset is similar to that of LD. However, characteristically, action myoclonus and tonic-clonic seizures are more easily controlled. There is no specific pathology. Finally, cognitive impairment is not a distinctive symptom of Unverricht-Lundborg disease and is usually mild (Minassian et al., 2001; Striano et al., 2008). Neuronal ceroid lipofuscinoses are heterogeneous conditions characterized by ceroid-lipofuscin lysosomal storage occurring in different organs, including the central nervous system and skin (see chapter 14). All NCLs exhibit ceroid lipofuscin accumulation, apart from LB, in various organs, including the skin. Most NCLs present in early childhood.

A juvenile form of NCL (Batten's disease, involving the *CLN3* gene) may have onset late enough to overlap with that of LD, but this form has a prolonged initial period of visual loss, resulting from retinal degeneration and mild seizures, which LD patients typically do not have. Some cases of the infantile form (Santavuori-Haltia disease, involving the *CLN1* gene) present late as a result of particular mutations, and there is a very rare form of adult-onset NCL (Kufs disease; gene unknown), however, these diseases are excluded by the presence of LB. Mitochondriopathies, such as MERRF and MELAS, usually exhibit maternal mtDNA transmission. Clinical presentation may be heterogeneous and includes a wide range of associated symptoms, such as deafness, low stature, myopathy, lactic acidosis and optic atrophy, with variable prognosis. Sialidosis is an extremely rare lysosomal disease with cherry red spot maculopathy and elevated urine oligosaccharides (Berkovic *et al.*, 1986).

Prognosis and evolution

The prognosis of LD is invariably progressive and fatal, leading to death 5-10 years after clinical onset. Genotype-phenotype correlations do not reveal substantial differences between patients carrying *EPM2A* and *EPM2B* mutations, but a few specific *EPM2B* mutations appear to correlate with a late onset and slow progressing LD (Boccella *et al.*, 2003; Minassian *et al.*, 2001; Franceschetti *et al.*, 2006; Striano *et al.*, 2008). At present, LD treatment remains palliative, with the best current therapies having limited success in the modulation of symptoms. Commonly used antiepileptic therapy for the management of myoclonus may improve symptoms during the early stages of the disease (Minassian *et al.*, 2001; Striano *et al.*, 2008). Hopefully, the work of many investigators, who are putting a massive effort into elucidating the pathophysiology, will result in focused treatments to control the deterioration of this otherwise devastating condition.

Epidemiology of Lafora disease and its genetic correlations

LD is a rare orphan disease. Based on all published reports of LD mutations, we estimate an overall frequency of ~4 cases per million individuals in the world. Over 250 patients and/or families have been described with LD (Fig. 2A). Of these, 42 per cent are caused by mutations in *EPM2A* and 58 per cent by *EPM2B* mutations (Fig. 2B). The ratio of *EPM2A* to *EPM2B* cases varies with population, with some regions having many more *EPM2A* cases than *EPM2B*, and vice versa, and this is, remarkably, not solely due to founder mutations (Gomez-Garre *et al.*, 2000; Franceschetti *et al.*, 2006). The most common *EPM2A* mutation is the R241X mutation, which accounts for approximately 17 percent of *EPM2A*-mediated LD. Large deletions make up 10-15 percent of *EPM2A* mutations, with the remainder ranging from those causing approximately eight percent of *EPM2A*-mediated cases of LD (*i.e.* R171H) to orphan mutations spread across the gene (Fig. 3A). For *EPM2B*, the two most common mutations are the missense mutation P69A and the frameshift mutation G158fs16 which affect ~15 and ~8 per cent of *EPM2B*-mediated LD, respectively. As with *EPM2A*, the remaining *EPM2B* mutations span the gene (Fig. 3B) and are rare, though some mutations (*i.e.* C26S and D146N) are more frequently observed. Because deletions can be overlooked using conventional sequencing techniques, it is critical to consider deletion/duplication analysis in any suspected LD patients in whom initial sequencing of *EPM2A* and *EPM2B* reveals no change.

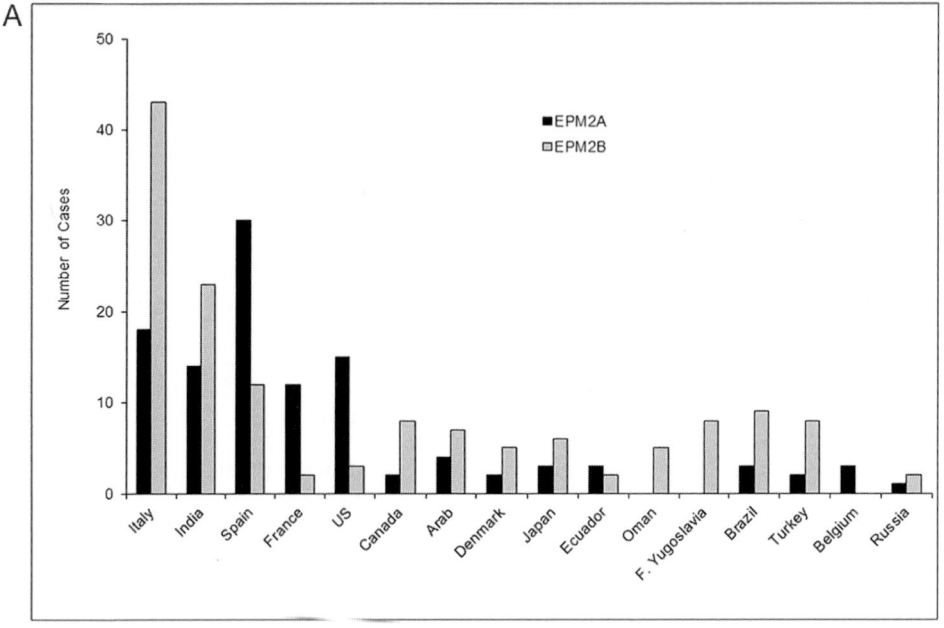

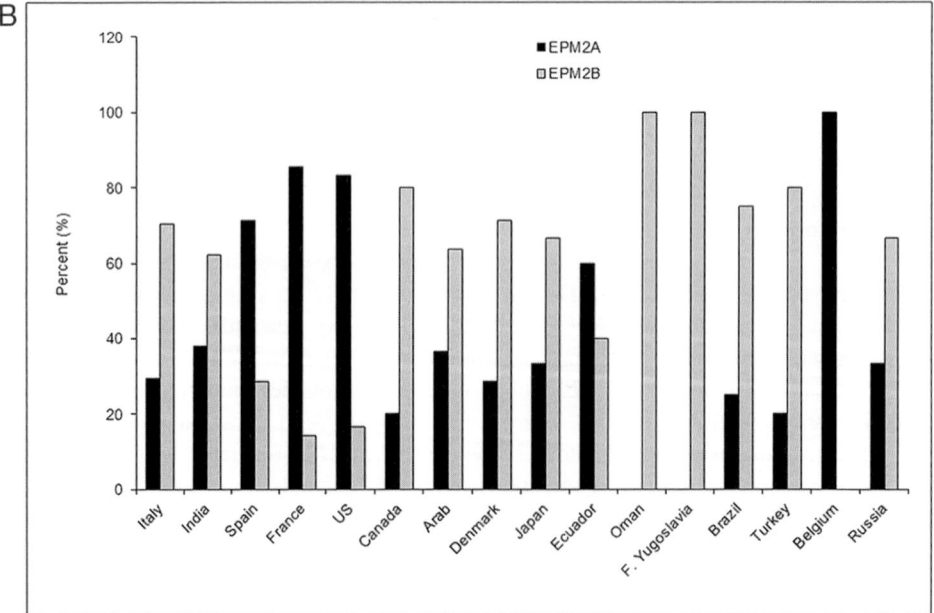

*Fig. 2. Number (**A**) and percentage (**B**) of EPM2A and EPM2B cases according to ethnicity/country, known to us at the time this chapter was prepared.*

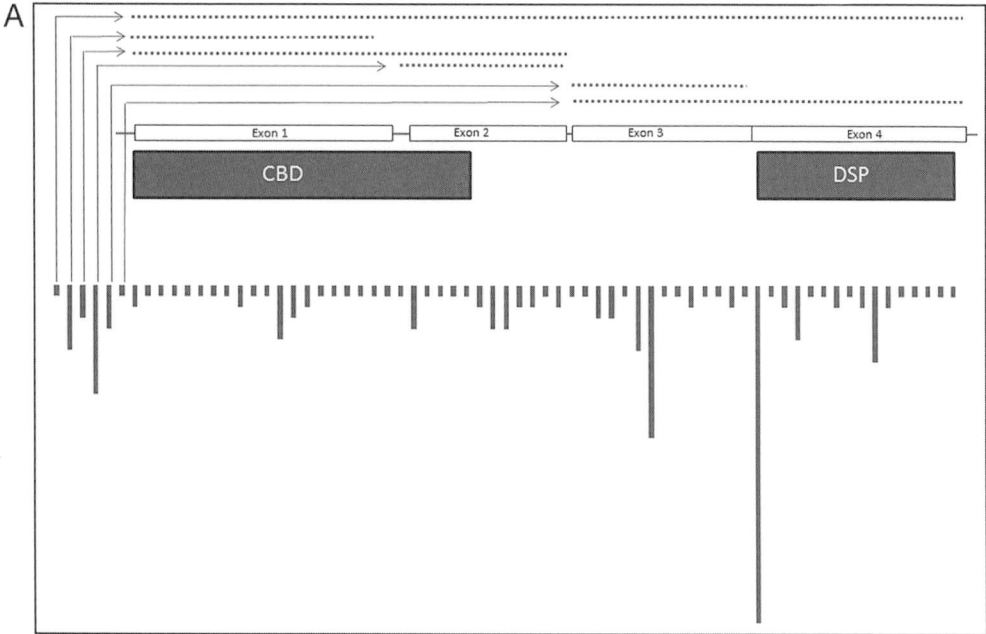

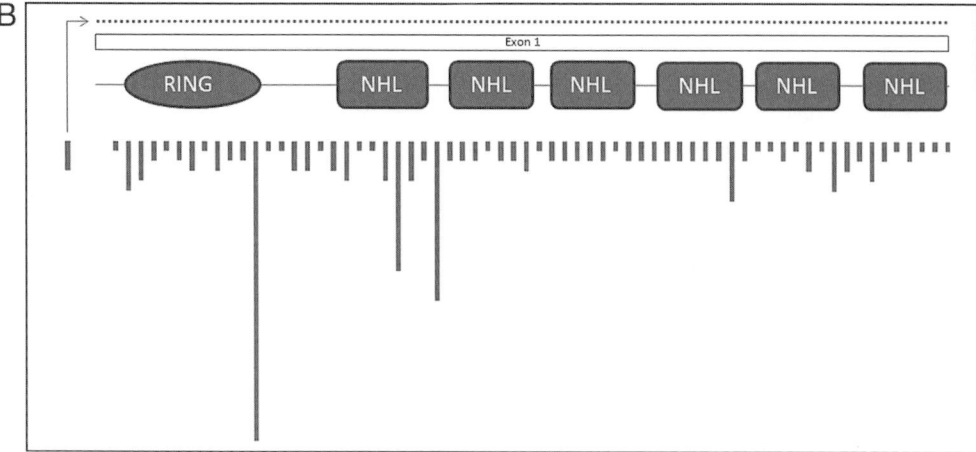

Fig. 3. Location and relative frequency of *EPM2A* (**A**) and *EPM2B* (**B**) mutations; dotted lines indicate deletion mutations.

Founder effects and recurrent mutations

Certain mutations appear to be specific to particular ethnic groups and/or geographical locations. For example, LD affects French Canadians from a geographically isolated area of eastern Quebec with an unusually high frequency, which is likely to be due to the ancestral *EPM2B* C26S mutation (Chan *et al.*, 2003a, 2003b). One study has been published on LD in Oman, in which all cases in 5 separate, unrelated families resulted from a single ancestral mutational event in *EPM2B* (Turnbull *et al.*, 2008). Interestingly, the *EPM2A* R241X mutation commonly found in individuals of Spanish descent resulted from both recurrent events and founder effects (Gomez-Garre *et al.*, 2000; Ganesh *et al.*, 2002a). At least 5 unique haplotypes are associated with this mutation, indicating that a minimum of 5 separate mutational events have led to the prevalence of the R241X mutation. Accordingly, *EPM2A*-mediated LD is more common than *EPM2B*-mediated LD in Spain. The second most common mutation in *EPM2B*, the missense P69A mutation, appears to have occurred from multiple mutational events similar to the *EPM2A* R241X mutation (Gomez-Abad *et al.*, 2005). Only one common haplotype was found among 8 patients analyzed with P69A mutations, strongly indicative of a recurrent event.

Phenotypic hetero- and homogeneity

Clinically, LD is a fairly homogenous disease with onset in adolescence and neurological decline soon after, but the timing and severity of symptoms can be variable, even within families. Both phenotypic heterogeneity and homogeneity have been noted in LD (see below) and with the large number of mutations in both *EPM2A* and *EPM2B*, genotype-phenotype correlations have been difficult to ascertain. Nonetheless, some associations between the two have been made. Gomez-Abad *et al.* identified three Arabic families with a complete deletion of the *EPM2A* gene (Gomez-Abad *et al.*, 2007). Haplotype analysis and breakpoint mapping established a shared haplotype among the patients, suggesting a common ancestral origin for this mutation. Of the 7 confirmed LD patients in the pedigrees, there was great variability in both disease onset and severity of symptoms, which was unexpected, due to the founder effect of the mutation. Clearly, even with the same ancestral mutation, phenotypic heterogeneity is common. This has been shown with other ancestral founder mutations, including the recurrent R241X *EPM2A* mutation (Gomez-Garre *et al.*, 2000; Ganesh *et al.*, 2002a). However, in a genetic isolate, the same ancestral founder mutation within a population resulted in phenotypic homogeneity (Turnbull *et al.*, 2008). The uniformity of environmental and genetic background reinforces the idea that other genetic and/or environmental modifiers may influence the phenotypic spectrum in LD. Indeed, this has been shown within one family; an *EPM2B* patient harbouring a coding variant for the *PPP1R3C* gene, which encodes protein targeting to glycogen (PTG), exhibited a milder course of LD (Guerrero *et al.*, 2011). The resulting conclusion from reports of both clinical homogeneity and heterogeneity in LD is that even among families, the disease course may or may not be identical and each LD patient is just as likely to have a clinically diverse, rather than classic, disease course.

Genotype-phenotype correlations

'Atypical' LD with early-onset childhood learning disabilities has been reported (Ganesh *et al.*, 2002a; Annesi *et al.*, 2004). Here, the authors showed a significant association with exon 1 mutations in *EPM2A*, linked to the development of learning disabilities prior to the onset of classic neurological symptoms of LD. Exon 4 mutations were mainly associated with classic LD with no childhood-onset educational difficulties. The authors suggest that exon 1 mutations can result in the complete loss of laforin function, whereas exon 4 mutations may preserve some of its functionality. However, other studies have not shown the same association, even with patients with the same or similar mutations in exon 1. Atypical LD with childhood learning difficulties, as observed by Ganesh *et al.* and Annesi *et al.*, may prove to be a sub-syndrome of LD or could be due to as-yet-unknown genetic and/or environmental modifying factors (Lesca *et al.*, 2010).

One study identified a family with two siblings with LD, one of whom presented with severe liver failure as an initial symptom (Gomez-Garre et al., 2007). Liver function in the sibling was abnormal, although the patient remained asymptomatic. Upon further follow-up, both developed classic LD, and mutation screening revealed a homozygous *EPM2A* R241X mutation in both siblings. Interestingly, the liver disease resembled type IV glycogen storage disease (GSD; due to GBE1 deficiency). The two diseases (type IV GSD and LD) share very similar features, namely the presence of polyglucosan bodies. This suggests a role for modifier genes in LD and the authors propose that these defects may lie in the same metabolic pathway, *i.e.* the glycogen metabolic pathway. The *EPM2A* R241X mutation is a prevalent mutation, and no other cases of hepatic failure have been identified in patients with this mutation. It is likely that other modifying factors led to this presentation, but the similarity to type IV GSD is intriguing and, as the authors of the study mention, certain modifiers may influence the severity of non-neurological symptoms in LD.

Some studies have indicated that patients with malin-mediated LD have a slightly milder disease course than patients with laforin-mediated LD (Gomez-Abad et al., 2005; Baykan et al., 2005; Singh et al., 2006). However, others found no change in severity between the two (Brackmann et al., 2011; Franceschetti et al., 2006; Lesca et al., 2010; Traore, 2009; Lohi et al., 2007). Conclusive evidence involving large-scale comparisons is lacking, but it is clear that there exists one relatively common, milder, *EPM2B* mutation, which may be skewing the comparative results in some analyses. Patients with either heterozygous or homozygous D146N mutation in *EPM2B*, in all cases in our experience and in the literature, have an atypical milder LD consisting of a later onset of symptoms, longer disease course, and extended preservation of daily living activities (Chan et al., 2003b; Francheschetti, 2006; Gomez-Abad et al., 2005; Baykan et al., 2005; Couarch et al., 2011). It is likely that at least some of the functionality of malin is preserved in patients with D146N mutations, as it has been demonstrated that the mutation preserves both the E3 ubiquitin ligase activity and a weak interaction with laforin (Solaz-Fuster et al., 2008). Clinical heterogeneity is common in LD, even among patients with allelic homogeneity and while it is true that certain mutations, such as D146N, cause a milder disease course, most cases of malin-mediated LD have a devastating disease course which is comparable to that of laforin-mediated LD.

The pathology of Lafora disease and Lafora disease animal models

The primary morphological change in LD is the deposition of polyglucosans, which consists of discrete deposits of fibrillar polysaccharides composed of poorly-branched glucose polymers (LBs). They are typically found in the brain, in the periportal hepatocytes of the liver, skeletal and cardiac myocytes, and in the eccrine duct and apocrine myoepithelial cells of the sweat glands (Sakai et al., 1970; Barbieri et al., 1987; Shirozu et al., 1985; Carpenter & Karpati, 1981a).

In the brain, the largest LBs tend to have 2 layers of various proportions in haemotoxylin and eosin (H and E) -stained preparations, the outer layer being pale and the core basophilic (Fig. 4A). These large bodies are usually found in neuronal perikarya. The ratio of perikaryal LBs to neurons is highest in the substantia nigra, followed by the dentate nucleus and some thalamic nuclei (Fig. 4B). They are rare or absent in the anterior part of the spinal cord. In the cerebral cortex, perikaryal LBs are rather scant, but a periodic acid Schiff (PAS) stain reveals numerous small LBs in the cortical neuropil (Fig. 4C), the majority being found in dendrites. These are commonly referred to as 'dust-like' in appearance. The PAS positive material found

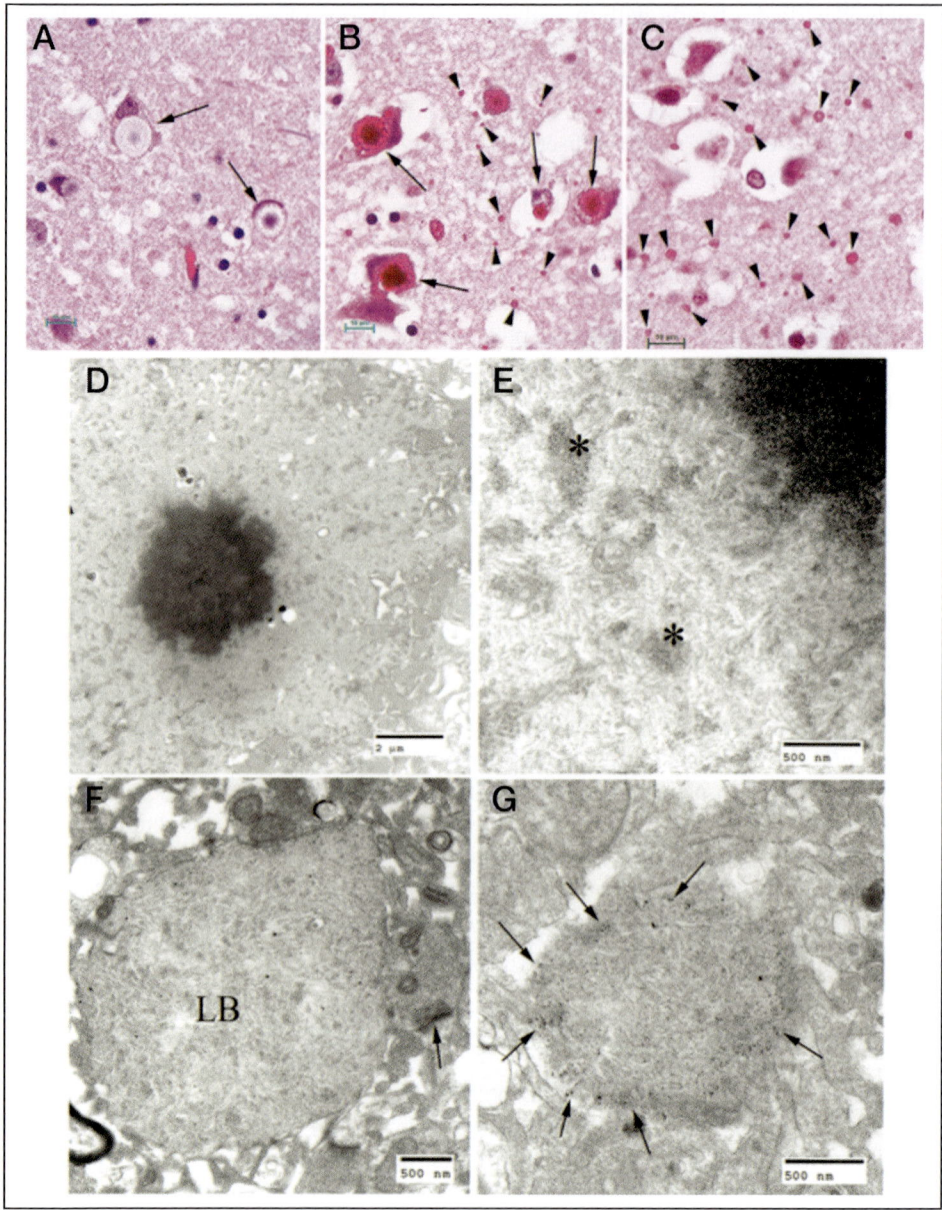

Fig. 4. Lafora disease in human brain. (**A**) Haematoxylin and eosin (H&E)-stained section of brain obtained from an LD patient at autopsy. Arrows indicate perikaryal LBs. Note the outer pale layer and the basophilic core. (**B**) Diastase-digested periodic acid Schiff (PASD) section of the substantia nigra from the same patient. Note the intense staining of the perikaryl LBs (arrows) and the 'dust-like' LBs (arrowheads). (**C**) PASD-stained cerebral cortex. Note the presence of numerous 'dust-like' LBs (arrowheads). (**D**) Low-power electron micrograph of a perikaryl LB. Electron dense core is the equivalent of the basophilic core seen in H&E-stained material. (**E**) Higher power of (**D**). As well as the filamentous polyglucosans, aggregates of 'glycogen-like' material was frequently seen (asterisks). (**F**) Electron micrograph of a dendritic LB. Note the synaptic density (arrow). (**G**) Electron micrograph of a tannic acid-stained LB. Note the presence of glycogen particles at the periphery (arrows).

in both perikaryal and 'dust-like' LBs, as well as LBs found in other tissues, are diastase-resistant, hence for all diagnoses of suspect LD patients, diastase-treated PAS (PASD) staining plays an integral role in the identification of the disease in both surgical biopsy and autopsy materials. Some patchy neuronal loss may be present in the later stages of the disease, but this is not a prominent feature (Sakai *et al.*, 1970; Carpenter & Karpati, 1981a).

Electron microscopy confirms the presence of fibrillary accumulations typical of polyglucosans within the LBs. Using electron tomography, we were recently able to identify an ordered structure where individual polyglucosan fibrils bifurcate at a regular periodicity, ranging from 50-125 nm, depending on the tissue of origin (unpublished observation). This is especially true of the perikaryal and 'dust-like' LBs found in the brain, in skeletal muscle myocytes, and all of the LBs in affected sweat glands. Along with the filaments, there is often poorly-defined granular material within the LB itself. In 2 extremely well preserved brain biopsy specimens, we observed 'glycogen-like' particles in the dendritic cytoplasm and the perykaryon of neurons in both perikaryal and 'dust-like' LBs (unpublished data) (Fig. 4D-G). Glycogen is rarely found in neurons because the sugars are rapidly metabolized. In skeletal muscle and cardiac myocytes, the fibrillary polysaccharide accumulates in membrane-bound spaces which are not lysosomal (Barbieri *et al.*, 1987; Carpenter & Karpati, 1981a; Yokoi *et al.*, 1975). There is variation in the morphology of the enclosed material, including some granular material, but the majority is fibrillar. Skeletal muscle can be used as a source for morphological diagnosis, but it is far from ideal, since the degree of involvement varies, and not all muscle fibre types are involved (Neville *et al.*, 1974; Turnbull *et al.*, 2011a) (Fig. 5A, B). This has been clearly demonstrated in a laforin knockout mouse model, and retrospective studies on human muscle biopsies are currently underway. Similar to the mouse, preliminary data suggest that humans do in fact produce LBs in type II fibres (Turnbull *et al.*, 2011a).

Hepatic insufficiency is an early event in rare LD patients (Tomimatsu *et al.*, 1985; Nishimura *et al.*, 1980; Gomez-Garre *et al.*, 2007). In the liver, PASD staining shows deposits of large portions of PASD positive material in many of the periportal hepatocytes, confining the nucleus and other organelles to one side of the cell. Liver biopsy has been used for diagnosis, but the pathology is not specific to LD alone (Nishimura *et al.*, 1980). Electron microscopy of periportal hepatocytes with LBs reveals lakes of loosely packed fibrillar material with some glycogen particles and/or rosettes within the LB. Although a few organelles such as mitochondria and peroxisomes can be found in the LB, the majority of the smaller organelles are confined to a thin layer of cytoplasm which is continuous with the thicker side of the cell which contains the nucleus, the majority of the endoplasmic reticulum, and the Golgi (Fig. 5C, D).

The occurrence of LBs in the sweat glands has become the gold standard in the pathological diagnosis of LD (Carpenter & Karpati, 1981b; Andrade *et al.*, 2003). Skin is the most accessible of the affected tissues and biopsy procedures are the least invasive. LBs can be found in the eccrine duct cells, close to the secretory coil or close to the surface. They are extremely PASD positive and are roughly the size of the cell nucleus. Under the electron microscope, LBs are almost 'starch-like' in appearance, however, this is not a diagnostic feature. The eccrine myoepithelial cells rarely contain LBs. The apocrine myoepithelial cells, in contrast, contain LNs in almost all cases. The apocrine secretory (luminal) cells never contain LBs, but do contain PASD-positive inclusions which can be misleading (Andrade *et al.*, 2003) (Fig. 6).

A third gene (*PRDM8*) has recently been discovered in a single family. As with *EPM2A* and *EPM2B* mutations, the patients have a progressive myoclonus epilepsy which is similar to typical LD, but also exhibits significant differences (Turnbull *et al.*, 2012). The sweat glands in these patients contain no LBs. At present, we have not been able to study the brain of these

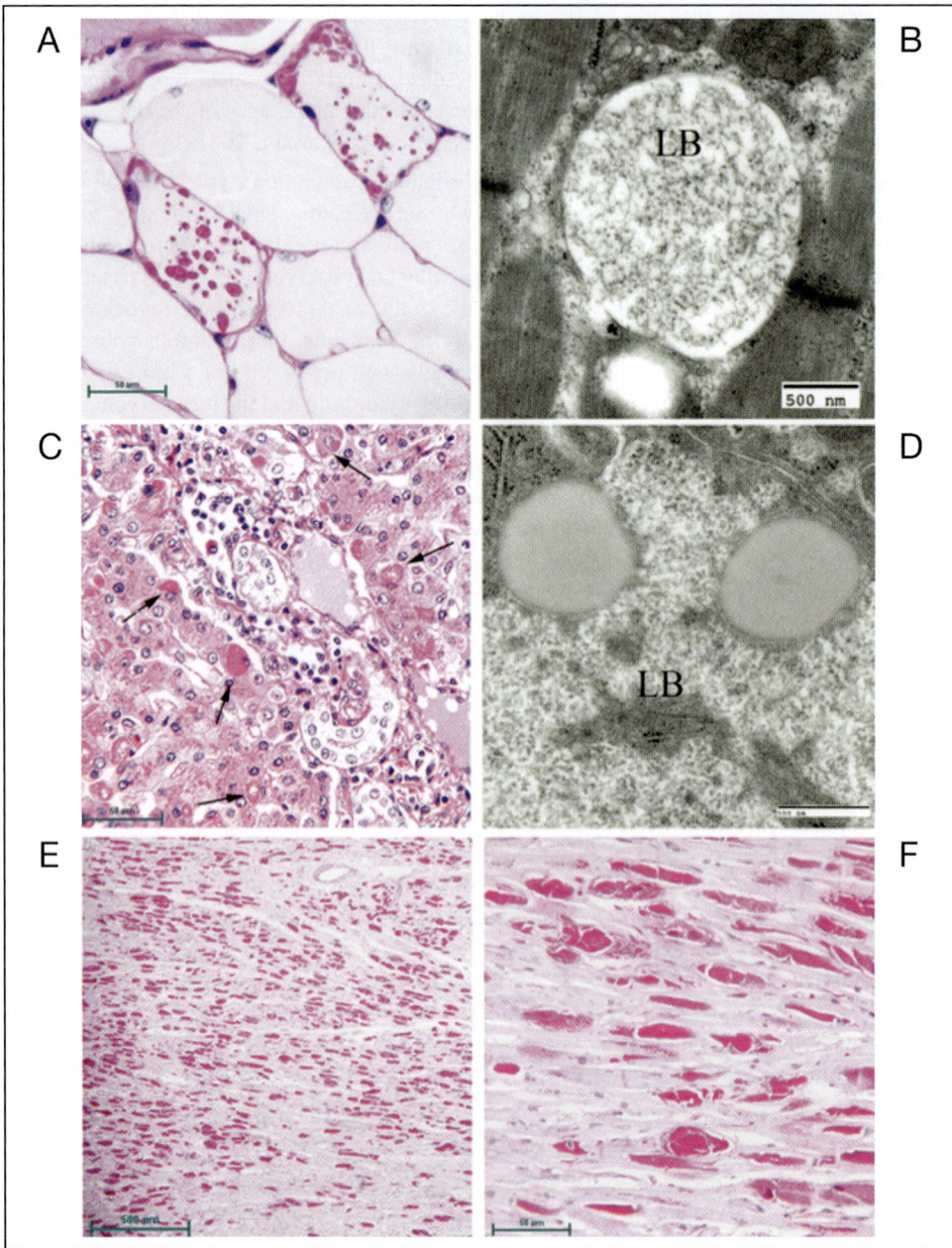

Fig. 5. Lafora disease in human muscle, liver, and heart. (**A**) PASD-stained formalin-fixed muscle biopsy from a patient. Two of the fibres contain LBs. (**B**) Electron micrograph of an LB (LB) in muscle. Note that it is membrane bound and contains both fibrillar and granular material. (**C**) PASD-stained hepatic periportal region of an LD patient at autopsy. Arrows indicate hepatocytes containing LBs. (**D**) Electron micrograph of a LB in liver from biopsy material. Note the thin cytoplasm (arrows) and the predominately granular, with some filamentous, material forming the LB. (**E**) Low power of a PASD-stained heart from a LD patient at autopsy. Note the numerous LDs. (**F**) Higher magnification of (**E**). LBs occupied a high percentage of the sarcoplasm of the cardiac myocyte.

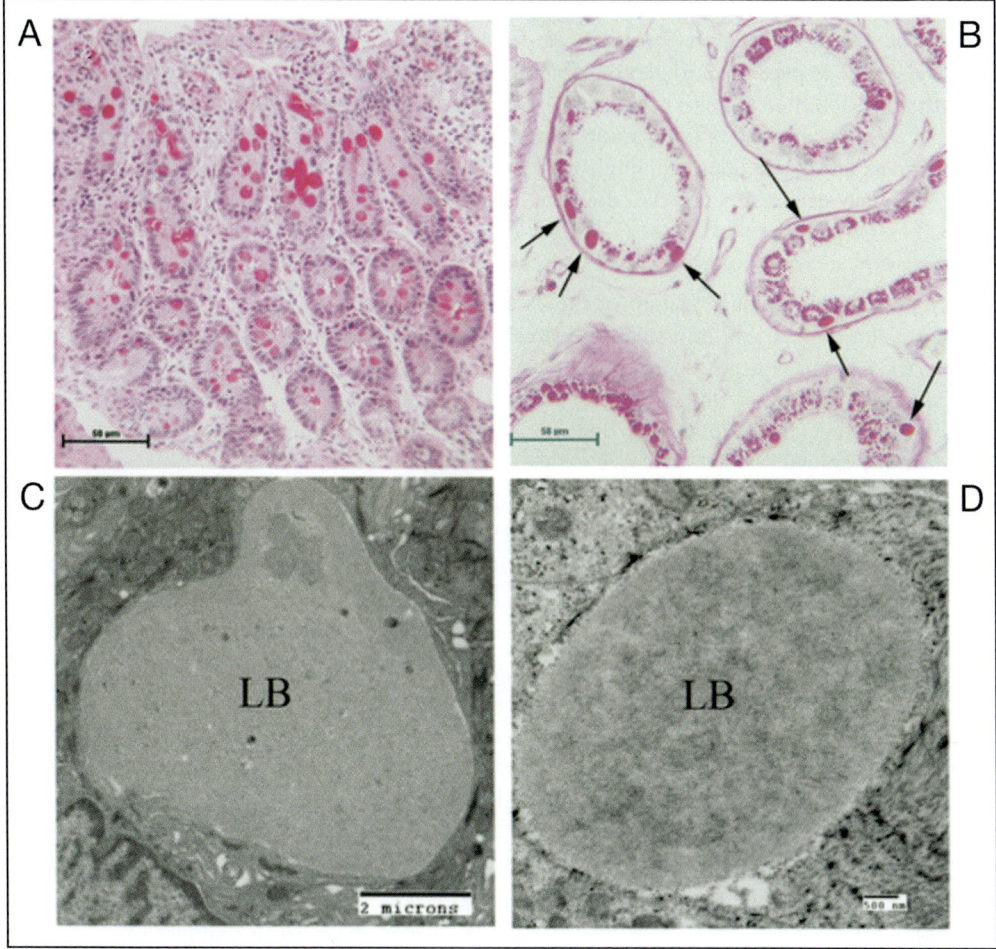

Fig. 6. Lafora disease in human sweat glands. (**A**) PASD staining of LBs in ductile cells in eccrine sweat glands. (**B**) PASD staining of LBs in the myoepithelial cells of apocrine sweat glands (arrows). (**C**) Electron micrograph of an LB from a ductile cell in an eccrine sweat gland. (**D**) Electron micrograph of an LB in a myoepithelial cell from an eccrine sweat gland.

patients for lack of material. Absence of LBs in the sweat glands of these patients could influence the current diagnostic algorithm. If a patient has all the clinical manifestations of LD, a new gene defect is detected, and there are no LBs found in the sweat glands in the skin biopsy, the physician should consider an open muscle biopsy, as LBs are readily found in the muscle.

In order to further our knowledge of LD, it is necessary to study animal models of this disease which could lead to breakthroughs in the understanding of the pathogenesis, which may subsequently lead to potential therapies. Polyglucosan storage disease with myoclonic epilepsy has been known to exist in animals since it was reported in a beagle in the early 1920s. Although it has only been reported in several breeds of dogs and other species of the Canidae class, as well as cockatiels, pigs and cattle, it has probably been overlooked in many other species, since it is rare for animals to be subjected to post mortem examination, especially non-domesticated animals. The most widely studied of these naturally occurring animal models is the pure bred dog. As these animals are bred from a limited gene pool, the potential for consanguinity is greatly increased. Fortunately, breeders are regulated by kennel clubs and in order for these dogs to be sold as pure bred, evidence of a known lineage and a stringent medical examination must first be submitted to these organizations, prior to a certificate being issued. As the majority of these animals are sold as companion animals, the dogs are routinely examined by qualified veterinarians and sometimes, although rarely, LD is detected in these dogs. LD in dogs can occur spontaneously in any breed of dog, but it particularly affects miniature wire-haired dachshunds, basset hounds, and beagles (Kaiser et al., 1991; Gredal et al., 2003; Lohi et al., 2005). The disease does not present in dogs until at least 5 years age (35 in human years).

Myoclonus is the dominant feature of the canine disease and this can be induced by flashing lights, sudden sounds, and movement. Generalized or complex partial seizures can be seen in some dogs. The disease progresses over many years and gradually other neurological deficits, such as ataxia, blindness, and dementia, occur. Unlike humans, affected animals have a near-normal life expectancy, though as quality of life diminishes, the owner may be forced to euthanize the animal.

Pathological examination of these dogs revealed distribution and frequency of LBs in the brain identical to that found in the human disease (Lohi et al., 2005). As with humans, the liver contains LBs only in periportal hepatocytes. Both cardiac and skeletal myocytes contain LBs. Dogs do not have sweat glands in the skin, except in the footpads, where both apocrine and merocrine sweat glands are present; the LBs are identical in size and structure to those of the human disease. They are found in the apocrine myoepithelial cells and in the merocrine ductile and myoepithelial cells (Fig. 7).

With the identification of two genes (EPM2A [laforin] and EPM2B [malin]) responsible for LD, it was only logical that transgenic mice technology be utilized to develop murine models of the disease, in order to further advance our knowledge of LD.

The first of the animal models developed was a laforin-deficient murine mutant (Ganesh et al., 2002b). This was achieved by deleting the dual-specificity phosphatase domain of the EPM2A gene. These null mutants developed LBs in the brain, specifically in the hippocampus, cerebellum, cortex, and brainstem. Neuronal degeneration was observed in younger mice, but the same phenomenon was observed in age-matched wild-type littermates, which is suggestive of neuronal remodelling during development. The onset of LB accumulation occurred at 2 months. The highest number of perikaryal LBs was found in the molecular layer of the cerebral cortex and, as with humans, perikaryal LBs had 2 layers of various proportions; the outer layer being pale and the core basophilic. 'Ground glass' LBs were found throughout. Mild focal neuronal degenerative changes were detected primarily in the Purkinje cells of the cerebellum and were particularly present in the later stages of the disease. Ultrastructural examination of these tissues revealed prominent LBs in many of the neurons in all of the affected areas. As with dogs, mice have no sweat glands in the skin, except in the footpads where LBs were found. LBs were also found in skeletal and cardiac myocytes. No LBs were detected in the liver using either PASD staining or electron microscopy, although they were reported to be present using an antibody against polyglucosan bodies.

A transgenic mouse was generated which overexpressed myc-tagged inactivated laforin, in order to trap the substrate of laforin (Chan et al., 2004). Myc-laforin was expressed 150 fold higher than endogenous laforin. LBs were formed in the neuronal perikarya and dendrites, liver, sweat glands in the footpad, and skeletal and cardiac myocytes. In the liver, hepatocytes with LBs were found in discrete clusters throughout zones 2 and 3. Using an antibody against

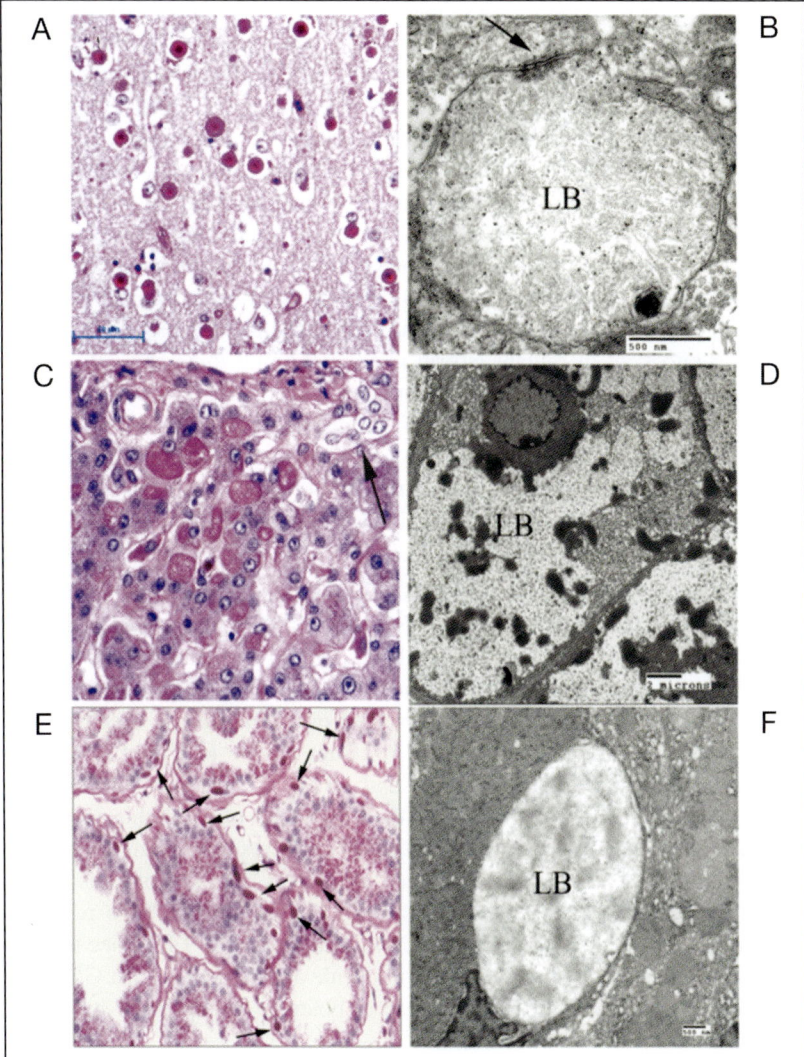

Fig. 7. Canine Lafora disease. (**A**) PASD-stained brain from a mini wire-haired dachshund. Numerous perikaryl and 'dust-like' LBs are seen. (**B**) Dendritic LB. Note the filamentous polyglucosans. Arrow indicates the synaptic density. (**C**) PASD staining of a liver from an affected dog. A cluster of hepatocytes containing LBs is seen in the portal tract. Arrow indicates a bile duct. (**D**) Low-power electron micrograph of a hepatocyte containing an LB (LB). Note how the majority of the cytoplasm has been pressed to the periphery of the cell. (**E**) PASD-stained sweat gland from the footpad of an affected dog. Note the numerous LBs confined to the myoepithelial cells. (**F**) Electron micrograph of an LB (LB) in a myoepithelial cell.

myc with immunperoxidase staining or immunogold labelling, we were able to determine both the cellular and subcellular distribution of myc-laforin. Particularly striking was the staining of the LBs in cerebellar Purkinje cell somas and dendrites and stellate neurons, as well as the presence of discrete punctate structures consistent with LBs throughout the molecular layer of the cortex, and in some hippocampal and cerebral neurons. Overall, however, LBs in the brain in this model were much lower in number than in the knockout mouse mentioned above.

In addition, a malin knockout mouse was developed. The malin exon was removed by *in vivo* recombination and an embryonic stem cell line (ESL) was created. The ESL was aggregated and a chimeric mouse was generated. These were bred into a C57B6 background and the malin null mouse line was established from the resultant heterozygous mice (Turnbull *et al.*, 2010). These mice, like the laforin knockout mice, developed LBs in the brain at around 2 months. These null mutants developed LBs in the brain in the hippocampus, cerebellum, cortex, and brain stem. As was the case for the laforin deficient mouse, the LBs consisted of two populations. The perikaryal LBs consisted of 2 layers; the outer layer being pale and mildly eosinophilic and the core basophilic. These were found primarily in the cell bodies of neurons in the cerebral cortex molecular layer. 'Dust-like' LBs were found throughout the grey matter. LBs were also found in the sweat glands of the footpads and in skeletal muscle and cardiac myocytes. Unlike the laforin knockout or mutant laforin mice, malin null mice had LBs in some of the periportal hepatocytes. Not unlike the human or canine liver LBs, they occupied the centre of the cells, pressing the nuclei and the majority of cytoplasm to one side, as well as the periphery of the cell. Under the electron microscope, the LBs formed lakes which consisted of clusters of 'glycogen-like' particles and fibrillar material. Other groups have also generated malin knockout animals with similar results. Pathological sample images from the third mouse model mentioned above are presented in Figs 8 to 10.

One of the most exciting developments in the study of LD using transgenic mice is the use of double knockouts. In LD, glycogen synthase (GS) over-activity is considered one of the primary culprits for the formation of polyglucosans (Vilchez, 2007). It has been hypothesized that the reduction in GS activity might prevent polyglucosan formation. Laforin-deficient mice were bred with mice deficient in PTG, a protein involved in activating GS, resulting in LD mice lacking the GS-activating effect of PTG. The resultant double knockout (DKO) mice have almost no polyglucosan or neurodegeneration, and no seizures (Turnbull *et al.*, 2011b). The development of this DKO mouse demonstrates the importance of using this approach to create strategies for therapeutic interventions which ultimately may result in a cure for this devastating disease. Due to the inability to use this approach in humans, results from this and knockouts of other glycolytic pathway constituents in other DKO mice are likely to reveal molecules which, when inactivated or eliminated, lead to the control or cure of LD. Once these molecules have been identified, the development of small molecule antagonists against GS, its activators, and potential GS up-regulators will be developed as potential therapies for human LD.

Pathogenesis of Lafora disease

Normal glycogen remains soluble in the cell due to its highly organized structure, whereas polygluosans precipitate in the cell due to disturbances in the structure of the carbohydrate, and aggregate into LB (Tagliabracci *et al.*, 2008). LBs are very similar in morphology to polyglucosan bodies seen in glycogen-branching enzyme deficiency, differing only in their cellular location. In both LD and glycogen-branching enzyme deficiency, polyglucosans form in neurons. In LD, they are exclusively seen in the cell bodies and dendrites. In glycogen-branching enzyme deficiency, they are seen in axons. The two diseases have markedly dissimilar clinical symptoms, which is most likely to be due to this difference in polyglucosan localization. LD is a progressive myoclonus epilepsy, whereas glycogen-branching enzyme deficiency patients suffer from an adult-onset motor neuron disease, similar to that seen in amyotrophic lateral sclerosis (ALS) (Bruno *et al.*, 1993).

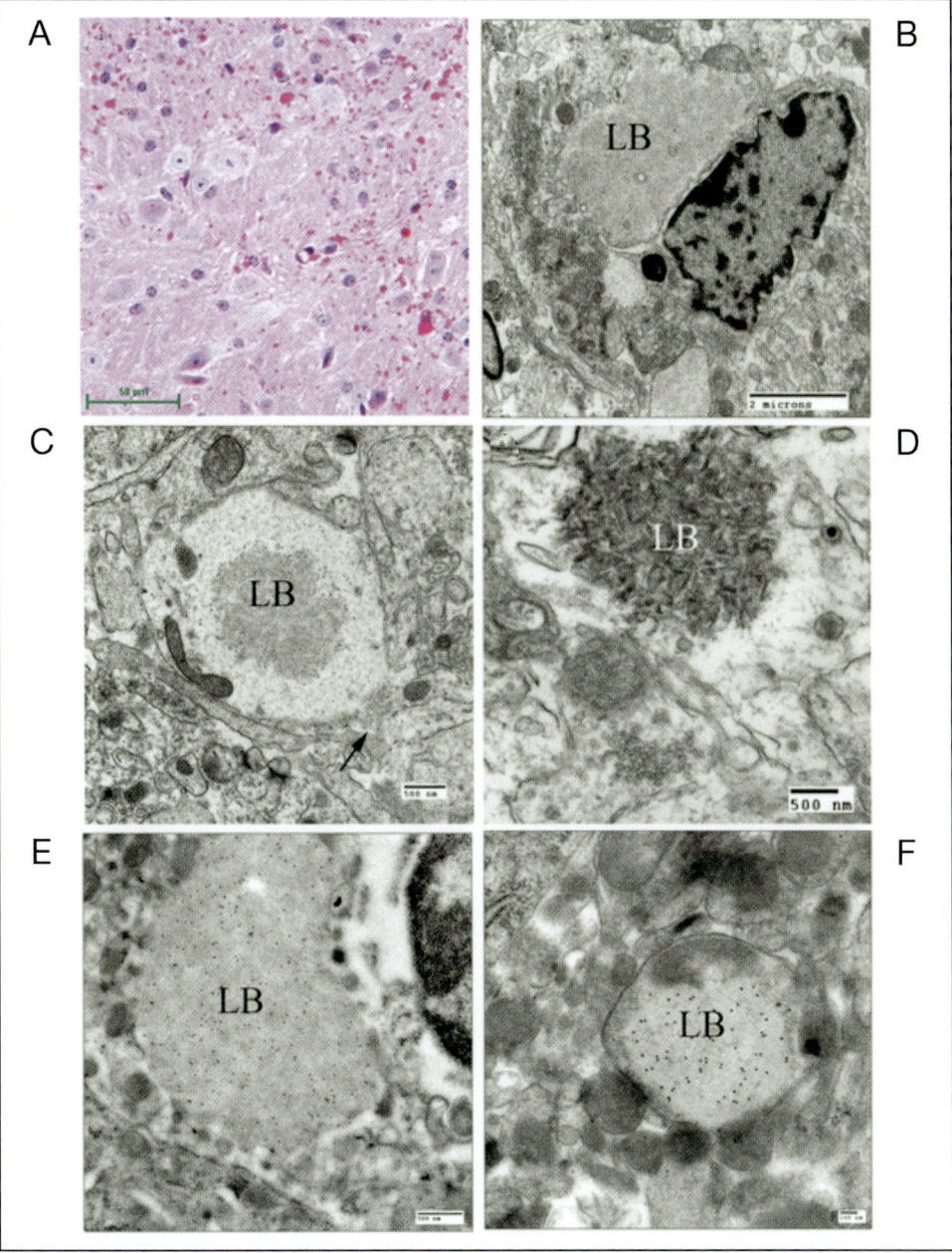

*Fig. 8. Lafora disease in the brain of a mouse model. (**A**) PASD-stained cortex from a malin-deficient mouse. Both perikaryal and 'dust-like' LBs are seen. (**B**) Electron micrograph of a juxtanuclear LB (LB) from a laforin knockout mouse. (**C**) Electron micrograph of a dendritic LB (LB) from a laforin deficient mouse. Note central location of the polyglucosans within the dendrite. Arrow indicates the synaptic density. (**D**) Electron micrograph of an LB (LB) from a malin-deficient mouse. Polyglucosans appear thicker and more electron opaque. (**E**) Electron micrograph of a perikaryal LB (LB) from a myc-tagged mutant laforin over-expressing mouse, which has been immunogold labelled for myc. Gold label is confined to the LB. (**F**) Electron micrograph of an LB from the same mouse line as (**D**). Gold label is confined to the LB.*

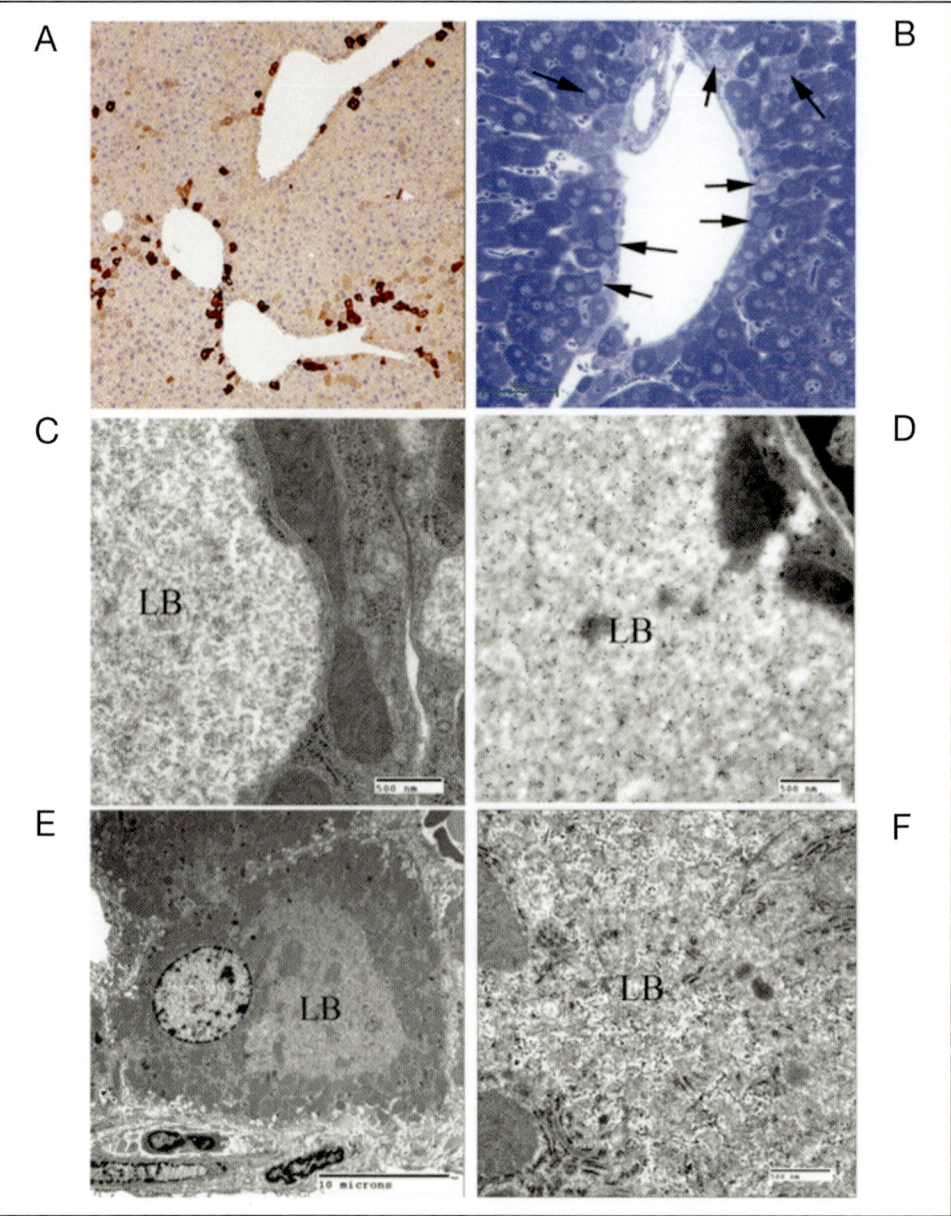

Fig. 9. Lafora disease in the liver of a mouse model. (**A**) Low power of myc immunoperoxidase-stained liver from a myc-tagged mutant laforin over-expressing mouse. Hepatocytes with LBs were only found in zone 2 or 3. (**B**) Toluidine blue stained section of a portal tract from a malin-deficient mouse. Arrows indicate hepatocytes containing LBs. (**C**) Electron micrograph of a LB (LB) from a myc tagged mutant laforin over-expressing mouse hepatocyte. Note how the cytoplasm has been pressed to one side. Note the predominately granular nature of the LB. (**D**) Electron micrograph of a LB (LB) from a myc-tagged mutant laforin over-expressing mouse hepatocyte that has been immunogold labelled with an antibody against myc. Label is confined to the LB. (**E**) Low-power electron micrograph of a malin-deficient periportal hepatocyte containing an LB (LB). (**F**) Higher power of (**E**) showing that the LB contains both granular and filamentous material (LB).

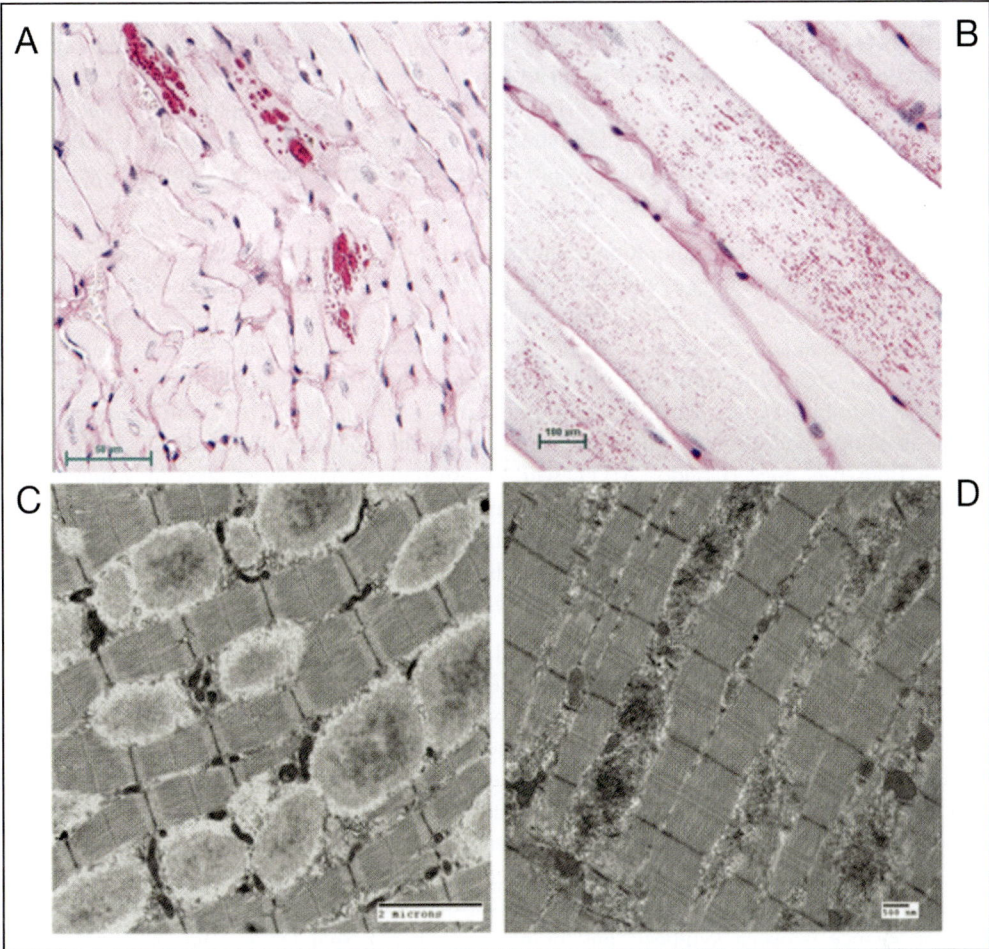

*Fig. 10. Lafora disease in the heart and skeletal muscle of a mouse model. (**A**) PASD staining of a laforin-deficient mouse heart. LBs were detected in some of the cardiac myocytes. (**B**) PASD staining of malin-deficient mouse skeletal muscle. Numerous LBs were detected in some of the muscle cells. (**C**) Electron micrograph of LBs in laforin-deficient mouse skeletal muscle. (**D**) Equivalent field in a malin-deficient mouse muscle. Note the overall electron opaque filamentous appearance of the LBs.*

EPM2A encodes a protein named laforin which contains a dual specificity phosphatase domain and a carbohydrate binding motif (Minassian *et al.*, 1998). The second LD gene, *EPM2B*, encodes malin, an E3 ubiquitin ligase (Chan *et al.*, 2004). Over a decade has passed since the second causative LD gene was identified. Since then, a number of hypotheses have been put forward as to the function of both malin and laforin in the pathogenesis of LD. The next decade will, most likely, unravel the complete pathway leading to LD and provide the knowledge which is necessary for finding a cure for this devastating disease.

LD has been speculated to be caused by defects in the clearance system(s) of the cell, similar to diseases such as Parkinson's and Alzheimer's. The presence of large inclusions and LBs, along with the finding that LBs contain a minor component of protein(s), suggested a defect in either autophagic processes and/or protein clearance. In keeping with this line of thought, defects in both autophagy and protein clearance have been reported in both Epm2a-/- and

Epm2b-/- mice (Aguado *et al.*, 2010; Criado *et al.*, 2011; Knecht *et al.*, 2010; Puri & Ganesh, 2010; Puri *et al.*, 2012; Garyali *et al.*, 2009; Rao *et al.*, 2010). Unexpectedly, the autophagic dysfunction in Epm2b-/- mice is different to that of Epm2a-/- mice, resulting from an mTor-independent pathway (Criado *et al.*, 2011). This suggests that if autophagic dysfunction is, indeed, at least partly causative of LD, mutations in malin and laforin may have separate and dissimilar disease mechanisms, which would be surprising, given the highly similar phenotypic outcomes in both laforin- and malin-deficient LD.

Malin has been reported to ubiquitinate a number of proteins, including laforin (Gentry *et al.*, 2005), glycogen-debranching enzyme (Cheng *et al.*, 2007), PTG/GS (Solaz-Fuster *et al.*, 2008; Vilchez, 2007; Worby *et al.*, 2008), neuronatin (Sharma *et al.*, 2011), AMPK (Moreno *et al.*, 2010), and dishevelled2 (Sharma *et al.*, 2012). However, only laforin and GS have been clearly shown to be increased in Epm2b-/- mice (Tagliabracci *et al.*, 2007, 2008; DePaouli-Roach *et al.*, 2010; Turnbull *et al.*, 2010; Valles-Ortega *et al.*, 2011), indicative of *in vivo* action of malin on laforin. Additionally, no changes affecting the ubiquitin-proteasomal system were seen in Epm2b-/- mice (Criado, 2011), while these defects have been seen in a number of laforin-deficient models. It therefore appears that these protein clearance defects are a secondary consequence of LB formation, which is supported by recent studies showing that removal of the major polyglucosan component of LB by downregulation of glycogen synthesis results in near-complete disease resolution (Turnbull *et al.*, 2011; Duran *et al.*, 2014).

A major prevailing hypothesis over the years in LD research has focused on the balance between glycogen synthesis and glycogen branching (Lohi *et al.*, 2006). Normally, GS synthesizes glycogen while the branching enzyme promotes the extension of the growing chain. This balance results in a soluble, highly ordered glycogen molecule. When this balance is disturbed in the direction of synthesis (*i.e.* when branching enzyme is deficient), polyglucosans form, as is seen in patients with glycogen-branching enzyme deficiency. The similarities between LBs and the accumulations seen in glycogen-branching enzyme deficiency, as well as data showing that over-expression of GS can also cause polyglucosan accumulation (Raben *et al.*, 2001), make this an appealing and logical hypothesis. More substance was added to this proposal that there is a misbalance between synthesis and branching, when Fernández-Sánchez and colleagues demonstrated an interaction between laforin and PTG, a glycogen-targeting subunit of protein phosphatase-1 (PP1) (Fernandez-Sanchez *et al.*, 2003). PTG directs PP1 to the glycogen-metabolizing enzymes, activating GS while inhibiting glycogen phosphorylase, and thus leading to a net increase in glycogen synthesis (Printen *et al.*, 1997). In addition to its interaction with PTG, laforin has also been shown to interact with other regulatory subunits of PP1, including GL and R6, members of the same family as PTG. Subsequent studies have confirmed the PTG interaction using cell over-expression systems *in vitro*, but no *in vivo* interaction studies have been reported, which is likely to be due to a lack of a suitable antibody to PTG. Interestingly, some disease-causing mutations in laforin specifically affect its interaction with PTG, indicating that disruption of this interaction is pathogenic. Dysregulation of PTG has been hypothesized to cause LD, primarily based on results from *in vitro* studies. Elegant work by Vilchez and colleagues showed that malin and laforin act together to control levels of glycogen synthesis by targeting PTG and/or GS for proteasomal degradation (Solar-Fuster, 2008; Vilchez, 2007; Worby *et al.*, 2008). When either laforin or malin is missing, levels of PTG, an indirect activator of GS, increase, causing GS over-activation. In this hypothesis, over-active GS would cause an imbalance between glycogen branching and extension, leading to the formation of LBs. Results from studies using animal models of LD showed no increases in PTG levels or GS activity, indicating that dysregulation of PTG may not be causative of LD (DePaouli-Roach *et al.*, 2010; Turnbull *et al.*, 2010; Valles-Ortega *et al.*, 2011). Nonetheless, the large amount of *in vitro* data, along with a study showing that removal of PTG from laforin deficient mice resulted in a dramatic reduction in LB and a cure for LD in the mouse, strongly supports the conclusion that PTG and laforin interact, and that both are involved in the same metabolic pathway.

The beginnings of an attractive hypothesis emerged from the laboratory of Jack Dixon when they reported that laforin was a carbohydrate phosphatase which could dephosphorylate amylopectin, a plant carbohydrate (Worby *et al.*, 2006). Following this, Tagliabracci and colleagues expanded on this work in a series of elegant experiments. First, they demonstrated that laforin could indeed dephosphorylate glycogen and, most importantly, that glycogen phosphate levels were present at a much higher level than normal in mice lacking laforin (Tagliabracci *et al.*, 2007, 2008). The covalently bound phosphate on glycogen was shown to be present at all available glucose carbons of glycogen, *i.e.* C2, C3 and C6 (Tagliabracci *et al.*, 2011; Nitschke *et al.*, 2013). Precisely where the phosphate on glycogen originates and how it results in glycogen becoming polyglucosan remains unknown. It was shown that laforin removes these phosphates during glycogen degradation (Irmia, 2015). This emerging phosphate hypothesis is compelling, but fails to identify a role for malin in LD. At 12 months of age, laforin-deficient mice have a 4.2-fold increase in muscle glycogen phosphate, whereas malin-deficient mice present a more modest increase of 2.8-fold over normal wild-type levels (Tagliabracci *et al.*, 2008; Tiberia *et al.*, 2012). The lack of a comparable phosphate increase in malin deficiency when laforin deficiency and malin deficiency are clinically equivalent raises the likelihood of other mechanisms at play in malin deficient LD. Based on our most recent results from malin-deficient mice, we showed that absence of malin leads to increased laforin, as an initial step prior to any LB formation, and then progressive accumulation of laforin in glycogen. We also found that the gradual accumulation of laforin in glycogen renders the latter progressively less soluble. In related work, we showed that over-expressing laforin in cell culture leads to a conversion of glycogen to polyglucosan masses. This phenomenon continues to occur when laforin mutants, which bind glycogen but are phosphatase-inactive, are used. This no longer occurs when laforin mutants which cannot bind glycogen are used. Collectively, these results suggest that malin functions to regulate the quantity of laforin, and excess laforin on glycogen is detrimental to glycogen, leading to glycogen conversion to polyglucosan and LB (Tiberia *et al.*, 2012).

The last decade has brought about a number of breakthroughs in the understanding of LD pathogenesis, though a clear picture has not yet formed. Each new hypothesis has come with its own weaknesses. The two main hypotheses of LB formation centre round the synthesis of glycogen and its structure. Compelling evidence has been presented for both, though each has their own caveats. Tiberia and colleagues attempted to propose a unifying hypothesis (Tiberia *et al.*, 2012). Firstly, they considered laforin's role as a glycogen phosphatase, which removes phosphate from glycogen allowing it to remain soluble in the cell. Secondly, malin acts on laforin, and is likely also to act on other glycogen metabolic enzymes, to remove them from the glycogen molecule. If laforin is missing, phosphate accumulates and causes glycogen to become structurally abnormal and precipitate. If malin is missing, laforin remains 'stuck' to glycogen, again disturbing the precise structure of glycogen and causing it to precipitate. This hypothesis answers a number of outstanding questions in LD research, foremost addressing the role of malin in LD. Here, malin has two roles; the first to control cytosolic amounts of laforin to keep it from inadvertently 'clogging up' the structure of glycogen, and second, to remove laforin (and probably other proteins, such as GS) from glycogen itself after laforin has removed the specific phosphate. Gentry and colleagues (Gentry *et al.*, 2005) had previously speculated that malin may play a role in the regulation of laforin levels, but the actual mechanism behind this was unknown. In this hypothesis, both laforin deficiency and malin deficiency lead to LB formation by means of foreign matter on the glycogen molecule itself (phosphate and protein, respectively). While this theory appeared to bring together disparate aspects of LD research, most recent results once again raised a new and serious challenge. It was shown that expressing a phosphatase-inactive laforin in laforin knockout mice can fully rescue LD in these mice (Gayarre *et al.*, 2014). This finding puts back into question the role of phosphate in polyglucosan formation, causing the field to be re-examined once more. The field has, however, been very rich in results since the genes for this disease were identified. It is hoped that a few new breakthroughs will lead to a comprehensive understanding of this deadly disease.

Disease management and therapy

Lafora disease (LD) is a devastating condition, with severely limited life expectancy and therapeutic options which continue to be limited. Its striking clinical and EEG features may lead to early diagnosis, but because it remains uncommon, few clinicians gain significant experience of this condition, and diagnosis is often delayed. Moreover, LD is a recessively inherited condition, with founder effects and increased prevalence associated with inbreeding, and thus LD is unevenly distributed across the world, which contributes to 'knowledge gaps' about the condition.

We will try here to delineate the practical steps that we recommend in the management of patients with LD. It is clear, in our eyes, that there is an intermediary stage: the clinical diagnosis of LD is now comparatively easy to confirm. Efficient anticonvulsants can be used to alleviate the burden of the attacks, but better insights into the mechanisms underlying the production of LBs and the progression of clinical symptoms have not yet produced ground-breaking therapeutic advances. Thus, dealing with LD patients and their families is not an easy task, because there is little hope to offer and the genetic nature of the condition raises many questions within the affected families.

Management: diagnosis and genetic counselling (Fig. 11)

Given the severity of the prognosis, a biological confirmation of the diagnosis of LD is necessary; this used to be made based on typical pathological findings (from a skin, muscle, or liver biopsy), but nowadays relies on genetics. It is our opinion that this procedure, which remains costly, should be justified by solid clinical and EEG evidence, and should not be performed together with a variety of tests, while screening for all possible genetic mechanisms in a poorly-assessed case with epilepsy and myoclonus.

The diagnosis of LD is based on three levels of evidence:

(1) The clinical evidence is a compound of history-taking (family background, circumstances, aspects and progression of seizures and myoclonus, and visual agnosia) and examination (including cognitive and psychological assessment, exclusion of associated symptoms such as sensory deficits, and video documentation of myoclonus and general behaviour). The most common clinical situation is one where idiopathic generalized epilepsy (IGE) or even juvenile myoclonic epilepsy (JME) has been diagnosed, with a re-assessment of the patient's situation because of a very unusual evolution which tends towards worsening; the clinical work-up should help exclude the possibility of aggravation of IGE by inappropriate AEDs, which may result in a pseudo-PME.

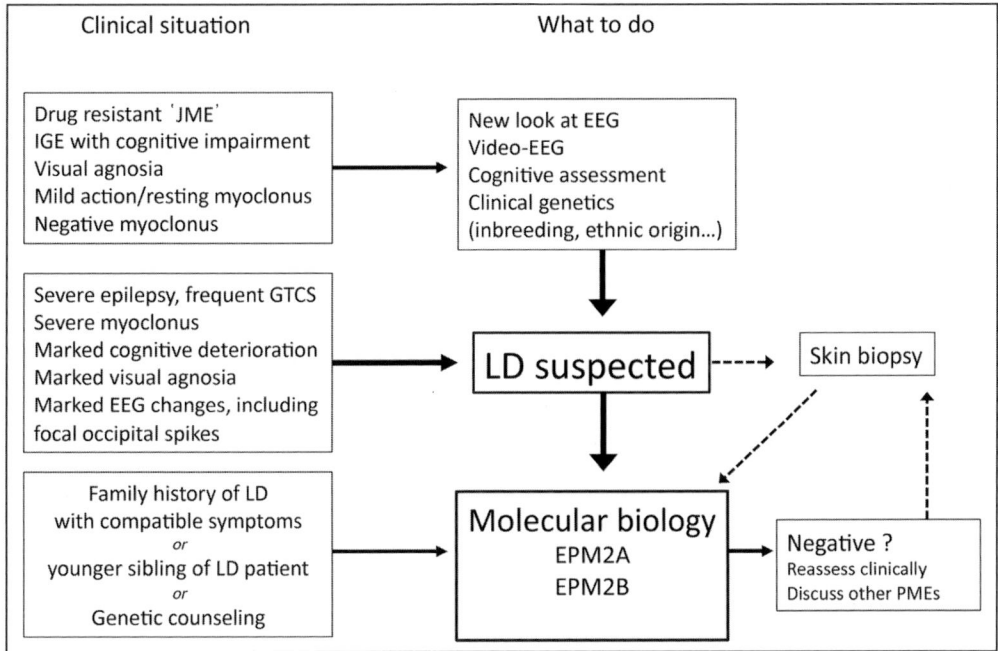

Fig. 11. Management of patients with LD: diagnosis.

(2) Complementary evidence is based on a thorough evaluation of the EEG, polygraphic EEG, and video-EEG (with an assessment of progression of changes over time). Neurophysiology may also help distinguish between LD and other adolescent-onset PMEs, *e.g.* Unverricht-Lundborg disease, in which the EEG changes are less pronounced, or juvenile ceroid-lipofuscinosis, in which prominent single-flash responses on the EEG are found. Other procedures may also help in the differential diagnosis (neuroimaging/MRI is not informative in LD). Pathological demonstration of LBs in sweat gland duct cells on axillary skin biopsy (or, less commonly, on liver or muscle biopsy) used to be the definitive diagnostic tool, but requires a highly trained pathologist; it may still render services as a supplementary element in favour of a diagnosis of LD when genetic testing is not available, or not entirely conclusive.

(3) The confirmation of diagnosis is nowadays provided by the demonstration of a pathogenic mutation in both alleles of one of the *EPM2* genes, with presence of heterozygous mutations in each of the clinically unaffected parents.

The diagnosis of LD can be made, or suspected, in various clinical settings, with, in our opinion, three typical situations:

At an advanced stage of the condition, in very typical patients and/or families who were not diagnosed earlier due to a lack of local expertise resulting from the rarity of LD in some settings, or due to the absence of molecular biological tools, *e.g.* in rural Africa (Traoré *et al.*, 2009). In such cases, genetic testing will show the genetic subtype, and contribute to the worldwide 'map' of mutations found in *EPM2A* and *EPM2B*.

A PME or LD should enter the differential diagnosis for any adolescent with a diagnosis of IGE, JME, or photosensitive epilepsy with not only failure to respond to antiepileptic drugs (AEDs), but also a condition that appears to worsen. In such patients, a thorough re-evaluation of the clinical data shows that the patient has resting and action myoclonus, often well-controlled/masked by medication, such as valproate (VPA), or, characteristically, negative myoclonus (Genton *et al.*, 2012), visual agnosia, and prominent, specific EEG changes. The search for a mutation in the known LD genes is warranted to confirm the diagnosis.

In other radically different situations within the context of a family with a confirmed diagnosis of LD in one of its members. Although LD is highly unlikely in asymptomatic adults, such adults will want to know whether they carry a heterozygous mutation; in younger asymptomatic siblings, LD may still manifest, and the emergence of 'preventive' treatment strategies may render the identification of the mutation useful in this context. As the pathogenic mutations have already been characterized in the proband, the cost of the investigations for other family members will be lower, and the importance of detecting preclinical cases will also be known.

It is evident that the diagnosis of LD should not be given to the family before a final and definitive confirmation, however, once it is confirmed, it should not be kept from the caregivers. Presenting the diagnosis to patients themselves is not advisable, as there is little hope to offer. Moreover, they may be too young or affected to understand the implications; at an early stage, some may still be able to understand and gain access, *e.g.* on the internet, to detailed information on LD, which might cause severe depression. In our experience, a diagnosis of 'severe, drug-resistant epilepsy' will satisfy the patient's curiosity and still offer some hope and a reason for accepting help. However, if significant progress occurs in the near future, this global attitude may have to change, for example, in order to accept pathogenetically-founded therapies.

The consequences of a diagnosis of LD for the family of the proband should not be underestimated. Time should be devoted to the change expected for patients and their families (see below), but also to counselling regarding the following topics:

– The legitimate feelings of guilt and resentment must be alleviated with a few simple statements, that the inheritance is bilateral (*i.e.* the disease does not come specifically from the father or from the mother, but from both sides), that the disease results from a very uncommon co-occurrence of abnormal genes (even in consanguineous marriages), and that persons with a single abnormal gene will not have the disease.

– The main concern is the possible occurrence of LD in other family members. The risk can be practically excluded in older, fully asymptomatic siblings, but cannot be excluded in younger asymptomatic siblings nor, *a fortiori*, in as yet unborn siblings, if the parents are young enough to have other children. Whether siblings, especially younger ones, should be subject to molecular screening is still debatable. There is no reliable, recommended treatment, in pre-symptomatic LD cases, to prevent or delay the appearance and progression of symptoms. However, new perspectives are opening up with new possible treatments. Knowledge of the type of causative mutation that affects the proband allows precise counselling in this matter. Having provided all the relevant information, the clinician in charge of the patient will come to an agreement with the family and obtain their informed consent for all the procedures performed on non-affected family members. If the family shows reluctance towards genetic testing, a simple EEG recording for a younger sibling may provide information on the potential risk of LD, as EEG changes may precede the first clinical symptoms by many years (Van Heycoptenhamm & De Jager, 1963). Concerning future pregnancies for the parents of a patient with LD, the risks are known (LD: 1/4; transmission of one pathogenic gene: 1/2; no risk: 1/4), and prenatal screening can also be proposed.

– The risk of carrying an abnormal gene and transmitting the condition to other generations is also a major concern in families with LD. We have no experience of patients with LD having children. Their siblings or parents (when they plan to have children with another spouse), as well as other family members, may benefit from molecular screening in order to assess the presence or absence of the pathogenic gene(s) found in the proband.

An important aspect of diagnosis and genetic counselling is financial; insurance and conditions of reimbursement (or, more basically, the availability for procedures, tests, and medications) differ greatly between countries and social systems. Families should always be informed about the costs involved; searching for a mutation is expensive, but the simple screening for a known mutation is less costly. Similarly, the regulations covering genetic diagnosis, screening, and counselling may differ between countries, and clinicians should always conform to local laws. Obtaining informed consent for the successive steps of diagnostic and screening procedures is a minimum requirement.

Management: treatment and social support (Fig. 12)

In this chapter, new therapeutic proposals are not discussed since these are covered in detail in the last chapter. We shall focus on the medical and social measures that are available for the care of present-day LD patients. It is clear that health systems vary greatly between countries, particularly between affluent and less developed societies. Moreover, in many developed countries, health coverage is not equal; some patients (*e.g.* public sector employees and their families) may benefit from a whole range of possibilities, while others (*e.g.* those informally employed in the private sector) do not. It is also clear that patients with LD should benefit from the maximum possible help provided by the available health system. LD is a rare condition which cannot be considered as a public health problem (as costs are limited by the small number of affected persons), but it has major consequences for patients and caregivers, and society should show solidarity and provide all available support.

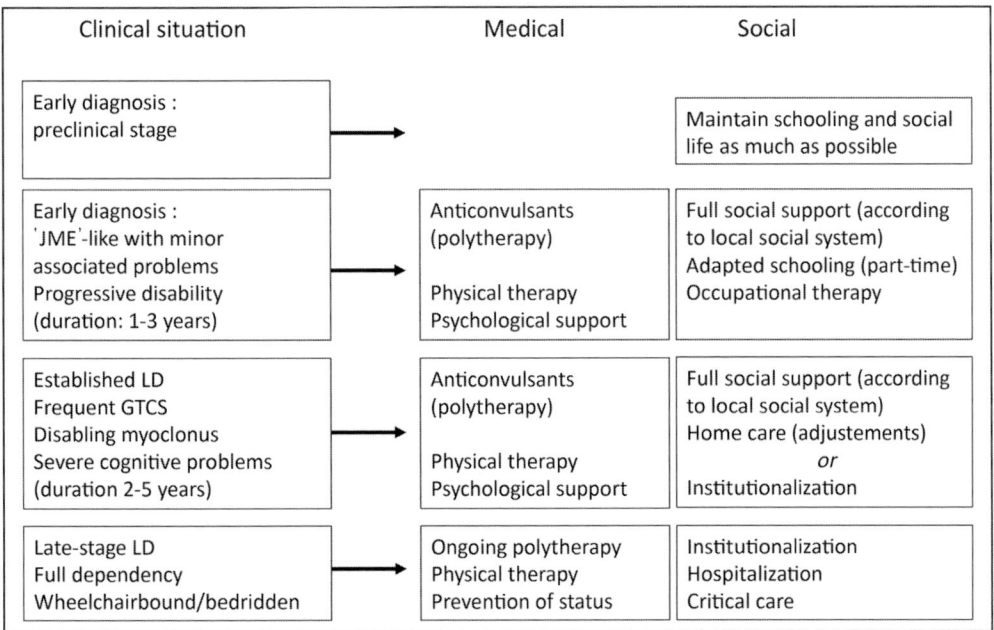

Fig. 12. Management of patients with LD: medical and social treatment.

With regards to AEDs, there are no specific antimyoclonic agents active against LD, to relieve seizures and myoclonus, and the effect is felt throughout the course of the disease. Unfortunately, their effect is partial and they have no major influence on the progression of cognitive and behavioural symptoms. Patients typically receive an AED, usually valproic acid, after the first generalized tonic-clonic seizure (GTCS). This is usually effective in suppressing, for some time, most GTCS, the symptoms associated with photic sensitivity, and some of the myoclonus. There are two unusual effects, which should lead to an early diagnosis of LD: first, the EEG shows rapidly increasing, permanent interictal changes, including focal occipital spikes, despite the apparent clinical remission; second, the patients develop negative myoclonus, which becomes prominent before the more characteristic myoclonic jerks. Other AEDs are used during this stage: lamotrigine (LTG) is not very advisable in the context of a myoclonic epilepsy, but may help transiently; phenobarbital (PB) and primidone (PRM) are effective, but are often used at high doses and their cognitive effects are added to those of the condition; and levetiracetam (LEV) is increasingly used early for adolescents with IGE, hence in LD cases, even before confirmation of the diagnosis. Other helpful drugs include topiramate (TPM) and zonisamide (ZNS), which both have marked antimyoclonic effects in some patients. Additional relief can be obtained, often transiently, with ethosuximide, felbamate, methsuximide, and benzodiazepines (BZD). The latter (usually clobazam, clonazepam, and diazepam) should be used with care since there is a marked initial effect followed by quick tolerance. Finally, there have been 2 recent single case reports of rather dramatic beneficial effects of perampanel (Schorlemmer *et al.*, 2013; Dirani *et al.*, 2014), and a larger study is presently underway.

With such a severe condition, the paradoxical aggravating effect of some AEDs may be difficult to pinpoint. There is no evidence that carbamazepine (CBZ), oxcarbazepine (OXC), phenytoin (PHT), eslicarbazepine, gabapentin, pregabalin, vigabatrin, or lacosamide are of any benefit. Often, withdrawal of one of these AEDs (especially CBZ or OXC) will bring some relief. However, we have experienced cases in which status epilepticus responds well to phenytoin loading. Phenytoin should not, however, be kept as maintenance medication subsequent to arresting the status.

With the progression of LD, AED treatment progresses to polytherapy, with a combination of several of the drugs quoted above (with the exclusion of LTG); the commonly used combinations are VPA+TPM or ZNS or LEV, with an additional BZD, a 3- to 5-drug combination being fairly common; one can switch between BZD when tolerance occurs. In case of severe, transient aggravation, with serial seizures or status epilepticus, there should be no abrupt changes to the usual regimen (except for the interruption of a potentially aggravating AED), and IV BZD should be used, as well as, for a limited period, IV PB or PHT. In our recent experience, the final progression of the disease no longer includes refractory status epilepticus, but more commonly involves non-specific complications, infectious or otherwise, in bedridden and demented patients. Thus, despite their lack of influence on the overall evolution of the disease, modern AEDs have partly changed the outcome, which is apparently no longer accompanied by severe, formerly often terminal, episodes of refractory convulsive status epilepticus.

In LD, social support is at least as important as medical treatment. Psychological support can be provided by patient organisations and there are several which are specifically devoted to LD (Table 2). Individual patients should also receive professional psychological support during the early stages of the condition. Physical therapy aims at maintaining a good overall muscular condition and at preserving ambulation, for as long as possible.

At the onset of seizures, patients are usually in secondary school and experiencing increasing difficulties with academic requirements. In order to enable them to maintain social contacts, it is best to maintain schooling for as long as possible, while negotiating with teachers about academic performance. However, this cannot be kept up for extensive periods. Some families will choose to keep patients at home with the best possible environment; this often requires adaptive measures, avoiding the use of stairs, setting up the patient close to the bathroom, and providing 24-hour presence at home with the help of a health professional to check medications. Other families will seek a specialized institution where patients are kept with other epilepsy patients in the same age group, with some amount of education and social activities. Re-evaluation at the specialized neurological department can be organized at 6- or 12-month intervals, with acute admissions in the event of complications, often due to intercurrent diseases (*e.g.* febrile infections) and/or worsening of epilepsy.

Table 2. Web-based family support organizations

Name	Site/address	Service
Association France-Lafora	http://www.Lafora.org 16, rue Amaudrut F- 53000 Laval	Patient organization Promotes self-help and research Collects funds for research
A.I.LA. Associazione Italiana Lafora	http://www.Lafora.it	Patient organization Promotes exchanges between families Identifies centres for diagnosis and treatment. Collects funds for research
Chelsea's Hope Lafora Children Research Fund	http://www.chelseashope.org	Family-based organization Connects families with LD worldwide Collects funds for research

The latter period is characterized by increasing dependency as the patient becomes wheelchair bound and, later, bedridden. According to local availability and the wishes and capacities of the caregivers, the patient is maintained at home, institutionalized or hospitalized. There should always be a connection between the reference specialized epilepsy team and the local caregiving structure.

Conclusion

For patients with LD, the present state of possible management includes a logical, effective approach to diagnosis, and the rational use of all available tools to help both the patients and their families. We hope that the management of LD patients will undergo a profound change in the near future, when effective, pathogenetically-oriented treatments become available.

Conflicts of interest: none.

References

Aguado, C., Sarkar, S., Korolchuk, V.I., *et al.* (2010): Laforin, the most common protein mutated in Lafora disease, regulates autophagy. *Hum. Mol. Genet.* **19,** 2867–2876.

Andrade, D.M., Ackerley, C.A., Minett, T.S., *et al.* (2003): Skin biopsy in Lafora disease: genotype-phenotype correlations and diagnostic pitfalls. *Neurology* **61,** 611–614.

Andrade, D.M., del Campo, J.M., Moro, E., Minassian, B.A. (2005): Nonepileptic visual hallucinations in Lafora disease. *Neurology* **64**, 1311–1312.

Annesi, G., Sofia, V., Gambardella, A., *et al.* (2004): A novel exon 1 mutation in a patient with atypical Lafora progressive myoclonus epilepsy seen as childhood-onset cognitive deficit. *Epilepsia* **45**, 294–295.

Barbieri, F., Santangelo, R., Gasparo-Rippa, P. & Santoro, M. (1987): Biopsy findings (cerebral cortex, muscle, skin) in Lafora disease. *Acta Neurol.* **9**, 81–94.

Baykan, B., Striano, P., Gionotti, S., *et al.* (2005): Late-onset and slow-progressing Lafora disease in four siblings with, EPM2B mutation. *Epilepsia* **46**, 1695–1697.

Berkovic, S.F., Andermann, F., Carpenter, S. & Wolfe, L.S. (1986): Progressive myoclonus epilepsies: specific causes and diagnosis. *N. Engl. J. Med.* **315**, 296–305.

Boccella, P., Striano P., Zara, F., *et al.* (2003): Bioptically demonstrated Lafora disease without *EPM2A* mutation: a clinical and neurophysiological study of two sisters. *Clin. Neurol. Neurosurg.* **106**, 55–59.

Brackmann, F.A., Kiefer, A., Agaimy, A., Gencik, M. & Trollmann, R. (2011): Rapidly progressive phenotype of Lafora disease associated with a novel *NHLRC1* Mutation. *Pediatr. Neurol.* **44**, 475–477.

Bruno, C., Servidei, S., Shanske, S., *et al.* (1993): Glycogen branching enzyme deficiency in adult polyglucosan body disease. *Ann. Neurol.* **33**, 88–93.

Canafoglia, L., Ciano, C., Visani, E., *et al.* (2010): Short and long interval cortical inhibition in patients with Unverricht-Lundborg and Lafora body disease. *Epilepsy Res.* **89**, 232–237.

Carpenter, S. & Karpati, G. (1981a): Ultrastructural findings in Lafora disease. *Ann. Neurol.* **10**, 63–64.

Carpenter, S. & Karpati G (1981b): Sweat gland duct cells in Lafora disease: diagnosis by skin biopsy. *Neurology* **131**, 1564–1568.

Chan, E.M., Bulman, D.E., Paterson, A.D., *et al.* (2003a): Genetic mapping of a new Lafora progressive myoclonus epilepsy locus (EPM2B) on 6p22. *J. Med. Genet.* **40**, 671–675.

Chan, E.M., Young, E.J., Ianzano, L., *et al.* (2003b): Mutations in *NHLRC1* cause progressive myoclonus epilepsy. *Nat. Genet.* **35**, 125–127.

Chan, E.M., Ackerley, C.A., Lohi, H., *et al.* (2004): Laforin preferentially binds the neurotoxic starch-like polyglucosans, which form in its absence in progressive myoclonus epilepsy. *Hum. Mol. Genet.* **13**, 1117–1129.

Cheng, A., Zhang, M., Gentry, M.S., *et al.* (2007): A role for AGL ubiquitination in the glycogen storage disorders of Lafora and Cori's disease. *Genes Dev.* **21**, 2399–2409.

Couarch, P., Vernia S., Gourfinkel-An, I., *et al.* (2011): Lafora progressive myoclonus epilepsy: *NHLRC1* mutations affect glycogen metabolism. *J. Mol. Med. (Berl)* **89**, 915–925.

Criado, O., Aguado, C., Gayarre, J., *et al.* (2011): Lafora bodies and neurological defects in malin-deficient mice correlate with impaired autophagy. *Hum. Mol. Genet.* **21**, 1521–1533.

DePaoli-Roach, A.A., Tagliabracci, V.S., Segvich, D.M., *et al.* (2010): Genetic depletion of the malin E3 ubiquitin ligase in mice leads to Lafora bodies and the accumulation of insoluble laforin. *J. Biol. Chem.* **285**, 25372–25381.

Dirani, M., Nasreddine, W., Abdulla, F. & Beydoun, A. (2014): Seizure control and improvement of neurological dysfunction in Lafora disease with perampanel. *Epilepsy Behav. Case Rep.* **29**, 164–166.

Duran, J., Gruart, A., García-Rocha, M., Delgado-García, J.M. & Guinovart, J.J. (2014): Glycogen accumulation underlies neurodegeneration and autophagy impairment in Lafora disease. *Hum. Mol. Genet.* **23**, 3147–3156.

Fernandez-Sanchez, M.E., Criado-Garcia, O., Heath, K.E., *et al.* (2003): Laforin, the dual-phosphatase responsible for Lafora disease, interacts with R5 (P.T.,G), a regulatory subunit of protein phosphatase-1 that enhances glycogen accumulation. *Hum. Mol. Genet.* **12**, 3161–3171.

Franceschetti, S., Gambardella, A., Canafoglia, L., *et al.* (2006): Clinical and genetic findings in 26 Italian patients with Lafora disease. *Epilepsia* **47**, 640–643.

Ganesh, S., Delgado-Escueta, A.V., Suzuki, T., *et al.* (2002a): Genotype-phenotype correlations for *EPM2A* mutations in Lafora's progressive myoclonus epilepsy: exon 1 mutations associate with an early-onset cognitive deficit subphenotype. *Hum. Mol. Genet.* **11**, 1263–1271.

Ganesh, S., Delgado-Escueta, A.V., Sakamoto, T., *et al.* (2002b): Targeted disruption of the Epm2a gene causes formation of Lafora inclusion bodies, neurodegeneration, ataxia, myoclonus epilepsy and impaired behavioral response in mice. *Hum. Mol. Genet.* **11**, 1251–1262.

Ganesh, S., Puri, R., Singh, S., Mittal, S. & Dubey, D. (2006): Recent advances in the molecular basis of Lafora's progressive myoclonus epilepsy. *J. Hum. Genet.* **51**, 1–8.

Garyali, P., Siwach, P., Singh, P.K., *et al.*. (2009): The malin-laforin complex suppresses the cellular toxicity of misfolded proteins by promoting their degradation through the ubiquitin-proteasome system. *Hum. Mol. Genet.* **18**, 688–700.

Gayarre, J., Duran-Trío, L., Criado Garcia, O., *et al.* (2014): The phosphatase activity of laforin is dispensable to rescue Epm2a-/- mice from Lafora disease. *Brain* **37,** 806–818.

Genton, P., Delgado Escueta, A., Serratosa, J.M., Michelucci, R. & Bureau, M. (2012): Progressive myoclonus epilepies. In: *Epileptic Syndromes in Infancy, Childhood and Adolescence, 5th edition*, eds. M. Bureau, P. Genton, A. Delgado Escueta, *et al*. Montrouge: John Libbey Eurotext, pp. 575–606.

Gentry, M.S., Worby, C.A. & Dixon, J.E. (2005): Insights into Lafora disease: malin is an E3 ubiquitin ligase that ubiquitinates and promotes the degradation of laforin. *Proc. Natl. Acad. Sci. USA* **102,** 8501–8506.

Gomez-Abad, C., Gomez-Garre, P., Gutiérrez-Delicado, E. *et al.* (2005): Lafora disease due to *EPM2B* mutations: a clinical and genetic study. *Neurology* **64,** 982–986.

Gomez-Abad, C., Afawi, Z., Korczyn, A.D., *et al.* (2007): Founder effect with variable age at onset in Arab families with Lafora disease and *EPM2A* mutation. *Epilepsia* **48,** 1011–1014.

Gomez-Garre, P., Sanz, Y., Rodriguez De Cordoba, S.R., & Serratosa, J.M. (2000): Mutational spectrum of the *EPM2A* gene in progressive myoclonus epilepsy of Lafora: high degree of allelic heterogeneity and prevalence of deletions. *Eur. J. Hum. Genet.* **8,** 946–954.

Gomez-Garre, P., Gutiérrez-Delcado, E., Gomez-Abad, C., *et al.* (2007): Hepatic disease as the first manifestation of progressive myoclonus epilepsy of Lafora. *Neurology* **68,** 1369–1373.

Gredal, H., Berendt, M. & Leifsson, P.S. (2003): Progressive myoclonus epilepsy in a beagle. *J. Small Anim. Pract.* **44,** 511–514.

Guerrero, R., Vernia, S., Sanz, R., *et al.* (2011): A PTG variant contributes to a milder phenotype in Lafora disease. *PLoS One* **6,** e21294.

Jennesson, M., Milh, M., Villeneuve, N., *et al.* (2010): Posterior glucose hypometabolism in Lafora disease: early and late, FDG-PET assessment. *Epilepsia* **51,** 708–711.

Kaiser, E., Krauser, K. & Schwartz-Porsche, D. (1991): Lafora disease (progressive myoclonic epilepsy) in the Bassett hound-possibility of early diagnosis using muscle biopsy? *Tierarztl Prax.* **19,** 290–295.

Knecht, E., Aguado, C., Sarkar, S., *et al.* (2010): Impaired autophagy in Lafora disease. *Autophagy* **6,** 991–993.

Lesca, G., Boutry-Kryza, N., de Touffol, B., *et al.* (2010): Novel mutations in *EPM2A* and *NHLRC1* widen the spectrum of Lafora disease. *Epilepsia* **51,** 1691–1698.

Lohi, H., Young, E.J., Fitzmaurice, S.N., *et al.* (2005): Expanded repeat in canine epilepsy. *Science* **307,** 81.

Lohi, H., Chan, E.M., Scherer, S.W. & Minassian, B.A. (2006): On the road to tractability: the current biochemical understanding of progressive myoclonus epilepsies. *Adv Neurol* **97,** 399–415.

Lohi, H., Turnbull, J., Zhao, X.C., *et al.* (2007): Genetic diagnosis in Lafora disease: genotype-phenotype correlations and diagnostic pitfalls. *Neurology* **68,** 996–1001.

Minassian, B.A. (2001): Lafora's disease: towards a clinical, pathologic, and molecular synthesis. *Pediatr. Neurol.* **25,** 21–29.

Minassian, B.A., Lee, J.R., Herbrick, J.A., *et al.* (1998): Mutations in a gene encoding a novel protein tyrosine phosphatase cause progressive myoclonus epilepsy. *Nat. Genet.* **20,** 171–174.

Moreno, D., Towler, M.C., Hardie, D.G., Knecht, E. & Sanz, P. (2010): The Laforin-Malin complex, involved in Lafora disease, promotes the incorporation of K63-linked ubiquitin chains into AMP-activated protein kinase beta subunits. *Mol. Biol. Cell.* **21,** 78–88.

Neville, H.E., Brooke, M.H. & Austin, J.H. (1974): Studies in myoclonus epilepsy (Lafora body form) I.V. Skeletal muscle abnormalities. *Arch. Neurol.* **30,** 466–474.

Nishimura, R.N., Ishak, K.G., Reddick, R., Porter, R., James, S. & Barranger, J.A., (1980): Lafora disease: diagnosis by liver biopsy. *Ann. Neurol.* **8,** 409–415.

Nitschke, F., Wang, P., Schmieder, P., *et al.* (2013): Hyperphosphorylation of glucosyl C6 carbons and altered structure of glycogen in the neurodegenerative epilepsy Lafora disease. *Cell Metab.* **17,** 756–767.

Pichiecchio, A., Veggiotti, P., Cardinali, S., Longaretti, F., Poloni, G.U. & Uggetti, C. (2008): Lafora disease: spectroscopy study correlated with neuropsychological findings. *Eur. J. Paediatr. Neurol.* **12,** 342–347.

Printen, J.A., Brady, M.J. & Saltiel, A.R. (1997): PTG, a protein phosphatase 1-binding protein with a role in glycogen metabolism. *Science* **275,** 1475–1478.

Puri, R. & Ganesh, S. (2010): Laforin in autophagy: a possible link between carbohydrate and protein in Lafora disease? *Autophagy* **6,** 1229–1231.

Puri, R., Suzuki, T., Yamakawa, K. & Ganesh, S. (2012): Dysfunctions in endosomal-lysosomal and autophagy pathways underlie neuropathology in a mouse model for Lafora disease. *Hum. Mol. Genet.* **21,** 175–184.

Raben, N., Danon, M., Lu, N., *et al.* (2001): Surprises of genetic engineering: a possible model of polyglucosan body disease. *Neurology* **56,** 1739–1745.

Rao, S.N., Maity, R., Sharma, J., *et al.* (2010): Sequestration of chaperones and proteasome into Lafora bodies and proteasomal dysfunction induced by Lafora disease-associated mutations of malin. *Hum. Mol. Genet.* **19**, 4726–4734.

Sakai, M., Austin, J., Witmer, F. & Trueb L. (1970): Studies in myoclonus epilepsy (Lafora body form). I.I. Polyglucosans in the systemic deposits of myoclonus epilepsy and in corpora amylacea. *Neurology* **20**, 160–176.

Schorlemmer, K., Bauer, S., Belke, M., *et al.* (2013): Sustained seizure remission on perampanel in progressive myoclonic epilepsy (Lafora disease). *Epilepsy Behav. Case Rep.* **1**, 118–121.

Sharma, J., Rao, S.N., Shankar, S.K., Satishchandra, P. & Jana, N.R. (2011): Lafora disease ubiquitin ligase malin promotes proteasomal degradation of neuronatin and regulates glycogen synthesis. *Neurobiol. Dis.* **44**, 133–141.

Sharma, J., Mulherkar, S., Mukherjee, D. & Jana, N.R. (2012): Malin regulates Wnt signalling pathway through degradation of dishevelled 2. *J. Biol. Chem.* **287**, 6830–6839.

Shirozu, M., Hashimoto, M., Tomimatsu, M., Nakazawa, Y., Anraku, S. & Nagata, M. (1985): Lafora disease diagnosed by skin biopsy. *Kurume Med. J.* **32**, 311–313.

Singh, S., Sethi, I., Francheschetti, S., *et al.* (2006): Novel *NHLRC1* mutations and genotype-phenotype correlations in patients with Lafora's progressive myoclonic epilepsy. *J. Med. Genet.* **43**, e48.

Solaz-Fuster, M.C., Gimeno-Alcañiz, J.V., Fernandez-Sanchez, M.E., *et al.*. (2008): Regulation of glycogen synthesis by the laforin-malin complex is modulated by the AMP-activated protein kinase pathway. *Hum. Mol. Genet.* **17**, 667–678.

Striano, P., Zara, F., Turnbull, J., *et al.* (2008): Typical progression of myoclonic epilepsy of the Lafora type, a case report. *Nat. Clin. Pract. Neurol.* **4**, 106–111.

Tagliabracci, V.S., Turnbull, J., Wang, W., Girard, J.M., Zhao, X., *et al.* (2007): Laforin is a glycogen phosphatase, deficiency of which leads to elevated phosphorylation of glycogen in vivo. *Proc. Natl. Acad. Sci. USA* **104**, 19262–19266.

Tagliabracci, V.S., Girard, J,M., Segvich, D., *et al.* (2008): Abnormal metabolism of glycogen phosphate as a cause for Lafora disease. *J. Biol. Chem.* **283**, 33816–33825.

Tagliabracci, V.S., Heiss, C., Karthik, C., *et al.* (2011): Phosphate incorporation during glycogen synthesis and Lafora disease. *Cell Metab.* **13**, 274–282.

Tiberia, E., Turnbull, J., Wang, T., *et al.* (2012): Increased laforin and laforin binding to glycogen underlie Lafora body formation in malin-deficient Lafora disease. *J. Biol. Chem.* **287**, 25650–25659.

Tomimatsu, M., Nakamura, J., Inoue, Y., Kojima, H., Anraku, S. & Noda, T. (1985): Lafora disease diagnosed by liver biopsy. *Kurume Med. J.* **32**, 307–309.

Traoré, M., Landouré, G., Motley, W., *et al.* (2009): Novel mutation in the *NHLRC1* gene in a Malian family with a severe phenotype of Lafora disease. *Neurogenetics* **10**, 319–323.

Turnbull, J., Kumar, S., Ren, Z.P., *et al.* (2008): Lafora progressive myoclonus epilepsy: disease course homogeneity in a genetic isolate. *J. Child Neurol.* **23**, 240–242.

Turnbull, J., Wang, P., Girard, J.M., *et al.* (2010): Glycogen hyperphosphorylation underlies Lafora body formation. *Ann. Neurol.* **68**, 925–933.

Turnbull, J., Girard, J.M., Pencea, N., *et al.* (2011a): Lafora bodies in skeletal muscle are fiber type specific. *Neurology* **76**, 1674–1676.

Turnbull, J., DePaoli-Roach, A.A., Zhao, X., *et al.* (2011b): PTG depletion removes Lafora bodies and rescues the fatal epilepsy of Lafora disease. *PLoS Genet.* **7**, e1002037.

Turnbull, J., Girard, J.M., Lohi, H., *et al.* (2012): Early-onset Lafora body disease. *Brain* **135**, 2684–2698.

Valles-Ortega, J., Duran, J., Garcia-Rocha, M., *et al.* (2011): Neurodegeneration and functional impairments associated with glycogen synthase accumulation in a mouse model of Lafora disease. *EMBO Mol. Med.* **3**, 667–681.

Van Heycoptenhamm, M.W. & De Jager, H. (1963): Progressive myoclonus epilepsy with Lafora bodies. Clinical-pathological features. *Epilepsia* **4**, 95–119.

Villanueva, V., Alvarez-Linera, J., Gómez-Garre, P., Gutiérrez, J. & Serratosa, J.M. (2006): MRI volumetry and proton MR spectroscopy of the brain in Lafora disease. *Epilepsia* **47**, 788–792.

Worby, C.A., Gentry, M.S. & Dixon, J.E. (2006): Laforin, a dual specificity phosphatase that dephosphorylates complex carbohydrates. *J. Biol. Chem.* **281**, 30412–30418.

Worby, C.A., Gentry, M.S. & Dixon, J.E. (2008): Malin decreases glycogen accumulation by promoting the degradation of protein targeting to glycogen (PTG). *J. Biol. Chem.* **283**, 4069–4076.

Yokoi, S., Aihara, Y. & Maeda, S. (1975): The myocardium in Lafora disease. *Acta Neuropathol.* **33**, 343–349.

Chapter 5

SCARB2/LIMP2 deficiency in action myoclonus-renal failure syndrome

Leanne M. Dibbens[1], Michael Schwake[2], Paul Saftig[3] and Guido Rubboli[4,5]

[1] *Epilepsy Research Group, School of Pharmacy and Medical Sciences, University of South Australia, and Sansom Institute for Health Research, University of South Australia, Adelaide 5000, South Australia, Australia*
[2] *Fakultät für Chemie, Universität Bielefeld, Universitätsstr. 25, D-33615 Bielefeld, Germany*
[3] *Biochemical Institute, Christian-Albrechts-University Kiel, Olshausenstr. 40, D-24098 Kiel, Germany*
[4] *Danish Epilepsy Center, Filadelfia/University of Copenhagen, Dianalund, Denmark*
[5] *IRCCS, Institute of Neurological Sciences, Bellaria Hospital, Bologna, Italy*
leanne.dibbens@unisa.edu.au
guru@filadelfia.dk

Summary

Action myoclonus-renal failure syndrome (AMRF) is an autosomal recessive progressive myoclonus epilepsy (PME) associated with renal dysfunction that appears in the second or third decade of life and is caused by loss-of-function mutations in the *SCARB2* gene encoding lysosomal integral membrane protein type 2 (LIMP2). Recent reports have documented cases with PME associated with *SCARB2* mutations without renal compromise. Additional neurological features can be demyelinating peripheral neuropathy, hearing loss and dementia. The course of the disease is relentlessly progressive. In this chapter we provide an updated overview of the clinical and genetic features of *SCARB2*-related PME and the functions of the LIMP2 protein.

Introduction

In 1986, Andermann *et al.* reported four French Canadian patients from three sibships with a condition characterized by the appearance of tremor in the fingers and hands and proteinuria at 17-18 years of age. Severe progressive action myoclonus, dysarthria, ataxia, infrequent generalized seizures, and renal failure ensued between 19 and 23 years of age. Despite severe neurological disability, due mainly to action myoclonus, intelligence remained normal in all four patients. They labelled this condition 'action myoclonus-renal failure (AMRF) syndrome'. Since this first description, it has been pointed out that the neurological picture was not caused merely by a metabolic encephalopathy due to renal failure, but rather was the result of a pathophysiological process that appeared to involve primarily both the brain and the kidneys (Andermann *et al.*, 1986). This syndrome was not recognized prior to the advent of dialysis and renal transplantation because of its rapidly fatal course if renal failure is untreated.

Discovery of *SCARB2* as the causative gene for AMRF

Three unrelated Australian families with a single proband were used to identify *SCARB2* as the causative gene for AMRF. Case A was of Turkish-Cypriot origin; her parents were first cousins. The ancestors of families B and C came from different regions of Britain and no inbreeding loops were known for either family. Case C was deceased, but stored brain tissue in paraffin blocks was available for DNA extraction.

A critical region of 5.3 cM (equivalent to 6.6 Mb) on chromosome 4 (4q13-21) was narrowed down by identifying an overlap of regions in which Case A and Case C were homozygous by descent. The region was reduced slightly in size by excluding a region in family B in which the affected individuals shared a segment identical by descent with an unaffected sibling.

The critical region on chromosome 4 contained 66 annotated genes of which approximately half are expressed in both the brain and kidney. In order to prioritize candidate genes for sequencing, it was hypothesized that the mRNA of the causative gene would be downregulated in affected subjects, possibly because of mutations causing RNA instability or removal by the process of nonsense-mediated decay. RNA from lymphoblastoid cell lines derived from two living affected subjects and from a healthy gender-matched sibling of each (families A and B) was analysed with Affymetrix U133 Plus2 arrays to look for RNAs with decreased abundance in the affected individuals in comparison to their unaffected sibling. RNA analysis was confined to the probe sets in the 6.6 Mb chromosome 4 region, defined by homozygosity mapping. *SCARB2* (*Scavenger Receptor B2*) emerged as a possible candidate gene. The amount of mRNA was reduced approximately 2-fold in the affected subjects compared to their healthy siblings.

The protein-coding regions of the *SCARB2* gene were analysed for mutations by direct Sanger sequencing. A homozygous splice-site mutation (c.1239+1G>T) in Case A was identified. RT-PCR analysis showed that this mutation leads to retention of intron 10 and the subsequent insertion of 20 amino acids, and premature truncation of the protein at residue 433. A homozygous mutation in Case C (c.435_436insAG W146SfsX161) was identified resulting in a frameshift predicted to truncate the SCARB2 protein to 160 amino acids. Case B was a compound heterozygote, carrying two different mutations in the *SCARB2* gene: a frameshift mutation (c.296 delA N99IfsX34) predicted to shorten the protein to 131 amino acids and a splice site mutation c.704+5G>A. These findings confirmed *SCARB2* as a causative gene for AMRF (Berkovic *et al.*, 2008).

The *SCARB2* gene encodes a 478 amino acid glycoprotein located in lysosomal membranes in a range of tissues including the brain and kidney. The function of *SCARB2* is not well understood, but it is thought to play a role in the biogenesis and maintenance of endosomal and lysosomal compartments. The human and mouse SCARB2/Limp2 proteins share 85 per cent amino acid identity.

Founder mutations of *SCARB2* in the French-Canadian and Scottish populations

A number of families were identified from Quebec, Canada, to have probands clinically diagnosed with AMRF. The Quebec population is known to have a high degree of consanguinity which results in a higher incidence of recessive disorders than other parts of the world. Molecular analysis of *SCARB2* found that all but one of the Quebec cases of AMRF were homozygous for the mutation c.862C>T, Q228X. Haplotype analysis using microsatellite markers on affected members and carriers was employed to determine whether *SCARB2* Q288X was a founder mutation inherited from a common ancestor. A shared haplotype spanning 0.6 cM encompassing the *SCARB2* mutation indicated the presence of a founder Q288X mutation for AMRF in the Quebec population. One family from Quebec was found to carry a second *SCARB2* mutation, c.1197+3insT.

Two subjects with AMRF from Scotland were found to be homozygous for the *SCARB2* mutation c.435_436insAG (W146S fs X161). This mutation is the same as that found in an Australian patient (Case C above) and in a Canadian patient (not French-Canadian). Haplotype analysis of the Australian, Canadian and the two Scottish cases, which were not previously known to be related, showed a shared haplotype of 0.6 cM, indicating that the mutation was inherited from a shared ancestor. The Scottish population, therefore, also contains a *SCARB2* founder mutation, W146S fs X161, causing AMRF.

Further cases of AMRF due to *SCARB2* mutations

Given that demyelinating neuropathy is seen in the mouse model deficient in functional SCARB2/Limp2 (Gamp *et al.*, 2003), a patient from the USA presenting with PME and asymptomatic neuropathy was hypothesized to carry a *SCARB2* mutation. This patient was found to be a compound heterozygote, carrying two different AMRF-causing mutations: the Q288X (Quebec) mutation on one chromosome and the second Quebec mutation c.1187+3insT on the other (Dibbens *et al.*, 2011). Since renal dysfunction is usually seen in AMRF, this patient is now undergoing tests for kidney function. Further cases of AMRF from Argentina, Turkey, Portugal and Spain (Balreira *et al.*, 2008; Perandones *et al.*, 2012) have been found to be caused by mutation of *SCARB2*, suggesting the syndrome is likely to be found worldwide.

Clinical features of action myoclonus-renal failure

Following the initial report by Andermann *et al.* (1986), several studies confirmed that the predominant clinical manifestations of AMRF are progressive myoclonus epilepsy and renal failure (Badhwar *et al.*, 2004; Vadlamudi *et al.*, 2006; Balreira *et al.*, 2008; Perandones *et al.*, 2012). Disease onset is typically in the late teens or early twenties, and the neurological features can be seen before, after, or simultaneously with the renal features. The neurological picture may present as a tremor, which is typically first noted in the fingers and hands, present at rest and exacerbated by fine motor activities. The tremor can later involve the head, trunk, lower extremities and sometimes the tongue and voice. As the disease progresses, involuntary spontaneous action-activated myoclonic jerks are seen, as well as asynchronous involuntary spontaneous myoclonic jerks at rest. A reflex myoclonus which is sensitive to touch on the extremities is also present. Action myoclonus, refractory to antimyoclonic drugs, is the most debilitating feature of the disease and, in the final stages, it renders the patients bedridden or wheelchair-bound with lap, trunk and leg belts. Diurnal or nocturnal generalized tonic-clonic seizures occur in the majority of patients.

Badhwar *et al.* (2004) reported that the convulsive seizures start with a generalized clonic phase with preserved consciousness proceeding to unconsciousness with tonic-clonic features. Antiepileptic drugs can control convulsive seizures without affecting ongoing active myoclonic jerks. Other common features appearing during the course of the disease include ataxia and dysarthria due to cerebellar dysfunction. Remarkably, despite the progression and severity of the neurological picture, cognitive function is preserved or only slightly affected until the final stages of the disease.

A demyelinating peripheral neuropathy has been reported in a number of patients (Rothdach et al., 2001; Dibbens et al., 2011; Hopfner et al., 2011), while electrophysiological findings indicating a predominantly axonal neuropathy have been observed in a patient without clinical evidence of involvement of the peripheral nervous system (Badhwar et al., 2004). Auditory defects ranging from abnormal brainstem auditory evoked potentials without clinical expression to severe hearing loss have been reported by Perandones et al., (2012, 2014) in a patient and two siblings with SCARB2 mutations and clinical features of AMRF. Interestingly, both these latter neurological manifestations correlate with the phenotype of the Limp2 knock-out mice whose neurological alterations consist of deafness and peripheral neuropathy, without features of progressive myoclonus epilepsy (Gamp et al., 2003). Finally, a dilated cardiomyopathy has been described in two patients (Hopfner et al., 2011).

Renal involvement in AMRF is heralded by the appearance of proteinuria that can relentlessly progress to a nephrotic syndrome and end-stage renal disease, requiring dialysis or renal transplantation. Detection of proteinuria usually occurs around the age of 20, although onset in childhood has been reported (Badhwar et al., 2004). No correlation has been observed between the ages of onset of proteinuria and tremor, nor between renal failure and onset of myoclonus.

The absence of renal involvement in PME associated with SCARB2 mutations has also been described. In 2009, Dibbens et al. reported SCARB2 mutations in 5 of 41 cases considered clinically to be 'Unverrich-Lundborg disease (ULD)-like' (Dibbens et al., 2009). The patients had disease onset between 14 and 26 years of age, with no evidence of renal failure during 5.5 to 15 years of follow-up, although one of them had slight proteinuria in the final stage of the disease. Death ensued in all five patients (the only surviving patient at the time of the report died later). Since this initial report, other cases have been reported and the clinical features of PME without renal failure associated with SCARB2 have been described (Rubboli et al., 2011; Guerrero-López et al., 2012; Higashiyama et al., 2013; Fu et al., 2014; Zeigler et al., 2014). Features seen in these patients included a variable severity of epilepsy; from uncontrolled seizures or status epilepticus with prominent photosensitivity in patients with adolescent onset, to infrequent or no major seizures in patients with a more delayed onset (Rubboli et al., 2011), late onset in adulthood (Higashiyama et al., 2013; Fu et al., 2014), and the occurrence of dementia (Fu et al., 2014). These findings suggest that SCARB2 mutations in patients with PME without renal complications might not be rare and that SCARB2 gene mutations should therefore be evaluated even in the absence of renal involvement.

The course of AMRF is fatal with relentless progression of neurological deterioration and increasing severity of myoclonus and renal impairment leading to death usually within 7 to 15 years after disease onset, due to renal failure, aspiration pneumonia, or septicaemia with multiorgan failure.

EEG and brain imaging

EEG and polygraphic recordings show generalized epileptiform abnormalities that at onset may resemble epileptic activity observed in idiopathic generalized epilepsy (Badhwar et al., 2004; Rubboli et al., 2011). Background activity is preserved at disease onset, slowing progressively over the years. In photosensitive patients, intermittent photic stimulation can trigger bursts of generalized spike-polyspike-wave discharges, often associated with massive myoclonic jerks that can evolve to myoclonic seizures. Polygraphic recordings show action myoclonus and erratic myoclonic jerks at rest, inconstantly associated with contralateral central spikes (Fig. 1). Back-averaging analysis of EEG discharges triggered from myoclonic jerks can reveal a cortical spike at the centroparietal electrodes (Fig. 1). Surface EMG recording of the fine tremor in the upper limbs showed quasirhythmic EMG bursts at a frequency of 12-20 Hz (Fig. 2). Analysis of the EEG-EMG relationship by coherence spectra of the tremor demonstrated a pattern consistent with a rhythmic myoclonic phenomenon of cortical origin, as in 'cortical tremor' (Rubboli et al., 2011).

Brain imaging studies are usually unremarkable or display diffuse cerebral atrophy, often associated with cerebrellar atrophy.

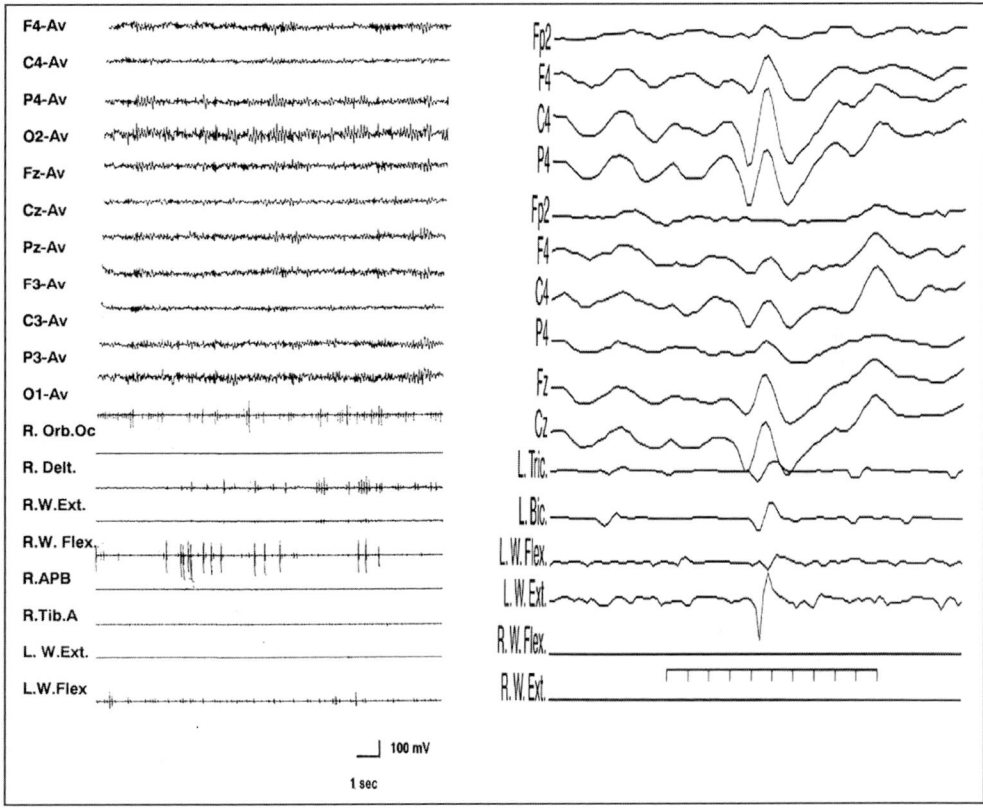

Fig. 1. Polygraphic recording in a 32-year-old patient with PME without renal failure associated with SCARB2 mutation. Left panel: the recoding shows preserved EEG background activity and erratic myoclonic jerks at rest without overt EEG correlate. Right panel: back-averaging triggered by myoclonia in the left wrist extensor reveals a cortical spike at the contralateral centroparietal electrodes.

Histology

Widespread deposition of abnormal, extraneuronal brown pigment in the brain, with no neuronal loss or significant gliosis, has been reported in AMRF patients (Andermann et al., 1986; Badhwar et al., 2004), and more recently in two patients with PME without renal failure associated with *SCARB2* mutations (Fu et al., 2014). Based on the staining characteristics, it has been suggested that the pigment consists of lipofuscin-like oxidized lipid or proteolipid (Badhwar et al., 2004). The deposits of pigment granules are extraneuronal, in astrocytes or in the extracellular space, especially in the cerebellar and cerebral cortices without any increase

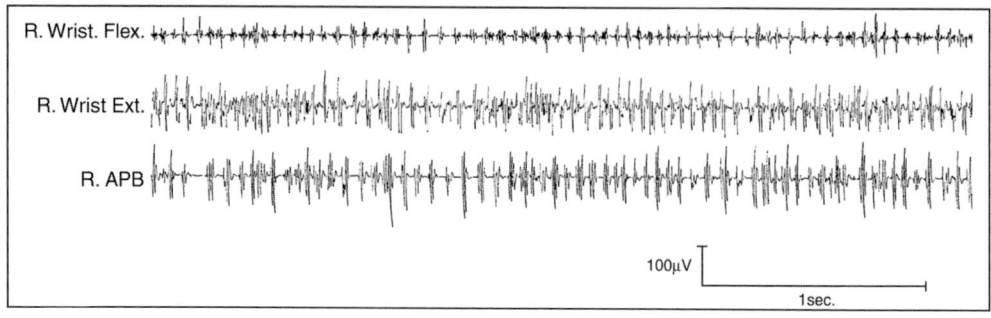

Fig. 2. Surface EMG recording of the tremor in the upper limbs shows quasirhythmic EMG bursts at a frequency of 12-20 Hz.

in intraneuronal lipofuscin (Badhwar *et al.*, 2004; Fu *et al.*, 2014). Interestingly, the patients without renal failure reported by Fu *et al.* (2014) also showed neurodegenerative changes, such as neuronal loss and gliosis in the brain, including the pallidoluysian and cerebello-olivary systems and the spinal cord. The authors speculate that the neuronal loss and gliosis in the pallidoluysian and cerebello-olivary systems may be responsible for the patients' involuntary movements and cerebellar dysfunction. Moreover, degenerative changes observed in the upper and lower motor neuronal systems, as well as in the dorsal root ganglia, strongly suggested that both the motor and sensory neuronal systems were also involved in the disease process.

Renal biopsy specimens have shown extensive tubular abnormalities with isometric vacuolization in distal and collecting tubules, the presence of granular material in cortical tubules without inflammatory infiltration (Chaves *et al.*, 2011), and focal glomerulosclerosis, with features of collapsing glomerulopathy (Badhwar *et al.*, 2004; Berkovic *et al.*, 2008).

Differential diagnosis

Differential diagnosis of AMRF primarily concerns other PMEs without dementia. At onset, since they share various clinical features, the correct diagnosis may be difficult on clinical grounds, particularly when renal impairment has not yet appeared or has not been diagnosed. Unverricht-Lundborg disease (ULD) is the paradigmatic example of PME with action myoclonus, ataxia, generalized seizures, and preserved intellect. The clinical suspicion of AMRF should be raised when a fine postural tremor in the upper limbs, which is generally not present in ULD, is detected on neurological examination at disease onset. Other rare causes of PME without dementia that should be considered in the differential diagnosis include sialidoses, distinguishable by macular cherry red spots, and PME, caused by mutations in *PRICKLE1*, the onset of which is generally earlier than that in AMRF and associated with early ataxia.

Concluding clinical remarks

The molecular analysis of patients clinically diagnosed with AMRF showed that mutations in *SCARB2* have been identified in many patients, confirming that the likelihood of identifying a *SCARB2* mutation in a patient presenting with PME and renal complications is fairly high. The French Canadian and Scottish populations have been shown to have founder mutations in *SCARB2* causing AMRF. Different *SCARB2* mutations have now been found in patients in many different countries, suggesting that *SCARB2*-associated PME is a world-wide disorder that is presently under recognized. Onset of PME due to mutations in *SCARB2* occurs in teenagers or young adults, and diagnosis is important in terms of providing counselling for the patient and family, particularly as the prognosis is worse than for classic ULD. Being informed about the carrier status of family members is particularly relevant in terms of the prevention of future disease in populations of known high consanguinity. In addition, in AMRF patients, an early diagnosis is of utmost importance as renal dysfunction can cause premature death in childhood or adolescence. Treatment with kidney dialysis or renal transplantation has been shown to prolong life by at least 10 years (Badhwar *et al.*, 2004). Furthermore, *SCARB2* mutations in patients with PME in the absence of renal complications are probably not rare, therefore mutations of the *SCARB2* gene should be considered in undiagnosed PME without renal involvement.

The LIMP-2 protein

The lysosome is the major degradative compartment of the cell. Its limiting membrane fulfils multiple functions, such as acidification of the interior, sequestration of active lysosomal enzymes, and transport of degradation products from the lysosomal lumen to the cytoplasm (Saftig & Klumperman, 2009). The lysosomal membrane contains several highly N-glycosylated proteins, the functions of which remain largely unknown (Eskelinen *et al.*, 2003).

LIMP-2, a major component of the lysosomal membrane

LIMP-2 (lysosomal integral membrane protein type 2), also known as SCARB2, is an abundant, highly glycosylated lysosomal membrane protein and belongs to the CD36 family (Calvo *et al.*, 1995). All family members share a common topology, transversing the membrane twice with an N-terminal transmembrane domain, a large luminal domain, and a second membrane-spanning domain preceding a 20-amino-acid cytoplasmic tail at the C-terminus (Fig. 3). Whereas in most tissues LIMP2 is found in lysosomes, other members of the CD36 superfamily are localized and function at the cell surface.

LIMP2 is a ubiquitously expressed protein with highest expression in the liver and spleen (Tabuchi *et al.*, 1997). It has a molecular weight of about 74 kDa, which includes a 54-kDa polypeptide backbone of 478 amino acids. The luminal domain contains 10 to 11 putative glycosylation sites (Fig. 3). The degree of the complex glycosylation of LIMP-2 depends on the species, tissue, and cell type. A leucine-isoleucine motif, within the C-terminal cytoplasmic tail, interacts with the heterotetrameric adaptor-complex 3 (AP3) and has been proposed to be responsible for the lysosomal localization of LIMP-2 (Honing *et al.*, 1998). In addition, based on antibody uptake experiments, a recycling of LIMP-2 between lysosomes and the plasma membrane has been described (Akasaki *et al.*, 1994). Furthermore, it has been demonstrated that distinct phosphatidylinositol 4-kinases influence the trafficking of LIMP-2 (Jović *et al.*, 2012).

Overexpression of LIMP-2 leads to altered cellular membrane trafficking

Overexpression of LIMP-2 causes an enlargement of early and late endosomes/lysosomes, which has not been observed for other abundant lysosomal membrane proteins. LIMP-2 overexpression impairs the endocytic membrane traffic out of these enlarged compartments and leads to an accumulation of cholesterol in these vacuole-like structures. Co-transfection of LIMP-2 and the dominant-negative form of Rab5b inhibits the formation of enlarged vacuoles,

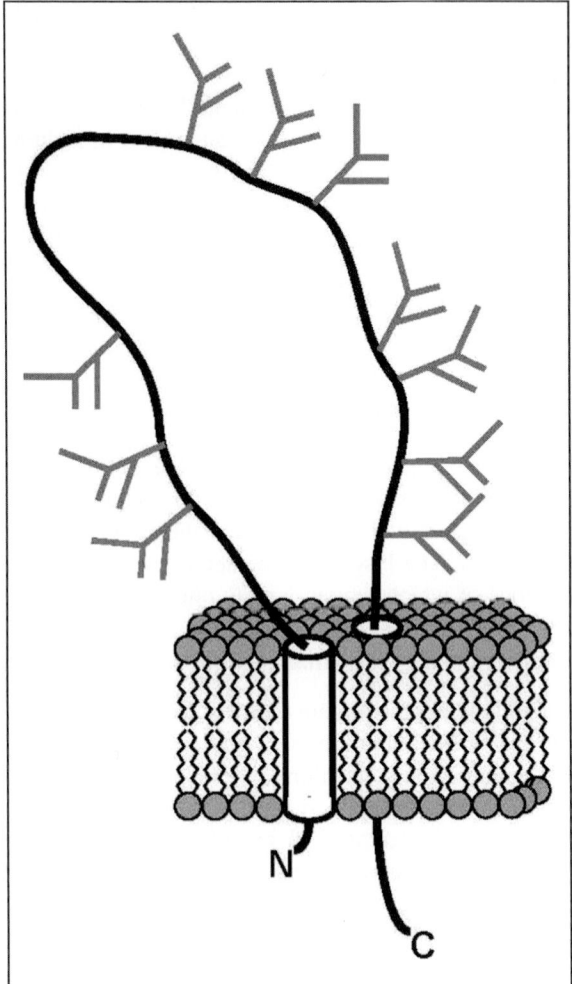

Fig. 3. Topology of the lysosomal membrane protein LIMP-2. LIMP-2 is a heavily N-glycosylated type III transmembrane protein with N- and C-termini located in the cytoplasm. The coiled-coil domain, which is necessary for GC binding, is located within the lumenal domain of LIMP-2.

suggesting that Rab5b function is necessary for the formation of such vesicles (Kuronita et al., 2002). Mutation experiments suggest that the N-terminal transmembrane and proximal lumenal domains of LIMP-2 are essential for the generation of the enlarged vesicular structures (Kuronita et al., 2005). These findings support the idea that LIMP-2 plays a role in the biogenesis and maintenance of the endo-lysosomal system.

LIMP-2 receptor functions

Similar to CD36, LIMP-2 appears to display a role as a multifunctional receptor at the plasma membrane. By using LIMP-2-GST fusion proteins and labelled thrombospondin, an interaction between both proteins was shown (Crombie & Silverstein, 1998).

In addition, LIMP-2 appears to be a cellular receptor for enterovirus 71 (EV71) and the coxsackie virus A16 (CVA16), which are most frequently associated with hand, foot and mouth disease (HFMD) (Yamayoshi et al., 2009). Although HFMD is considered to be a mild infection, it can progress to a severe neurological disease, associated with fatal encephalitis, aseptic meningitis, and acute flaccid paralysis.

It is well established that LIMP-2 has another important receptor function. It acts as a receptor for the lysosomal delivery of acid hydrolase β-glucocerebrosidase (GC) (Reczek et al., 2007). Mutations in the gene encoding this enzyme have been shown to cause Gaucher Disease, the most common lysosomal storage disorder, which is due to lysosomal accumulation of the glycosphingolipid glucosylceramide. LIMP-2 binds the enzyme, involving a helical domain in the luminal domain, early in the endoplasmic reticulum and transports it all the way to the lysosome (Reczek et al., 2007; Neculai et al., 2013, Blanz et al., 2015; Zunke et al., 2016) (Fig. 4a). Due to the acidic pH of the lysosome, the LIMP-2 receptor and its ligand dissociate (Reczek et al., 2007; Zachos et al., 2012), leading to the active lysosomal enzyme. All analyzed clinical AMRF-causing mutations described for LIMP-2 thus far have led to retention of the mutated protein in the endoplasmic reticulum (Fig. 4b). However, the binding to GC is differentially affected by the various AMRF-causing mutations (Blanz et al., 2010). It will be interesting to study whether the lack of lysosomal transport of GC contributes to the pathology of AMRF syndrome. Interestingly, the structure of the extracellular domain of LIMP-2 was recently revealed, showing an exposed helical bundle where GC binds. In addition, a cavity within the protein suggests a possible lipid transport function (Neculai et al., 2013).

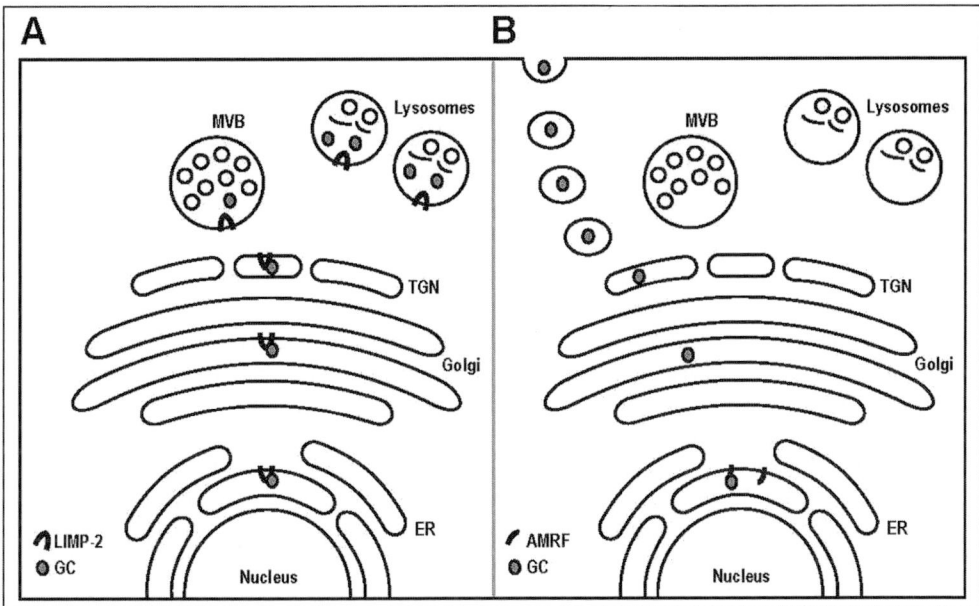

Fig. 4. LIMP-2-dependent targeting of GC to the lysosome. (**A**) In wild-type cells, GC is transported to the lysosome by LIMP-2. After binding between LIMP-2 and GC in the ER, GC leaves the receptor-ligand complex in the ER and moves via the Golgi apparatus to multivesicular bodies and lysosomes, where they dissociate due to the acidic pH. (**B**) All clinical AMRF-causing mutations described for LIMP-2 thus far have led to retention of the mutated protein in the ER. Therefore, in cells derived from AMRF patients, GC is retained in the ER and/or secreted to the extracellular space, depending on the effect of the AMRF-causing LIMP-2 mutation on binding to GC.

LIMP-2-deficiency in mice reveals major roles in the inner ear, kidney and myelinization of peripheral nerves

The different roles of LIMP-2 as a receptor may also contribute to the phenotype of mice engineered with a deletion of the mouse LIMP-2 gene. LIMP-2-deficient mice are characterized by the development of deafness, a unilateral or bilateral hydronephrosis, proteinuria, and a peripheral demyelinating neuropathy (Gamp et al., 2003).

The development of deafness was indicated by deficits in acoustic startle responses, in brainstem-evoked auditory potentials, and a reduced endochondral potential. A massive decline of spiral ganglia in the cochlea, concomitant with that of the inner and outer hair cells, and a progressive atrophy of the stria vascularis are typical pathological changes which start shortly after birth (Gamp et al., 2003). Hearing loss is temporally linked to a loss of the potassium channel subunits KCNQ1/KCNE1 and the endocytic receptor megalin in the luminal surface membrane of marginal cells of the stria vascularis (Knipper et al., 2006). A role of LIMP-2 in the regulation of the correct surface expression of these proteins through vesicular transport can be anticipated. This is also supported by the in-depth analysis of the development of a unilateral or bilateral hydronephrosis caused by an obstruction of the ureteropelvic junction. An impairment of the membrane transport processes is suggested by an abnormal accumulation of lysosomes in the epithelial cells of the ureter, adjacent to the ureteral lumen and a disturbed apical expression of uroplakin (Gamp et al., 2003). It is speculated that the pathology in the urothelium leads to the obstruction of the urinary tract between the renal pelvis and the ureter. In addition to this obstruction, kidney functions are affected. Decreased osmolality and altered urine parameters in LIMP-2-deficient mice point towards renal dysfunction. The high quantity of albumin in the urine of LIMP-2 knockout mice may be explained by glomerular filtration damage. Both the hydronephrosis and subtle glomerular changes may explain the kidney pathology in these mice (Berkovic et al., 2008). Interestingly, renin and LIMP-2 are co-regulated in renin-producing cells, although LIMP-2 does not play a role in the direct regulation of renin synthesis or release (Schmid et al., 2013).

The development of a peripheral demyelinating neuropathy in LIMP-2-deficient mice is an additional phenotypic hallmark and is most likely caused by a downregulation of peripheral myelin proteins (Gamp et al., 2003). Interestingly, lysosomal enzymes are upregulated in LIMP-2-deficient Schwann cells, suggesting that peripheral myelin proteins are missorted and degraded in the lysosomal compartment. Finally, Berkovic and colleagues observed in the LIMP-2-deficient mice, intracellular inclusions in cerebral and cerebellar cortex neurons accompanied by hyperactivity and ataxic gait behaviour (Berkovic et al., 2008). A recent study also revealed that the loss of LIMP-2 in the brain led to an almost complete loss of neuronal GC. This caused a substrate accumulation, followed by a secondary accumulation of neurotoxic a-synuclein. In cell-based assays, it was shown that an increased expression of LIMP-2 also led to a reduction in a-synuclein, suggesting a putative therapeutic role of LIMP-2 in synucleopathies (Rothaug et al., 2014).

Miscellaneous functions

Additional studies analysing the LIMP-2 homologue in *Dictyostelium discoideum* (DdLIMP) revealed a role as an effective suppressor of the profilin-minus phenotype (Karakesisoglou et al., 1999; Temesvari et al., 2000). Profilin is a ubiquitous G-actin binding protein which is involved in multiple cellular processes, such as cytokinesis, phagocytosis, and micripinocytosis. Profilin-deficient *Dictyostelium discoideum* cells show defects in pinocytosis, macropinocytosis, exocytosis, secretion of hydrolases, and an increased rate of phagocytosis. Interestingly, the infection of mice deficient in LIMP-2 revealed that phagocytosis is also compromised. When such mice were infected with *Listeria monocytogenes* (LM), it was found that they were highly susceptible to infection and displayed defective macrophage activation (Carrasco-Marin *et al.*, 2011). This defect increased the amount of pathogen, which is able to escape to the cytosol, increased the production of early acute phase pro-inflammatory cytokines, and enhanced the ability of LM phagosomes to interact with MIIC vesicles. These experiments suggested that in concert with active Rab5a, LIMP-2 regulates the phagosomal fusion machinery of the late endosomes-lysosomes and the cytosolic levels of the pathogen (Carrasco-Marin *et al.*, 2011).

Conclusions

Although the exact molecular role of LIMP-2 in the various cellular events is still incompletely understood, a central role for this lysosomal membrane protein in health and disease has emerged. Future studies will help to further understand the role of LIMP-2 in various tissues, including the central nervous system. It will be of particular importance to link the multitude of cellular functions with the phenotypic alterations seen in knockout mice and the clinical presentations in human AMRF patients. This will most likely also shed light onto the hitherto poorly understood role of the endocytic pathway in the central nervous system and the development of progressive myoclonus epilepsy disorders.

Acknowledgments and disclosures: This work was supported by the Deutsche Forschungsgemeinschaft (GRK 1459) (M.S and P.S).

None of the authors have any conflict of interest to disclose.

References

Akasaki, K., Michihara, A., Fukuzawa, M., Kinoshita, H. & Tsuji H. (1994): Cycling of an 85-kDa lysosomal membrane glycoprotein between the cell surface and lysosomes in cultured rat hepatocytes. *J. Biochem.* **116**, 670–676.

Andermann, E., Andermann, F., Carpenter, S., *et al.* (1986): Action myoclonus-renal failure syndrome: a previously unrecognized neurological disorder unmasked by advances in nephrology. *Adv. Neurol.* **43**, 87–103.

Badhwar, A., Berkovic, S.F., Dowling, J.P., *et al.* (2004): Action myoclonus-renal failure syndrome: characterization of a unique cerebro-renal disorder. *Brain* **127**, 2173–2182.

Balreira, A., Gaspar, P., Caiola, D., *et al.* (2008): A nonsense mutation in the LIMP-2 gene associated with progressive myoclonic epilepsy and nephrotic syndrome. *Hum. Mol. Genet.* **17**, 2238–2243.

Berkovic, S.F., Dibbens, L.M., Oshlack, A., *et al.* (2008): Array-based gene discovery with three unrelated subjects shows SCARB2/LIMP-2 deficiency causes myoclonus epilepsy and glomerulosclerosis. *Am. J. Hum. Genet.* **82**, 673–684.

Blanz, J., Groth, J., Zachos, C., Wehling, C., Saftig, P. & Schwake, M. (2010): Disease-causing mutations within the lysosomal integral membrane protein type 2 (LIMP-2) reveal the nature of binding to its ligand beta-glucocerebrosidase. *Hum. Mol. Genet.* **19** 563–572.

Blanz, J., Zunke, F., Markmann, S., *et al.* (2015): Mannose 6-phosphate-independent lysosomal sorting of LIMP-2. *Traffic.* **16**, 1127–1136.

Calvo, D., Dopazo, J. & Vega, M.A. (1995): The CD36, CLA-1 (CD36 L1), and LIMPII (CD36 L2) gene family: cellular distribution, chromosomal location, and genetic evolution. *Genomics* **25**, 100–106.

Carrasco-Marin, E., Fernandez-Prieto, L., Rodriguez-Del Rio, E., *et al.* (2011): LIMP-2 links late phagosomal trafficking with the onset of the innate immune response to Listeria monocytogenes: a role in macrophage activation. *J. Biol. Chem.* **286**, 3332–3341.

Chaves, J., Beirão, I., Balreira, A., *et al.* (2011): Progressive myoclonus epilepsy with nephropathy C1q due to SCARB2/LIMP-2 deficiency: clinical report of two siblings. *Seizure* **20**, 738–740.

Crombie, R. & Silverstein, R. (1998): Lysosomal integral membrane protein II binds thrombospondin-1. Structure-function homology with the cell adhesion molecule CD36 defines a conserved recognition motif. *J. Biol. Chem.* **273,** 4855–4863.

Dibbens, L.M., Michelucci, R., Gambardella, A., *et al.* (2009): SCARB2 mutations in progressive myoclonus epilepsy without renal failure. *Ann. Neurol.* **66,** 532–536.

Dibbens, L.M., Karakis, I., Bayly, M.A., Costello, D.J., Cole, A.J. & Berkovic, S.F. (2011): Mutation of *SCARB2* in a patient with progressive myoclonus epilepsy and demyelinating peripheral neuropathy. *Arch. Neurol.* **68,** 812–813.

Eskelinen, E.L., Tanaka, Y. & Saftig, P. (2003): At the acidic edge: emerging functions for lysosomal membrane proteins. *Trends Cell Biol.* **13,** 137–145.

Fu, Y.J., Aida, I., Tada, M., *et al.* (2014): Progressive myoclonus epilepsy: extraneuronal brown pigment deposition and system neurodegeneration in the brains of Japanese patients with novel *SCARB2* mutations. *Neuropathol. Appl. Neurobiol.* **40,** 551–563.

Gamp, A.C., Tanaka, Y., Lullmann-Rauch, R., *et al.* (2003): LIMP-2/LGP85 deficiency causes ureteric pelvic junction obstruction, deafness and peripheral neuropathy in mice. *Hum. Mol. Genet.* **12,** 631–646.

Guerrero-López, R., García-Ruiz, P.J., Giráldez, B.G., *et al.* (2012): New *SCARB2* mutation in a patient with progressive myoclonus ataxia without renal failure. *Mov. Disord.* **27,** 1826–1827.

Higashiyama, Y., Doi, H., Wakabayashi, M., *et al.* (2013): A novel *SCARB2* mutation causing late-onset progressive myoclonus epilepsy. *Mov. Disord.* **28,** 552–553.

Honing, S., Sandoval, I.V. & von Figura, K. (1998): A di-leucine-based motif in the cytoplasmic tail of LIMP-II and tyrosinase mediates selective binding of AP-3. *EMBO J.* **17,** 1304–1314.

Hopfner, F., Schormair, B., Knauf, F., *et al.* (2011): Novel *SCARB2* mutation in action myoclonus-renal failure syndrome and evaluation of *SCARB2* mutations in isolated AMRF features. *BMC Neurol.* **11,** 134.

Jović, M., Kean, M.J., Szentpetery, Z., *et al.* (2012): Two phosphatidylinositol 4-kinases control lysosomal delivery of the Gaucher disease enzyme, β-glucocerebrosidase. *Mol. Biol. Cell* **23,** 1533–1545.

Karakesisoglou, I., Janssen, K.P., Eichinger, L., Noegel, A.A. & Schleicher, M. (1999): Identification of a suppressor of the Dictyostelium profilin-minus phenotype as a CD36/LIMP-II homologue. *J. Cell Biol.* **145,** 167–181.

Knipper, M., Claussen, C., Ruttiger, L., *et al.* (2006): Deafness in LIMP2-deficient mice due to early loss of the potassium channel KCNQ1/KCNE1 in marginal cells of the stria vascularis. *J. Physiol.* **576,** 73–86.

Kuronita, T., Eskelinen, E.L., Fujita, H., Saftig, P., Himeno, M. & Tanaka, Y. (2002): A role for the lysosomal membrane protein LGP85 in the biogenesis and maintenance of endosomal and lysosomal morphology. *J. Cell Sci.* **115,** 4117–4131.

Kuronita, T., Hatano, T., Furuyama, A., *et al.* (2005): The NH(2)-terminal transmembrane and lumenal domains of LGP85 are needed for the formation of enlarged endosomes/lysosomes. *Traffic.* **6,** 895–906.

Neculai, D., Schwake, M., Ravichandran, M., *et al.* (2013): Structure of LIMP-2 provides functional insights with implications for SR-BI and CD36. *Nature* **504,** 172–176.

Perandones, C., Micheli, F.E., Pellene, L.A., Bayly, M.A., Berkovic, S.F. & Dibbens, L.M. (2012): A case of severe hearing loss in action myoclonus renal failure syndrome resulting from mutation in *SCARB2*. *Mov. Disord.* **27,** 1200–1201.

Perandones, C., Pellene, L.A. & Micheli, F.A. (2014): New *SCARB2* mutation in a patient with progressive myoclonus ataxia without renal failure. *Mov. Disord.* **29,** 158–159.

Reczek, D., Schwake, M. & Schroder, J. (2007): LIMP-2 is a receptor for lysosomal mannose-6-phosphate-independent targeting of beta-glucocerebrosidase. *Cell* **131,** 770–783.

Rothaug, M., Zunke, F. & Mazzulli, J.R. (2014): LIMP-2 expression is critical for β-glucocerebrosidase activity and β-synuclein clearance. *Proc. Natl. Acad. Sci. USA* **111,** 15573–15578.

Rothdach, A.J., Dietl, T. & Kumpfel, T. (2001): Familial myoclonus-renal failure syndrome. *Nervenarzt* **72,** 636–640.

Rubboli, G., Franceschetti, S., Berkovic, S.F., *et al.* (2011): Clinical and neurophysiologic features of progressive myoclonus epilepsy without renal failure caused by *SCARB2* mutations. *Epilepsia* **52,** 2356–2363.

Saftig, P. & Klumperman, J. (2009): Lysosome biogenesis and lysosomal membrane proteins: trafficking meets function. *Nature Rev.* **10,** 623–663.

Schmid, J., Oelbe, M., Saftig, P., Schwake, M. & Schweda, F. (2013): Parallel regulation of renin and lysosomal integral membrane protein 2 in renin-producing cells: further evidence for a lysosomal nature of renin secretory vesicles. *Pflugers Arch.* **465**(6): 895–905.

Tabuchi, N., Akasaki, K., Sasaki, T., Kanda, N. & Tsuji, H. (1997): Identification and characterization of a major lysosomal membrane glycoprotein, LGP85/LIMP II in mouse liver. *J. Biochem.* **122,** 756–763.

Temesvari, L., Zhang, L., Fodera, B., Janssen, K.P., Schleicher, M. & Cardelli, J.A. (2000): Inactivation of lmpA encoding a LIMPII-related endosomal protein, suppresses the internalization and endosomal trafficking defects in profilin-null mutants. *Mol. Biol. Cell* **11,** 2019–2031.

Vadlamudi, L., Vears, D.F., Hughes, A., Pedagogus, E. & Berkovic, S.F. (2006): Action myoclonus-renal failure syndrome: a cause for worsening tremor in young adults. *Neurology* **67,** 1310–1311.

Yamayoshi, S., Yamashita, Y., Li, J., *et al.* (2009): Scavenger receptor B2 is a cellular receptor for enterovirus 71. *Nat. Med.* **15**, 798–801.

Zachos, C., Blanz, J., Saftig, P. & Schwake, M.A. (2012): Critical histidine residue within LIMP-2 mediates pH sensitive binding to its ligand β-glucocerebrosidase. *Traffic.* **13**, 1113–1123.

Zeigler, M., Meiner, V., Newman, J.P., *et al.* (2014): A novel *SCARB2* mutation in progressive myoclonus epilepsy indicated by reduced β-glucocerebrosidase activity. *J. Neurol. Sci.* **339**, 210–213.

Zunke, F., Andresen, L., Wesseler, S., *et al.* (2016): Characterization of the complex formed by β-glucocerebrosidase and the lysosomal integral membrane protein type-2. *Proc. Natl. Acad. Sci.* **113**, 3791–3796.

Chapter 6

Neuronal ceroid lipofuscinoses

Dragos A. Nita[1], Sara E. Mole[2] and Berge A. Minassian[1]

[1] Division of Neurology, The Hospital for Sick Children, University of Toronto,
And Center for Brain and Mental Health, Sick Kids Research Institute,
555 University Avenue, Toronto, ON M5G 1X8, Canada
[2] MRC Laboratory for Molecular Cell Biology, UCL Institute of Child Health
and Department of Genetics, Evolution and Environment,
University College London, London WC1E 6BT, UK
berge.minassian@sickkids.ca

Summary

The neuronal ceroid lipofuscinoses (NCL) are neurodegenerative conditions that associate cognitive decline, progressive cerebellar atrophy, retinopathy, and myoclonic epilepsy. NCL result from the excessive accumulation of neuronal and extraneuronal lipopigments, despite having diverse underlying biochemical aetiologies. Here we review the clinical presentation, pathophysiology and genetics of these conditions as well as the approach to diagnosis and management.

Introduction

The neuronal ceroid lipofuscinoses (NCLs) represent a heterogeneous group of genetically-determined neurodegenerative conditions that are characterized by a progressive decline of cognitive and motor capacities, retinopathy evolving into blindness, variable cerebellar atrophy, and myoclonic epilepsy, leading to significantly decreased life expectancy (Jalanko & Braulke, 2009; Santavuori *et al.*, 2000; Mitchison *et al.*, 1998, Warrier *et al.*, 2013). They are the most prevalent neurodegenerative disorders of childhood with an incidence in the USA estimated at 1.6-2.4/100,000, while in Scandinavian countries the incidence varies between 2-2.5/100,000 in Denmark, 2.2/100,000 in Sweden, 3.9/100,000 in Norway, 4.8/100,000 in Finland, and 7/100,000 in Iceland (Uvebrant & Hagberg, 1997; also reviewed in Mole *et al.*, 2011).

The first description in the medical literature was probably by Otto Christian Stengel (1795-1890), a German physician who served in the mining community of Røros, Norway, between 1821 and 1882. He described a juvenile-onset disorder with blindness and progressive dementia (Stengel, 1826). In 1903, Frederick Eustace Batten (1865-1918), an English neurologist and paediatrician, described a similar clinical disorder and was the first to describe the neuropathology of cerebral degeneration with ocular macular changes in 2 members of a family (Batten, 1903). In 1905, Walther Spielmeyer (1879-1935), who had succeeded Aloïs Alzheimer as director of neurology and clinical psychiatry laboratory in Munich and Heinrich Vogt

(1875-1936) reported a similar disorder (Spielmeyer, 1905; Vogt, 1905). At this time, juvenile neuronal ceroid lipofuscinosis was referred to as Batten-Spielmeyer-Vogt disease. Later, Jan Janský (1873-1921) and Max Bielschowsky (1869-1940) described a similar disorder, but with a 'late-infantile' onset (Janský, 1908; Bielschowsky, 1913). This form came to be known as 'Janský-Bielschowsky disease' or 'late-infantile NCL'.

Hugo Kufs (1871-1955), from Leipzig, Germany, published 4 reports between 1925 and 1931 in which he described an adult-onset disease with similar pathological characteristics, but without the loss of vision that was so prominent in juvenile NCL and late-infantile NCL (Kufs, 1925). This came to be known as adult-onset NCL or Kufs disease. More recently, Matti Haltia (b. 1939) and Pirkko Santavuori (1933-2004), while investigating a child suspected to have GM1 gangliosidosis type II, concluded by identifying a novel type of NCL with early onset (Santavuori et al., 1973; Haltia et al., 1973a; Haltia et al., 1973b). Classic infantile NCL is also known as Haltia-Santavuori disease.

Traditionally, NCLs were classified according to the age at onset as: infantile (INCL), late-infantile (LINCL), juvenile (JNCL) and adult (ANCL), but were also known by their eponyms Haltia-Santavuori disease, Jansky-Bielschowsky disease, Batten-Spielmeyer-Vogt disease, and Kufs disease, respectively (Table 1 and Fig. 1). Moreover, the term 'Batten disease' was used in the literature to designate both the whole group of NCL and JNCL in particular. As less common forms of NCL began to be discovered, these were often referred to by the country of origin of the first described patients (Table 1).

Table 1. Historical NCL classification

Disease	Clinical phenotype	Abbreviated name	Eponym
CLN1	Infantile classic	INCL	Haltia-Santavuori
CLN2	Late-infantile classic	LINCL	Janský-Bielschowsky
CLN3	Juvenile	JNCL	Batten-Spielmeyer-Sjögren
CLN4	Adult autosomal dominant	ANCL	Parry
CLN5	Late-infantile variant	vLINCL	Finnish variant late infantile
CLN6	Early-juvenile / late-infantile	vLINCL	Lake-Cavanagh/Indian variant/Kufs (adult)
CLN7	Late-infantile variant	vLINCL	Turkish variant late infantile
CLN8	EPMR late-infantile variant	vLINCL	Northern epilepsy/EPMR

Today, at least 14 affected genes are implicated, from *CLN1* to *CLN14*, 13 of which have been identified (*CLN1-8* and *CLN10-14*). *CLN9* refers to the predicted locus in a family who do not appear to have mutations in any of the known genetic forms (Schulz et al., 2004). The currently genetically identified types of NCL are listed in Table 2.

Very recently, a new nomenclature has been discussed internationally and subsequently proposed which is gene-based and specific to phenotypic variation arising from different mutations. This is an axial diagnostic classification system that includes 7 axes: 1) affected gene (CLN gene symbol); 2) mutation diagnosis; 3) biochemical phenotype; 4) clinical phenotype; 5) ultra-structural features; 6) level of functional impairment; and 7) other remarks (additional genetic, environmental, or clinical features) (Mole & Williams, 2013). In reality, NCL classed according to the affected gene, combined with the age at onset, is sufficient for general use (*e.g.* classic infantile CLN1 disease, or adult CLN1 disease).

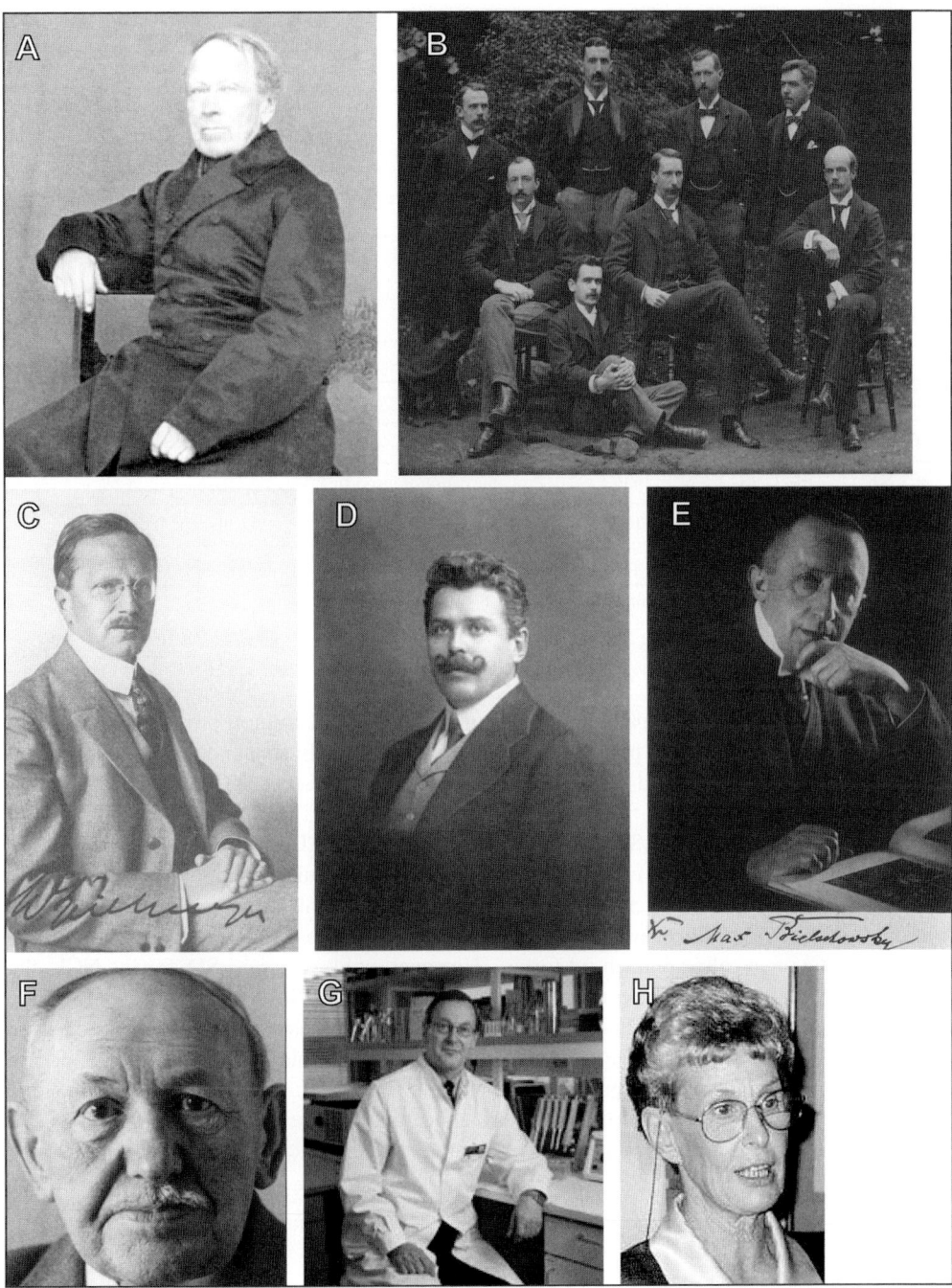

Fig. 1. (**A**) *Otto Christian Stengel;* (**B**) *Frederick Eustace Batten (first from the left, bottom row);* (**C**) *Walther Spielmeyer;* (**D**) *Jan Janský;* (**E**) *Max Bielschowsky;* (**F**) *Hugo Kufs;* (**G**) *Matti Haltia;* and (**H**) *Pirkko Santavuori.*

Table 2. Genetic classification of NCL

Locus name	Gene symbol	Locus	Protein name	Phenotypic spectrum
CLN1	PPT1	1p34.2	Palmitoyl protein thioesterase 1	I, LI, J, A
CLN2	TPP1	11p15.4	Tripeptidyl peptidase 1	LI, J, P
CLN3	CLN3	16p11.2	CLN3	J, P
CLN4	DNAJC5	20q13.33	DnaJ homolog	A (Parry disease) subfamily C member 5
CLN5	CLN5	13q22.3	CLN5	LI, J, P, A
CLN6	CLN6	15q23	CLN6	LI, P, A (Kufs type A)
CLN7	MFSD8	4q28.2	Major facilitator superfamily	LI, J domain-containing protein 8
CLN8	CLN8	8p23.3	CLN8	LI, P
CLN9	n/a	unknown	unknown	
CLN10	CTSD	11p15.5	Cathepsin D	C, LI, J, A
CLN11	GRN	17q21.31	Granulins	A
CLN12	ATP13A2	1p36.13	Probable cation-transporting	J ATPase 13A2
CLN13	CTSF	11q13.2	Cathepsin F	A (Kufs type B)
CLN14	KCTD7	7q11.21	BTB/POZ domain-containing	I protein KCTD7

A: adult; C: congenital; I: infantile; J: juvenile; LI: late-infantile; P: protracted.

Pathophysiology

NCL are grouped together on pathological grounds due to the common presence of neuronal and extraneural autofluorescent pigment accumulations, despite diverse underlying biochemical aetiologies. They are considered lysosomal storage diseases, however, NCLs also exhibit characteristics that distinguish them from lysosomal storage diseases (Mink, 2010). Consistent with lysosomal storage disorders (LSD), many of the identified NCL proteins are present in the lysosomes, and lipofuscin-like ceroid lipopigments also accumulate in the lysosomes. Under the electron microscope, the accumulated material takes different forms: granular osmiophilic deposits (GRODs), curvilinear profiles (CLP), fingerprint profiles (FPP), as well as rectilinear complex (RLC) or so called 'condensed forms'. However, unlike classic LSD, for the NCL, the 'stored' material is not disease-specific. While the major clinical NCL subtypes (CLN1, CLN2 and CLN3 diseases) were formerly each associated with characteristic inclusions under electron microscopy (GRODs, CLP, and FPP, respectively) (Fig. 2), the ultrastructural findings do not absolutely correlate with clinical presentation, and the same NCL may contain more than one pattern of inclusion (Table 3). Furthermore, the appearance of the pathological inclusions can depend on the tissue examined. Vacuolated lymphocytes are typically seen in classic juvenile CLN3 disease.

Table 3. Typical electron microscopy findings and enzyme activity according to NCL genotype

Disease	EM	Lymphocytes	Enzyme activity
CLN1	GROD	Non-vacuolated	PPT1 deficiency
CLN2	CLP	Non-vacuolated	TPP1 deficiency
CLN3	FPP	Vacuolated	Not applicable
CLN4	GROD, mixed	Non-vacuolated	Not applicable
CLN5	FPP, CLP, GROD	Non-vacuolated	Not applicable
CLN6	CLP, FPP, RLC	Non-vacuolated	Not applicable
CLN7	CLP, FPP, RLC	Non-vacuolated	Not applicable
CLN8	CLP, FPP, GROD	Non-vacuolated	Not applicable
CLN9	GROD, CLP	Non-vacuolated	Not applicable
CLN10	GROD	Non-vacuolated	CTSD deficiency
CLN11	FPP	Non-vacuolated	Not applicable
CLN12	GROD, mixed	Non-vacuolated	Not applicable
CLN13	FPP or none	Non-vacuolated	CTSF deficiency
CLN14	GROD, FPP	Non-vacuolated	Not applicable

GROD: granular osmophilic deposits; CLP: curvilinear profiles; FPP: fingerprint profiles; RLC: rectilinear complex.

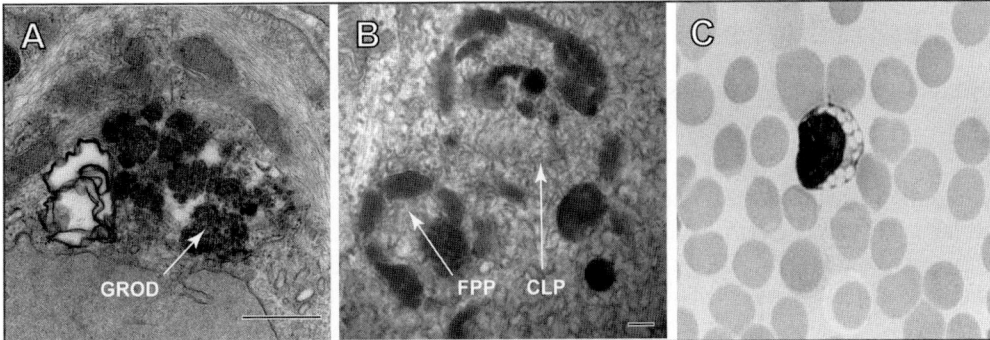

*Fig. 2. Electron microscopy and pathology findings in NCL. (**A**) Granular osmophilic deposits (GROD) in a conjunctival biopsy from a patient with CLN1 mutations (bar is 500 nm); (**B**) Fingerprint profiles (FPP) and curvilinear profiles (CLP) in a conjunctival biopsy from a patient with CLN2 mutations (bar is 100 nm). The predominance of curvilinear profiles and the comparative scarcity of fingerprint bodies were consistent with CLN2. Should fingerprint profiles predominate, the biopsy would be more consistent with CLN3; (**C**) Vacuolated lymphocytes in a patient with CLN3 disease.*

CLN1

Genetics

In CLN1 disease, the underlying defect is the lack of activity of the lysosomal palmitoyl protein thioesterase (PPT1), an enzyme that removes palmitate residues from proteins (Vesa *et al.*, 1995). The main protein component of the storage material is saposins A and D, with a characteristic ultrastructure of GRODs. To date, 64 mutations have been described in *CLN1* (for updated information on NCL mutations see the online database at http://www.ucl.ac.uk/ncl/). The exact physiological function and *in vivo* substrates of PPT1 are unknown, but it is proposed that PPT1 is required to maintain various cellular processes, including apoptosis, endocytosis, vesicular trafficking, synaptic function, and intracellular signalling (Greaves & Chamberlain, 2007). In neurons, PPT1 is found also outside the lysosomal compartment in presynaptic terminals (Ahtiainen *et al.*, 2006), suggesting that PPT1 is not exclusively confined to lysosomes, and the disease is not due solely to the abnormal storage.

Clinical presentation

The first symptoms of classic infantile CLN1 disease manifest in the second half of the first year of life, with irritability, followed by rapid psychomotor deterioration, central hypotonia, and deceleration of head growth. These are quickly followed by myoclonic jerks (and other seizures types) and blindness with optic atrophy. The ERG (electroretinogram) is unrecordable by age 4 years. Hand-wringing often develops during the disease course, which, along with the slowing of head growth and developmental regression, raises the differential for Rett syndrome, but unlike the latter, CLN1 disease does not stabilize, continuing instead to deteriorate until death in early childhood (Mole *et al.*, 2005). Most children die at around 10 years of age.

Of all the NCLs, CLN1 disease has the widest range of age at onset, determined by the combination of particular mutations. Although the majority of patients have infantile onset, some have late-infantile, juvenile, and even adult-onset, as late as 40 years of age (Van Diggelen *et al.*, 2001, Ramadan *et al.*, 2007).

Diagnosis

Historically, the diagnosis was made based on the ultrastructural finding of GRODs, together with the presence of suggestive clinical features. The diagnosis can now be made rapidly and specifically by demonstrating a lack of PPT1 activity, even in adult-onset forms.

Brain MRI usually demonstrates a variable degree of cerebral atrophy: signal change in the thalami and basal ganglia and thin, hyperintense, periventricular high-signal rims of white matter (Riikonen *et al.*, 2000). A progressive diffuse brain atrophy on MRI is seen in children during the first 4 years of life which then usually stabilizes. MR spectroscopy shows a decrease in the N-acetyl aspartate (NAA) peak and increased choline, however, with the rapid progression of the disease, all peaks completely disappear by the age of 6 years (Vanhanen *et al.*, 2004).

Neurophysiological findings in CLN1 disease are non-specific and include decreased reactivity of the posterior dominant rhythm to eye opening and eye closure, loss of sleep spindles by the age of 2 and an evolution towards an isoelectric electroencephalography (EEG) after the age of 3, which parallels the neuronal degeneration and brain atrophy.

Differential diagnosis

Differential diagnosis should include other progressive neurodegenerative disorders with onset from birth to age 2 years: Rett syndrome, hexosaminidase A deficiency, leukodystrophies, peroxisomal disorders, Niemann-Pick disease types A and B, and Leigh syndrome. While some of these disorders are associated with cortical blindness, retinal involvement is rarely seen (Mole & Williams, 2013).

Treatment

Treatment of CLN1 disease is symptomatic. As the enzyme cleaves fatty acid thioesters in plasma membranes, it was suggested that the drug cysteamine, a simple aminothiol used for the treatment of cystinosis, may have some effect. A clinical trial in children did not show any significant improvements (Levin et al., 2014) and in vitro studies also cast doubt on this concept (Lu & Hofmann, 2006). A phase I trial of intracerebral injection of human foetal neuronal stem cells has been performed (Guillaume et al., 2008; Mole, 2014) and enzyme replacement therapy has been considered (Lu et al., 2010).

CLN2

Genetics

CLN2 encodes the lysosomal enzyme tripeptidyl peptidase (TPP1), a member of the serine carboxyl proteinase family (Rawlings & Barrett, 1999). This group of enzymes removes tripeptides from the N termini of small polypeptides such as the subunit c of mitochondrial ATP synthase. To date, more than 109 mutations have been described, the 2 most common being the splice site mutation c.509-1G>C and the nonsense mutation p.Arg208* resulting in broadly similar clinical phenotypes (Mole et al., 2005). The majority of the protein component of the storage bodies is subunit c of mitochondrial ATP synthase, as well as low amounts of saposins A and D (Jalanko & Braulke, 2009; Lake & Hall, 1993).

Clinical presentation

Classic late-infantile CLN2 disease presents around the third year of life, with intractable epilepsy and an arrest of cognitive development. Myoclonus and ataxia are commonly seen early in the course, followed by progressive cognitive and motor decline. Retinopathy is often not prominent early in the course and may be overlooked after progression to more severe neurological deficits. Spasticity, truncal hypotonia, loss of head control, near-continuous myoclonus, frequent seizures, and an extended vegetative state are characteristic, until death in early adolescence. Death is often due to aspiration pneumonia. A few cases presenting late (8 years) have been reported, exhibiting slow regression with death as late as 40 years of age (Sleat et al., 1999).

Diagnosis

Historically, diagnosis was made based on the presence of clinical features and the ultrastructural demonstration of curvilinear bodies. However, the diagnosis can now be reached rapidly and specifically by demonstrating a lack of TPP1 activity using blood, skin biopsy, saliva, or dried blot spot.

Brain MRI in CLN2 disease shows progressive cerebral atrophy that predominates in the infratentorial region. Hypointense thalami on T2-weighted images were also reported (Seitz et al., 1998). MR spectroscopy demonstrates a reduction in the NAA peak and an increase in myoinositol and glutamate/glutamine in the white matter (Seitz et al., 1998).

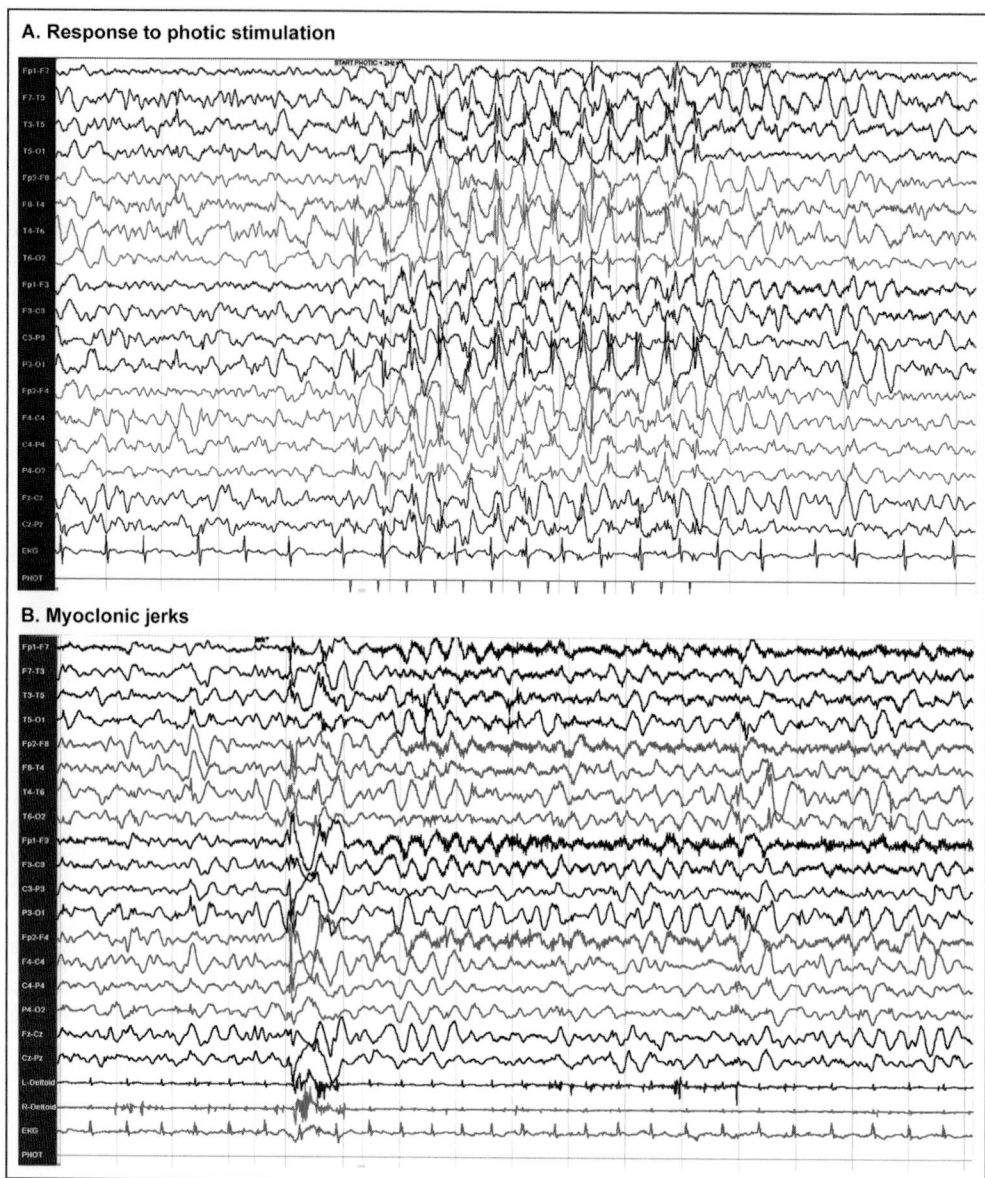

Fig. 3. Classic EEG findings in CLN2 disease.

EEG includes characteristic occipital spike responses to slow flash (1-2 Hz) stimulation which precede the onset of seizures and which increase as the disease progresses (Fig. 3). Electroretinogram is diminished even before noticeable visual loss (Wisniewski *et al.*, 1998; Wisniewski *et al.*, 2001; Goebel & Wisniewski, 2004). Visual evoked potentials are also enhanced at the onset of the disease.

Differential diagnosis

Other progressive neurological diseases with onset from ages 2 to 4 years should be considered, including epileptic encephalopathies, lysosomal storage disorders, mitochondrial diseases, and leukodystrophies. Other rarer NCL variants, such as CLN5, CLN6, CLN7 and CLN8 diseases, should also be considered if TPP1 activity is normal.

Treatment

Treatment is symptomatic. An experimental treatment approach uses intracerebral injection of viral vectors containing normal coding segments of the *CLN2* gene. In a mouse model of CLN2 disease, this procedure resulted in cerebral enzyme expression, reduced brain pathology, and increased survival. A small number of human patients have recently been treated in the same way (Worgall *et al.*, 2008), but the trial was too small to determine efficacy. A phase I trial of intracerebral injection of human foetal neuronal stem cells has been performed (Mink, 2010). Enzyme replacement therapy was efficacious in mice and dogs (Passini *et al.*, 2006; Chang *et al.*, 2008; Whiting *et al.*, 2014) and a phase 1 trial is well underway in Europe (Biomarin).

CLN3

Genetics

CLN3 encodes a membrane protein of unknown function. Whilst generally considered to be present predominantly in the endolysosome system, this protein has been reported to localize to membrane lipid rafts in synaptosomes, Golgi, and the cell membrane, as well as in mitochondria (Phillips *et al.*, 2005). Currently more than 57 mutations have been characterized in the *CLN3* gene. Most cases world-wide, which can be traced to a northern European origin, are due to a common ancestral 1-kb deletion founding mutation (Munroe *et al.*, 1997) shown to retain partial activity (Kitzmuller *et al.*, 2008).

Numerous roles have been attributed to the gene product of *CLN3*, and much work is needed to reconcile these disparate functions. In mitochondria, the gene product of *CLN3* was suggested to aid the processing of mitochondrial membrane proteins, such as ATPase subunit c, which accumulates in this condition as a result of synaptic vesicle transport (Margraf *et al.*, 1999). The *CLN3* gene product has been implicated in the regulation of lysosomal pH, transport of basic amino acids into the lysosome, and lysosomal size (Golabek *et al.*, 2000; Holopainen *et al.*, 2001; Ramirez-Montealegre & Pearce, 2005). An antiapoptotic role has been ascribed to the gene product of *CLN3*; the C-terminus appears to participate in cell cycle regulation, and mutations of this region result in slow growth and increased apoptosis (Puranam *et al.*, 1999). *CLN3* knockout mice show neutralizing antibodies against glutamic acid decarboxylase (GAD65), suggesting that an autoimmune response against GAD65 might contribute to preferential loss of GABAergic neurons in this disease. However, it is not understood whether these autoantibodies contribute to the pathogenesis or whether they are secondary entities arising during neurodegeneration, although their presence may influence excitotoxic mechanisms (Chattopadhyay *et al.*, 2002). Recently, an enzymatic function has been associated with the *CLN3* gene product, namely palmitoyl-protein D-9 desaturase activity (Narayan *et al.*, 2006). Another group showed a correlation between *CLN3* expression and the synthesis of bis monoacylglycerol phosphate (BMP) and suggested that the *CLN3* gene product may play a role in the biosynthesis of BMP (Hobert & Dawson, 2007).

Clinical presentation

Classic juvenile CLN3 disease presents between the ages of 4 to 8 years (mean of 5 years) with a progressive loss of vision due to retinal degeneration, followed by progressive dementia. Ocular pathology is initially a pigmentary retinopathy often misdiagnosed as retinitis pigmentosa or cone dystrophy. During adolescence, epilepsy and extrapyramidal/parkinsonian signs (rigidity, hypokinesia, shuffling gait, impaired balance) are more prominent. Neuropsychiatric symptoms, such as anxiety and aggression, are common (Marshall *et al.*, 2005). The clinical course is variable but inexorably progressive toward death in the second or third decade. CLN3 disease may present in adulthood with visual failure sometimes later accompanied with heart failure (Eksandh *et al.*, 2000).

Diagnosis

Ultrastructurally, CLN3 disease cases exhibit fingerprint profiles. These may be the only apparent feature within the lysosomal residual body, or may occur in conjunction with curvilinear or rectilinear profiles, or as a small component within large membrane-bound lysosomal vacuoles. The diagnostic hallmark of this frequent NCL type is conspicuous vacuoles in the cytoplasm of lymphocytes which are detectable on a regular blood smear (Anderson *et al.*, 2005). Diagnosis is based on clinical suspicion, the presence of vacuolated lymphocytes, and ultrastructural studies or combined with genetic testing.

Brain MRI shows cerebral and cerebellar atrophy in the later stages (age > 15 years) and is normal before the age of 10 years. MR spectroscopy has not shown specific abnormalities.

The EEG shows non-specific progressive background disorganization and spike-and-slow-wave complexes. The predominant seizure type is generalized tonic-clonic, however, partial complex seizures can occur as well. Enhanced somatosensory evoked potentials may be seen, supporting the presence of a myoclonic component even before myoclonus is clinically present.

Differential diagnosis

Differential diagnosis is limited given that juvenile CLN3 disease has a unique presentation. Peroxisomal, mitochondrial and other lysosomal disorders that are associated with retinopathy can be considered.

Treatment

Treatment is symptomatic. Autoimmunity against GAD65 has been used as the basis for investigation of immunomodulatory treatments (Pearce *et al.*, 2004).

CLN4

Genetics

The *CLN4* gene encodes DNAJC5, which underlies the autosomal dominant adult form of NCL, known as 'Parry disease'. The gene symbol *CLN4* was also used in the past to account for a heterogeneous group of adult forms of NCL which were recessively inherited (collectively recognised as Kufs disease) without known genetic loci at that time. Some of these forms were later identified as being secondary to mutations in *CLN6* and *CLN13*.

Other NCL genes that may present with adult-onset are *CLN1*, *CLN5*, *CLN10*, *CLN10* and *CLN13* (Table 2). While for most NCLs there is a specific phenotype associated with the loss of function of a particular *CLN* gene, for some NCLs that arise from mutations that have an incomplete effect of the gene function, the associated phenotypes are protracted or have a later age of onset (reviewed in Mole & Cotman [2015]).

Clinical presentation

Adult-onset NCL can present with 2 different clinical phenotypes: Kufs type A with marked myoclonus, progressive epilepsy, dementia and ataxia; and Kufs type B, marked by behavioural changes and dementia, as well as peculiar facial dyskinesia. Vision is not impaired in primary adult forms of NCL.

Diagnosis

Ultrastructural patterns include granular, curvilinear, or fingerprint profiles in different cell types and organs of the same patient, or a combination of patterns. Vacuolated lymphocytes were not reported.

Differential diagnosis

All NCL with possible onset in adulthood should be included in the differential diagnosis. The pattern of inheritance may point towards an autosomal recessive or autosomal dominant form.

Treatment

Treatment is symptomatic.

CLN5

Genetics

CLN5 encodes a soluble protein that is directed to the lysosome. It is reported to interact with the gene products of *CLN2* and *CLN3* (Vesa et al., 1995). These observations suggest that there may be common molecular pathways or important interactions between pathways in various types of NCLs. Currently, more than 36 different mutations have been described in *CLN5*. The most common mutation, occurring in patients of Finnish origin, is a 2-base pair deletion in exon 4 (c.1175_1176delAT) that results in an early stop codon (p.Tyr392*).

Clinical presentation

The first symptoms of the disease typically begin between 4 and 7 years of age (slightly older than the range in CLN2 disease), although cases are reported that present in adulthood. The usual course is motor clumsiness followed by progressive visual failure and blindness, dementia, motor decline, myoclonus, and seizures. The rate of progression is variable, but ultimately death occurs between the ages of 14 and 36 years (Mink, 2010). First reported in Finland, this type of NCL has recently been observed in many other European countries (UK, Czech Republic, Netherlands, Portugal, Italy), in North America (Canada, USA), South America (Argentina, Colombia), and other countries including Afghanistan and Pakistan. It should be considered in any exhaustive diagnostic approach of a patient with suspected NCL, especially with onset in late infancy but also up to adulthood (Santavuori et al., 1991).

Diagnosis

Ultrastructurally, lipopigments are distributed in the central nervous system and extracerebrally, and include fingerprint bodies, curvilinear profiles, lamellar inclusions, and occasionally condensed fingerprint images associated with lipid droplets. The major stored material is subunit c of the mitochondrial ATP synthase (Tyynela et al., 1997). Similar to CLN3-defective fibroblasts, CLN5-deficient fibroblasts also exhibit elevated intralysosomal pH (Kyttala et al., 2006). Brain imaging shows prominent cerebellar atrophy and in addition, on T2-weighted images, the thalamic signal intensity is low compared to that of the caudate, while increased signal intensity is seen in the periventricular white matter and the posterior limb of the internal capsule (Autti et al., 1992). Neurophysiological examination shows giant visual evoked potentials, exaggerated somatosensory potentials, and occipital spikes in response to photic stimulation, similar to CLN2. Ultimately, CLN5 can only be confirmed by DNA analysis.

Differential diagnosis

The clinical presentation with dementia, motor clumsiness and visual failure is strongly suggestive of a neurodegenerative disease. The probability of NCL is further supported by the electrophysiological and imaging studies.

Treatment

Treatment is symptomatic. The experimental finding that at least a portion of the *CLN5* gene product is trafficked via the manose-6-phosphate pathway (Sleat et al., 2005) means that therapeutic approaches that depend upon cross-correction, including enzyme replacement therapy, gene therapy, and stem cell transplantation are likely to be tested in the near future (Selden et al., 2013).

CLN6

Genetics

CLN6 encodes a protein of unknown function with 7 transmembrane domains localizing to the endoplasmic reticulum (ER) (Heine et al., 2004; Sharp et al., 2003). Currently, more than 68 different mutations have been described in CLN6 disease. Patients are found all over the world, with particular concentrations in Costa Rica and Portugal, arising from a founder effect, as well as a range of mutations in Turkey and Newfoundland.

Clinical presentation

Age at onset of CLN6 disease straddles the ages at onset of CLN1, CLN2, and CLN3 diseases, ranging from 18 months to 8 years, with the majority between 3 and 5 years. Early visual failure occurs in about 50 per cent of patients. The most prominent symptoms are motor impairment, including developmental delay, dysarthria, and ataxia. Seizures occur in the majority of patients, and usually begin before age 5 years. Deterioration is rapid after diagnosis and most children die between the ages of 5 and 12 years.

Diagnosis

Diagnosis is based on clinical suspicion and genetic testing. Ultrastructurally, a mix of rectilinear profiles and fingerprint profiles are seen. The stored material contains subunit c of mitochondrial ATP synthase (Elleder *et al.*, 1997). There is marked neuronal loss in layer V of the cerebral cortex and the extent of cerebral atrophy in CLN6 patients has been shown to be proportionate to the duration of symptoms based on post-mortem data (Elleder *et al.*, 1997).

MR imaging shows progressive cerebral and cerebellar atrophy. As in CLN2 disease, EEG shows progressive background slowing and high-amplitude discharges in the posterior head regions in response to the photic stimulation.

Differential diagnosis

Other NCL variants should be considered in the differential diagnosis of CLN6 disease. CLN1, CLN2 and CLN10 diseases can be excluded easily by enzyme analysis of PPT1, TPP1 and CTSD. Lymphocyte vacuolation, a hallmark of CLN3, is not seen in CLN6 disease.

Treatment

Treatment is symptomatic. As the function of the CLN6 protein remains unknown, no experimental therapeutic studies have yet been initiated.

CLN7

Genetics

The *CLN7* gene product belongs to the large major facilitator superfamily (MFS) that transports specific classes of substrates, including sugars, drugs, inorganic and organic cations, and various metabolites (Jalanko & Braulke, 2009). CLN7 is also referred to as MFSD8. CLN7 is localized to lysosomes (Kousi *et al.*, 2009). At present, more than 31 disease-causing mutations have been reported.

Clinical presentation

Age at onset is usually between 2 and 7 years. Psychomotor regression or seizures are the initial presenting signs. Progressive cognitive and motor deterioration, myoclonus, personality changes and blindness occur later. The disease has a rapidly progressing course. A Rett syndrome-like onset has also been reported (Craiu *et al.*, 2015).

Diagnosis

Ultrastructural examination reveals both fingerprint patterns and rectilinear patterns. This form can be diagnosed by ultrastructural pathological analysis of peripheral lymphocytes where dense fingerprint profiles are observed. Vacuolations are not usually present in lymphocytes. Diagnosis is based on clinical suspicion and genetic testing.

Brain MR studies are abnormal from the early stages of the disease and show progressive cerebral and cerebellar atrophy, thinning of the corpus callosum, and hypointensity of the thalami on T2-weighted images.

Neurophysiological studies show diffuse background slowing of the EEG with occipital spikes, more prominent during sleep, which may evolve into electrical status epilepticus during slow-wave sleep.

Differential diagnosis

Differential diagnosis includes mainly CLN3 and CLN6 diseases. Condensed fingerprint profiles in the lymphocytes and the absence of vacuolation is characteristic for CLN7 disease.

Treatment

Clinical management is supportive. No experimental therapeutic trials have been initiated so far.

CLN8

Genetics

CLN8 encodes a polytopic membrane protein that is localized to the ER and shuttles between the ER and ER-Golgi intermediate complex. The exact function is unknown, but it belongs to the TRAM-Lag1p-CLN8 (TLC) family of proteins, which are suggested to have roles in biosynthesis, metabolism, transport, and detection of lipids (Jalanko & Braulke, 2009). More than 24 mutations have been described.

Clinical presentation

Depending on the mutation, CLN8 disease presents with childhood-onset (5-10 years), intractable epilepsy, followed by progressive cognitive decline or mild developmental delay in late infancy, followed by a florid PME with progressive myoclonus, seizures, retinopathy, and psychomotor regression starting between 3 and 6 years. This typical late-infantile NCL phenotype leads to loss of vision (Topcu *et al.*, 2004).

In the very specific subtype of Progressive Epilepsy with Mental Retardation or Northern Epilepsy, caused by a defined missense mutation p.Arg24Gly, age at onset is 5 to 10 years and seizures are the first symptom. All patients have generalized tonic-clonic seizures with frequent episodes of status epilepticus. As patients pass through puberty, the frequency of seizures decreases but progressive dementia and motor impairment continues (Ranta & Lehesjoki, 2000). Patients with Northern Epilepsy may survive until 50-60 years of age.

Diagnosis

Diagnosis is based on clinical suspicion and genetic testing. GROD, curvilinear, and fingerprint profiles have been reported on electron microscopy, in various tissues, including lymphocytes, however, the stored material consists mostly of subunit c of mitochondrial ATP synthase.

MR studies show progressive cerebral and cerebellar atrophy with thinning of the corpus callosum. Neurophysiological testing is similar to other NCLs. Diagnosis can only be confirmed by DNA analysis.

Treatment

Treatment is supportive, and no experimental therapeutic trials have been attempted so far.

CLN9

Genetics

CLN9 has been proposed as a specific NCL entity, but no gene has yet been identified. Fibroblasts from affected families have a distinctive phenotype (rapid growth, sensitivity to apoptosis, manifestation of a cell adhesion defect, and reduced levels of ceramide, dihydroceramide, and sphingomyelin) (Schulz et al., 2004). Little is known of the function of the unidentified CLN9 protein.

Clinical presentation

CLN9 is clinically indistinguishable from juvenile CLN3 disease, but perhaps with a more rapid course.

Diagnosis

Ultrastructure is characterized by GRODs and curvilinear bodies. Diagnosis is one of exclusion. For patients presenting with typical features of CLN3 disease who have characteristic ultrastructural abnormalities, but no mutation in *CLN3,* possible CLN9 disease should be considered.

CLN10

Genetics

The affected gene encodes cathepsin D (CTSD), a lysosomal enzyme thought to be important for neuronal stability (Siintola et al., 2006; Steinfeld et al., 2006), which is also secreted and exerts effects in the extracellular environment. More than 7 mutations have been described. Alterations in a macroautophagy-lysosomal degradation pathway appear to mediate neurodegeneration in this disease.

Clinical presentation

CLN10 disease is characterized (in the congenital form) by primary microcephaly, neonatal (possibly already intrauterine) epilepsy, respiratory insufficiency, and rigidity. Death occurs within hours to weeks after birth. Late-onset forms of this NCL may be seen in juveniles and adults (Steinfeld et al., 2006). In one patient, missense mutations caused a childhood onset neurodegenerative disease with ataxia, retinopathy, severe cognitive decline, and apparently no seizures at age 17. The pathological correlate was GRODs (Steinfeld et al., 2006).

Diagnosis

Diagnosis is based on clinical presentation and enzymatic testing for CTSD in fibroblasts or blood. Genetic testing for mutations in *CLN10* is also available. On post-mortem examination, massive loss of neurons in the cerebral cortex, extensive gliosis, absence of myelin, and autofluorescent storage bodies with a GROD ultrastructure have been described.

Treatment

Treatment is symptomatic and mainly targets quality of life.

CLN11

CLN11 disease is characterized by rapidly progressive visual loss due to retinal dystrophy, seizures, cerebellar ataxia, and cerebellar atrophy. Two disease-causing mutations, present as compound heterozygous in the *GRN* gene, have been reported in 2 Italian siblings from nearby villages in Lombardy, Italy. The transmission pattern of adult-onset NCL in the family was consistent with an autosomal recessive inheritance. Electron microscopic examination of a skin biopsy demonstrated numerous fingerprint profiles in membrane-bound structures in eccrine secretory cells and in endothelium, consistent with NCL. EEG results showed polyspike-wave discharges with a posterior emphasis, and MRI indicated cerebellar atrophy. Heterozygous mutations in this gene were previously known to cause frontotemporal lobe dementia (Smith *et al.*, 2012).

CLN12

CLN12 disease was reported recently in a Belgian family. The index case had unsteady gait, myoclonus, and mood disturbance from age 11 to 13, progressing to clear extrapyramidal involvement with akinesia and rigidity, as well as dysarthric speech. There was no retinal involvement. Exome sequencing identified a single homozygous mutation in *ATP13A2* that fully segregated with the disease within the family. Muscle biopsy showed numerous subsarcolemmal autofluorescence bodies with a fingerprint appearance under electron microscopy, suggestive of neurogenic muscular atrophy. Mutations in *ATP13A2* are better known to cause Kufor-Rakeb syndrome (KRS), a rare parkinsonian phenotype with juvenile onset (Bras *et al.*, 2012).

CLN13

Five disease-causing mutations have been reported in *CLN3* (Smith *et al.*, 2013). CLN13 disease is an adult-onset neuronal ceroid lipofuscinosis with cathepsin F (CTSF) deficiency, without vacuolated lymphocytes. The clinical phenotype (Kufs type B) is characterized by behaviour abnormalities and dementia, which may be associated with motor dysfunction, ataxia, extrapyramidal signs, and bulbar signs. Electron microscopy has showed fingerprint profiles in some cases. The protein product, CTSF, is part of the papain family of cysteine proteinases that represent a major component of the lysosomal proteolytic system.

CLN14

One disease-causing mutation has been reported in a Mexican family with vision loss, cognitive and motor regression, premature death, and prominent NCL-type storage material (Staropoli et al., 2012). The gene product, BTB/POZ domain-containing protein KCTD7, is a potassium channel tetramerization domain-containing protein 7. Other mutations in this protein cause infantile PME or opsoclonus-myoclonius ataxia-like syndromes.

Diagnostic approach

NCL have a recognizable phenotype that correlates with the progressive grey matter neurodegenerative process involving the cortex, deep grey nuclei, cerebellum, and retina. The first approach to diagnosis should consider age at onset and type of clinical presentation, and has been well summarised recently (Schulz et al., 2013).

Presentation in a neonate with severe epilepsy and microcephaly should suggest CLN10 disease as a possible diagnosis. Enzyme testing for CTSD (CLN10) should be the first step. If this is negative, further or concurrent enzyme testing for PPT1 and TTP1 should be attempted before more invasive biopsies.

In young children (> 6 months) with otherwise unexplained epilepsy and developmental arrest, CLN1 and CLN2 diseases are the most likely considerations. If enzyme testing for PPT1 and TTP1 are negative and electron microscopy demonstrates typical storage material, genetic testing for *CLN5*, *CLN6*, *CLN7/MFSD8*, *CLN8* and *CLN14/KCTD7* should be considered.

A school-aged child presenting with rapid visual loss between ages 4 and 7 should be tested for CLN3 disease, first looking for lymphocyte vacuoles. If no lymphocyte vacuolization is present and testing for PPT1, TPP1 and CTSD is also negative, skin biopsy is indicated to assess if typical NCL storage material is present. If so, genetic testing for *CLN5*, *CLN6*, *CLN7/MFSD8*, *CLN8*, and *CLN12/ATP13A2* is indicated.

The NCL variants CLN5, CLN6, CLN7, or CLN8 should be considered in a child who phenotypically and ultrastructurally has an NCL, but testing for the more common entities is negative.

In adults with non-specific mental, motor, or behavioural abnormalities in which NCL is suspected, the first line of investigation includes the enzymatic assays for PPT1, TTP1, CTSD and CTSF which, if normal, should prompt ultrastructural examination. If storage material is present, genetic testing for autosomal recessive (*CLN6*, *CLN11/GRN*, *CLN13/CTSF*) and autosomal dominant NCL (*CLN4/DNAJC5*) should be initiated, and if negative, all other remaining NCL genes should be investigated.

Generally speaking, enzyme testing should be performed first. Ultrastructural examination of skin or lymphocytes should be performed prior to gene sequencing, however, gene 'chips' or other new DNA approaches that test concurrently for multiple NCL genes in the near future will reverse this approach. If there is no storage material, NCL is highly unlikely, although possible.

Symptomatic treatment for children with NCL

Patients with NCL require symptomatic treatment for a constellation of neurological manifestations, including seizures, sleep problems, extrapyramidal symptoms, behavioural problems, anxiety, and psychosis.

Routine medical management of children and young adults with complex neurological disability is relevant to all those affected by NCL, including clinical surveillance for sialorrhea, swallowing difficulties, gastroesophageal reflux, aspiration pneumonia, and X-ray surveillance of hips and spine.

Seizures may not require early treatment if generalized convulsions are rare and epileptic myoclonus is not obvious. As seizures progress, antiepileptic drugs of choice are valproic acid and lamotrigine, alone or in combination. However, lamotrigine may exacerbate seizures in CLN2 disease. Topiramate and levetiracetam are also effective. Benzodiazepines are useful in combination therapy, but they may cause problems due to sialorrhea. Carbamazepine, phenytoin, and gabapentin should be avoided as they may worsen myoclonic seizures. The ultimate goal must always be to improve the quality of life, and for this disease, the aim is not focussed on becoming seizure-free. Sleep disturbance is common and is likely to worsen with age. In general, a calm environment and set routines before going to bed are helpful. Benzodiazepines and sedatives are commonly used. Melatonin was found to have limited effect. Benzodiazepines may also benefit anxiety and spasticity. Trihexyphenydil improves dystonia and sialorrhea.

Emotional, behavioural and psychotic problems are common. Delusions and hallucinations may be managed using newer atypical neuroleptics, such as risperidone or olanzapine. If depression is thought to be the underlying problem, selective serotonin reuptake inhibitors may be considered which have been found to be beneficial. In all cases, medication should be kept to a minimum in order to avoid side effects or worsening disease progression.

Genetic counselling and genetic testing

The NCLs are inherited in an autosomal recessive manner with the exception of adult NCL, which can be inherited in either an autosomal recessive or an autosomal dominant manner. The parents of an affected child are obligate heterozygotes and are asymptomatic. The siblings of a proband have a 25 per cent chance of being affected, a 50 per cent chance of being an asymptomatic carrier, and a 25 per cent chance of being unaffected and not a carrier.

Prenatal testing is possible in high-risk pregnancies (if biochemical studies in the proband have revealed deficient activity of the enzymes CTSD, PPT1, or TPP1, or mutations defined in any NCL gene). In these instances, testing is performed on foetal cells obtained by chorionic villus sampling at 10-12 weeks of gestation or amniocentesis usually performed between 15-18 weeks of gestation (Mole & Williams, 2013).

Acknowledgments: We would like to especially thank Dr. Cameron A. Ackerley for the micrographs used in the figures. We thank the many clinicians whose experience we have drawn upon and those scientists whose original work has not been cited due to lack of space. The authors are not aware of any conflicts of interest. D.A.N. is supported through the Canadian League against Epilepsy Fellowship Award and University of Toronto Postgraduate Research Awards (Chisholm Memorial Fellowship, Elizabeth Arbuthnot Dyson Fellowship and the Joseph M. West Family Memorial Fund). B.A.M. holds the Michael Bahen Chair in Epilepsy Research and is supported by the Ontario Brain Institute and Genome Canada.

Conflicts of interest: none.

References

Ahtiainen, L., Luiro, K., Kauppi, M., Tyynela, J., Kopra, O. & Jalanko, A. (2006): Palmitoyl protein thioesterase 1 (PPT1) deficiency causes endocytic defects connected to abnormal saposin processing. *Exp. Cell Res.* **312**, 1540–1553.

Anderson, G., Smith, V.V., Malone, M. & Sebire, N.J. (2005): Blood film examination for vacuolated lymphocytes in the diagnosis of metabolic disorders; retrospective experience of more than 2,500 cases from a single centre. *J. Clin. Pathol.* **58**, 1305–1310.

Autti, T., Raininko, R., Launes, J., Nuutila, A. & Santavuori, P. (1992): Jansky-Bielschowsky variant disease: CT, MRI, and SPECT findings. *Pediatr. Neurol.* **8**, 121–126.

Batten, F.E. (1903): Cerebral degeneration with symmetrical changes in the maculae in two members of a family. *Trans. Ophthalmol. Soc. UK* **23**, 386–390.

Bielschowsky, M. (1913): Über spätinfantile familiäre amaurotische Idiotie mit Kleinhirnsymptonen. *Deutsche Zeitschrift für Nervenheilkunde* **50**, 7–29.

Bras, J., Verloes, A., Schneider, S.A., Mole, S.E. & Guerreiro, R.J. (2012): Mutation of the parkinsonism gene *ATP13*A2 causes neuronal ceroid-lipofuscinosis. *Hum. Mol. Genet.* **21**, 2646–2650.

Chang, M., Cooper, J.D., Sleat, D.E., et al. (2008): Intraventricular enzyme replacement improves disease phenotypes in a mouse model of late infantile neuronal ceroid lipofuscinosis. *Mol. Ther.* **16**, 649–656.

Chattopadhyay, S., Kriscenski-Perry, E., Wenger, D.A. & Pearce, D.A. (2002): An autoantibody to GAD65 in sera of patients with juvenile neuronal ceroid lipofuscinoses. *Neurology* **59**, 1816–1817.

Craiu, D., Dragostin, O., Dica, A., et al. (2015): Rett-like onset in late-infantile neuronal ceroid lipofuscinosis (CLN7) caused by compound heterozy ous mutation in the *MFSD8* gene and review of the literature data on clinical onset signs. *Eur. J. Paediatr. Neurol.* **19**, 78–86.

Eksandh, L.B., Ponjavic, V.B., Munroe, P.B., et al. (2000): Full-field ERG in patients with Batten/Spielmeyer-Vogt disease caused by mutations in the *CLN3* gene. *Ophthalmic Genet.* **21**, 69–77.

Elleder, M., Franc, J., Kraus, J., Nevsimalova, S., Sixtova, K. & Zeman, J. (1997): Neuronal ceroid lipofuscinosis in the Czech Republic: analysis of 57 cases. Report of the 'Prague NCL group'. *Eur. J. Paediatr. Neurol.* **1**, 109–114.

Goebel, H.H. & Wisniewski, K.E. (2004): Current state of clinical and morphological features in human NCL. *Brain Pathol.* **14**, 61–69.

Golabek, A.A., Kida, E., Walus, M., Kaczmarski, W., Michalewski, M. & Wisniewski, K.E. (2000): CLN3 protein regulates lysosomal pH, and alters intracellular processing of Alzheimer's amyloid-beta protein precursor and cathepsin D in human cells. *Mol. Genet. Metab.* **70**, 203–213.

Greaves, J. & Chamberlain, L.H. (2007): Palmitoylation-dependent protein sorting. *J. Cell Biol.* **176**, 249–254.

Guillaume, D.J., Huhn, S.L., Selden, N.R. & Steiner, R.D. (2008): Cellular therapy for childhood neurodegenerative disease. Part I: rationale and preclinical studies. *Neurosurg. Focus* **24**, E22.

Haltia, M., Rapola, J. & Santavuori, P. (1973a): Infantile type of so-called neuronal ceroid-lipofuscinosis. Histological and electron microscopic studies. *Acta Neuropathol.* **26**, 157–170.

Haltia, M., Rapola, J., Santavuori, P. & Keranen, A. (1973b): Infantile type of so-called neuronal ceroid-lipofuscinosis 2. Morphological and biochemical studies. *J. Neurol. Sci.* **18**, 269–285.

Heine, C., Koch, B., Storch, S., Kohlschutter, A., Palmer, D.N. & Braulke, T. (2004): Defective endoplasmic reticulum-resident membrane protein CLN6 affects lysosomal degradation of endocytosed arylsulfatase A. *J. Biol. Chem.* **279**, 22347–22352.

Hobert, J.A. & Dawson, G. (2007): A novel role of the Batten disease gene *CLN3*, association with BMP synthesis. *Biochem. Biophys. Res. Commun.* **358**, 111–116.

Holopainen, J.M., Saarikoski, J., Kinnunen, P.K. & Jarvela, I. (2001): Elevated lysosomal pH in neuronal ceroid lipofuscinoses (NCLs). *Eur. J. Biochem.* **268**, 5851–5856.

Jalanko, A. & Braulke, T. (2009): Neuronal ceroid lipofuscinoses. *Biochim. Biophys. Acta* **1793**, 697–709.

Janský, J. (1908): Dosud nepopsaný pripad familiárniamaurotické idiotie komplikované s hypoplasii mozeckovou. *Sborn Lék* **13**, 165–196.

Kitzmuller, C., Haines, R.L., Codlin, S., Cutler, D.F. & Mole, S.E. (2008): A function retained by the common mutant CLN3 protein is responsible for the late onset of juvenile neuronal ceroid lipofuscinosis. *Hum. Mol. Genet.* **17**, 303–312.

Kousi, M., Siintola, E., Dvorakova, L., et al. (2009): Mutations in *CLN7/MFSD8* are a common cause of variant late-infantile neuronal ceroid lipofuscinosis. *Brain* **132**, 810–819.

Kufs, H. (1925): Über eine Spätform der amaurotischen Idiotie und ihre heredofamiliären Grundlagen. *Z. Ges. Neurol. Psychiatr.* **95**, 168–188.

Kyttala, A., Lahtinen, U., Braulke, T. & Hofmann, S.L. (2006): Functional biology of the neuronal ceroid lipofuscinoses (NCL) proteins. *Biochim. Biophys. Acta* **1762,** 920–933.

Lake, B.D. & Hall, N.A. (1993): Immunolocalization studies of subunit c in late-infantile and juvenile Batten disease. *J. Inherit. Metab. Dis.* **16,** 263–266.

Levin, S.W., Baker, E.H., Zein, W.M., et al. (2014): Oral cysteamine bitartrate and N-acetylcysteine for patients with infantile neuronal ceroid lipofuscinosis: a pilot study. *Lancet Neurol.* **13,** 777–787.

Lu, J.Y. & Hofmann, S.L. (2006): Inefficient cleavage of palmitoyl-protein thioesterase (PPT) substrates by aminothiols: implications for treatment of infantile neuronal ceroid lipofuscinosis. *J. Inherit. Metab. Dis.* **29,** 119–126.

Lu, J.Y., Hu, J. & Hofmann, S.L. (2010): Human recombinant palmitoyl-protein thioesterase-1 (PPT1) for preclinical evaluation of enzyme replacement therapy for infantile neuronal ceroid lipofuscinosis. *Mol. Genet. Metab.* **99,** 374–378.

Margraf, L.R., Boriack, R.L., Routheut, A.A., et al. (1999): Tissue expression and subcellular localization of CLN3, the Batten disease protein. *Mol. Genet. Metab.* **66,** 283–289.

Marshall, F.J., de Blieck, E.A., Mink, J.W., et al. (2005): A clinical rating scale for Batten disease: reliable and relevant for clinical trials. *Neurology* **65,** 275–279.

Mink, J.W. (2010): *Neuronal Ceroid Lipofuscinoses (Batten's Disease)*. In: American Academy of Neurology Annual Meeting.

Mitchison, H.M., Hofmann, S.L., Becerra, C.H., et al. (1998): Mutations in the palmitoyl-protein thioesterase gene (PPT; CLN1) causing juvenile neuronal ceroid lipofuscinosis with granular osmiophilic deposits. *Hum. Mol. Genet.* **7,** 291–297.

Mole, S.E. (2014): Development of new treatments for Batten disease. *Lancet Neurol.* **13**(8), 749–751.

Mole, S.E. & Williams, R.E. (2013): *Neuronal Ceroid Lipofuscinoses*. In: Pagon R.A., Adam M.P., Ardinger H.H., Wallace S.E., Ameniya A., Bean L.J.H., Bird T.D., Fong C.T., Mefford H.C., Smith R.J.H., Stephens K. (eds). GeneReviews® [Internet], Seattle (WA), 2001 Oct. 10 [updated 2013 Aug. 1].

Mole, S.E. & Cotman, S.L. (2015): Genetics of the neuronal ceroid lipofuscinoses (Batten disease). *Biochim. Biophys. Acta* **1852**(10B), 2237–2241.

Mole, S.E., Williams, R.E. & Goebel, H.H. (2005): Correlations between genotype, ultrastructural morphology and clinical phenotype in the neuronal ceroid lipofuscinoses. *Neurogenetics* **6,** 107–126.

Mole, S., Williams, R. & Goebel, H. (2011): *The Neuronal Ceroid Lipofuscinoses (Batten Disease)* 2nd edition. Oxford: Oxford University Press.

Munroe, P.B., Mitchison, H.M., O'Rawe, A.M., et al. (1997): Spectrum of mutations in the Batten disease gene, *CLN3*. *Am. J. Hum. Genet.* **61,** 310-316.

Narayan, S.B., Rakheja, D., Tan, L., Pastor, J.V. & Bennett, M.J. (2006): CLN3 P the Batten's disease protein, is a novel palmitoyl-protein delta-9 desaturase. *Ann. Neurol.* **60,** 570-577.

Passini, M.A., Dodge, J.C., Bu, J., et al. (2006): Intracranial delivery of CLN2 reduces brain pathology in a mouse model of classical late infantile neuronal ceroid lipofuscinosis. *J. Neurosci.* **26,** 1334–1342.

Pearce, D.A., Atkinson, M. & Tagle, D.A. (2004): Glutamic acid decarboxylase autoimmunity in Batten disease and other disorders. *Neurology* **63,** 2001–2005.

Phillips, S.N., Benedict, J.W., Weimer, J.M. & Pearce, D.A. (2005): CLN3, the protein associated with Batten disease: structure, function and localization. *J. Neurosci. Res.* **79,** 573–583.

Puranam, K.L., Guo, W.X., Qian, W.H., Nikbakht, K. & Boustany, R.M. (1999): CLN3 defines a novel antiapoptotic pathway operative in neurodegeneration and mediated by ceramide. *Mol. Genet. Metab.* **66,** 294–308.

Ramadan, H., Al-Din, A.S., Ismail, A., et al. (2007): Adult neuronal ceroid lipofuscinosis caused by deficiency in palmitoyl protein thioesterase 1. *Neurology* **68,** 387–393.

Ramirez-Montealegre, D. & Pearce, D.A. (2005): Defective lysosomal arginine transport in juvenile Batten disease. *Hum. Mol. Genet.* **14,** 3759–3773.

Ranta, S. & Lehesjoki, A.E. (2000): Northern epilepsy, a new member of the NCL family. *Neurol. Sci.* **21,** S43-S47.

Rawlings, N.D. & Barrett, A.J. (1999): Tripeptidyl-peptidase I is apparently the CLN2 protein absent in classical late-infantile neuronal ceroid lipofuscinosis. *Biochim. Biophys. Acta* 1**429,** 496–500.

Riikonen, R., Vanhanen, S.L., Tyynela, J., Santavuori, P. & Turpeinen, U. (2000): CSF insulin-like growth factor-1 in infantile neuronal ceroid lipofuscinosis. *Neurology* **54,** 1828–1832.

Santavuori, P., Haltia, M., Rapola, J. & Raitta, C. (1973): Infantile type of so-called neuronal ceroid-lipofuscinosis 1. A clinical study of 15 patients. *J. Neurol. Sci.* **18,** 257–267.

Santavuori, P., Rapola, J., Nuutila, A., et al. (1991): The spectrum of Jansky-Bielschowsky disease. *Neuropediatrics* **22,** 92–96.

Santavuori, P., Lauronen, L., Kirveskari, K., Aberg, L. & Sainio, K. (2000): Neuronal ceroid lipofuscinoses in childhood. *Suppl. Clin. Neuro. Physiol.* **53**, 443–451.

Schulz, A., Dhar, S., Rylova, S., *et al.* (2004): Impaired cell adhesion and apoptosis in a novel CLN9 Batten disease variant. *Ann. Neurol.* **56**, 342–350.

Schulz, A., Kohlschütter, A., Mink, J., Simonati, A. & Williams, R. (2013): NCL diseases - clinical perspectives. *Biochim. Biophys. Acta* **1832**, 1801–1803.

Seitz, D., Grodd W., Schwab, A., Seeger, U., Klose, U. & Nagele, T. (1998): MR imaging and localized proton MR spectroscopy in late infantile neuronal ceroid lipofuscinosis. *Am. J. Neuroradiol.* **19**, 1373–1377.

Selden, N.R., Al-Uzri, A., Huhn, S.L., *et al.* (2013): Central nervous system stem cell transplantation for children with neuronal ceroid lipofuscinosis. *J. Neurosurg. Pediatr.* **11**, 643–652.

Sharp, J.D., Wheeler, R.B., Parker, K.A., Gardiner, R.M., Williams, R.E. & Mole, S.E. (2003): Spectrum of *CLN6* mutations in variant late infantile neuronal ceroid lipofuscinosis. *Hum. Mutat.* **22**, 35–42.

Siintola, E., Partanen, S., Stromme, P., *et al.* (2006): Cathepsin D deficiency underlies congenital human neuronal ceroid-lipofuscinosis. *Brain* **129**, 1438–1445.

Sleat, D.E., Gin, R.M., Sohar, I., *et al.* (1999): Mutational analysis of the defective protease in classic late-infantile neuronal ceroid lipofuscinosis, a neurodegenerative lysosomal storage disorder. *Am. J. Hum. Genet.* **64**, 1511–1523.

Sleat, D.E., Lackland, H., Wang, Y., *et al.* (2005): The human brain mannose 6-phosphate glycoproteome: a complex mixture composed of multiple isoforms of many soluble lysosomal proteins. *Proteomics* **5**, 1520–1532.

Smith, K.R., Damiano, J., Franceschetti, S., *et al.* (2012): Strikingly different clinicopathological phenotypes determined by progranulin-mutation dosage. *Am. J. Hum. Genet.* **90**, 1102–1107.

Smith, K.R., Dahl, H.H., Canafoglia, L., *et al.* (2013): Cathepsin F mutations cause Type B Kufs disease, an adult-onset neuronal ceroid lipofuscinosis. *Hum. Mol. Genet.* **22**, 1417–1423.

Spielmeyer, W. (1905): Über familiäre amaurotische Idiotien. *Neurol. Cb.* **24**, 602–621.

Staropoli, J.F., Karaa, A., Lim, E.T., *et al.* (2012): A homozygous mutation in *KCTD7* links neuronal ceroid lipofuscinosis to the ubiquitin-proteasome system. *Am. J. Hum. Genet.* **91**, 202–208.

Steinfeld, R., Reinhardt, K., Schreiber, K., *et al.* (2006): Cathepsin D deficiency is associated with a human neurodegenerative disorder. *Am. J. Hum. Genet.* **78**, 988–998.

Stengel, O.C. (1826): Beretnig om et maerkeligt Sygdomstilfaelde hos fire Sødskende I Nærheden af Roraas. *Eyr.*, **1**, 347–352.

Topcu, M., Tan, H., Yalnizoglu, D., *et al.* (2004): Evaluation of 36 patients from Turkey with neuronal ceroid lipofuscinosis: clinical, neurophysiological, neuroradiological and histopathologic studies. *Turk. J. Pediatr.* **46**, 1–30.

Tyynela, J., Suopanki, J., Santavuori, P., Baumann, M. & Haltia, M. (1997): Variant late infantile neuronal ceroid-lipofuscinosis: pathology and biochemistry. *J. Neuropathol. Exp. Neurol.* **56**, 369–375.

Uvebrant, P. & Hagberg, B. (1997): Neuronal ceroid lipofuscinoses in Scandinavia. Epidemiology and clinical pictures. *Neuropediatrics* **28**, 6–8.

Van Diggelen, O.P., Thobois, S., Tilikete, C., *et al.* (2001): Adult neuronal ceroid lipofuscinosis with palmitoyl-protein thioesterase deficiency: first adult-onset patients of a childhood disease. *Ann. Neurol.* **50**, 269–272.

Vanhanen, S.L., Puranen, J., Autti, T., *et al.* (2004): Neuroradiological findings (MRS, MRI, SPECT) in infantile neuronal ceroid-lipofuscinosis (infantile CLN1) at different stages of the disease. *Neuropediatrics* **35**, 27–35.

Vesa, J., Hellsten, E., Verkruyse, L.A., *et al.* (1995): Mutations in the palmitoyl protein thioesterase gene causing infantile neuronal ceroid lipofuscinosis. *Nature* **376**, 584–587.

Vogt, H. (1905): Über familiäre amaurotische Idiotie und verwandte Krankheitsbilder. *Mschr. Psychiatr. Neurol.* **18**, 161–171.

Warrier, V., Vieira, M. & Mole, S.E. (2013): Genetic basis and phenotypic correlations of the neuronal ceroid lipofusinoses. *Biochim. Biophys. Acta* **1832**, 1827–1830.

Whiting, R.E., Narfström, K., Yao, G., *et al.* (2014): Enzyme replacement therapy delays pupillary light reflex deficits in a canine model of late infantile neuronal ceroid lipofuscinosis. *Exp. Eye. Res.* **125**, 164–172.

Wisniewski, K.E., Connell, F., Kaczmarski, W., *et al.* (1998): Palmitoyl-protein thioesterase deficiency in a novel granular variant of LINCL. *Pediatr. Neurol.* **18**, 119–123.

Wisniewski, K.E., Zhong, N. & Philippart, M. (2001): Pheno/genotypic correlations of neuronal ceroid lipofuscinoses. *Neurology* **57**, 576–581.

Worgall, S., Sondhi, D., Hackett, N.R., *et al.* (2008): Treatment of late infantile neuronal ceroid lipofuscinosis by CNS administration of a serotype 2 adeno-associated virus expressing CLN2 cDNA. *Hum. Gene Ther.* **19**, 463–474.

Chapter 7

Sialidoses

Silvana Franceschetti and Laura Canafoglia

Fondazione I.R.C.C.S. Istituto Neurologico Carlo Besta, via Celoria 11, 20133 Milan, Italy
franceschetti@istituto-besta.it
canafoglia@istituto-besta.it

Summary

Sialidosis was first recognized as a specific neurological disorder in a patient presenting with muscular hypotonia and hypotrophy, ataxia, myoclonus, and seizures, who was later confirmed to have neuraminidase deficiency (Cantz *et al.*, 1977; Spranger *et al.*, 1978). However, it was first recognized as a clear causative factor for progressive myoclonus epilepsy (PME) by Rapin *et al.* (1978) who reported this disorder as 'cherry-red spot-myoclonus syndrome' because of the characteristic aspect of the fundus oculi, resulting from storage material in perifoveal ganglionic cells.

Aetiology

The disease presents with variable phenotypes, giving rise to at least two main age-related conditions: sialidosis type I and II. Both conditions exhibit autosomal recessive inheritance and are caused by mutations of the same gene, *NEU1*, localized on chromosome 6p21.3 (Bonten *et al.*, 1996; Pshezhetsky *et al.*, 1997), which encodes lysosomal neuraminidase (sialidase). Different mutations may account for the variable severity of the disease (Bonten *et al.*, 2000). Indeed, patients with the severe infantile type II disease typically have inactive sialidase, while patients with the milder type I disease have some residual activity.

Sialidase is part of a multienzyme complex containing other lysosomal enzymes such as cathepsin A, b-galactosidase, and N-acetylgalactosamine-6-sulfate sulfatase. The integrity of the multi-enzyme complex ensures the normal catalytic activity of sialidase and protects it against proteolysis.

NEU1 gene mutations can directly affect the active site or the central core of sialidase, leading to folding defects and retention of sialidase in the endoplasmic reticulum/Golgi compartment, but may also affect the surface region involved in binding to the multienzyme lysosomal complex (Lukong *et al.*, 2001; Pattison *et al.* 2004).

Sialidase has a central role in removing terminal sialic acid molecules from oligosaccharides and glycoproteins, and its deficiency therefore leads to sialic acid-rich macromolecular storage and urinary sialyl-oligosaccharide excretion.

Neuropathology

Light and electron microscopy reveal cytoplasmic vacuolation involving neurons and perineuronal and interfascicular oligodendroglia, and endothelial and perithelial cells. Vacuolations are associated with diffuse neuronal intracytoplasmic storage of lipofuscin-like pigment which is detectable in the neocortex, basal ganglia, thalamus, brainstem, and spinal cord, as well in extra-nervous organs (Allegranza et al., 1989).

The accumulation of the sialic acid-rich substrates prominently contributes to the pathogenesis of the disease, however, other 'indirect' mechanisms are possibly involved. For instance, it was recently discovered that neuraminidase is a negative regulator of the lysosomal exocytosis of catalytically-active hydrolases (Yogalingam et al., 2008). The resulting increase in extracellular proteolytic activity may lead to premature degradation of other molecules implied in various cellular activities.

Laboratory findings

The laboratory diagnosis is usually supported by increased urinary bound sialic acid excretion and confirmed by genetic analysis or the demonstration of neuraminidase enzyme deficiency in cultured fibroblasts (Lowden & O'Brien, 1979).

Clinical presentation

Sialidosis type I presents with the typical features characterizing PMEs (Rapin et al., 1978; Lowden & O'Brien, 1979), while the phenotype of sialidosis type II includes dysmorphic features (coarse facial features, short trunk, barrel chest, spinal deformity, and skeletal dysplasia), sometimes associated with corneal clouding, hepatomegaly, and inner ear hearing loss. The characteristic macular change found in this metabolic disorder, leading to the definition of 'cherry-red spot', may lead to late visual failure resulting from ganglionic degeneration. The cherry-red spot can, however, be clinically undetectable for many years and may, moreover, disappear in later stages of the disease (Kivlin et al., 1985). Young-onset cataract formation was also identified in a few patients with type I sialidosis (Thomas et al., 1979).

Both types of sialidosis present with progressively worsening multifocal myoclonus, usually occurring in the second decade of life and variably associated with seizures and ataxia (Lowden & O'Brien, 1979).

Recently, we observed 6 adult patients from 2 different families, presenting high-frequency myoclonus, but no seizures. The disorder progressed slowly and myoclonus was recognized after an interval of many years, although patients displayed a prominent gait disorder with occasional but repeated falls. At the time of our initial diagnostic observation, none of the patients had the cardinal signs suggesting sialidoses, such as macular cherry-red spot or significant urinary sialic acid excretion. Diagnosis resulted from the detection of *NEU1* mutation through genome-wide screening (Canafoglia et al., 2014). Our observation, together with a recent similar report (Schene et al., 2015), points towards the possibility that mild and late forms present with 'cortical myoclonus' and are possibly misdiagnosed.

Most of the patients, with either sialidosis type I or II, become wheelchair-bound within a few years due to severe motor impairment, mainly resulting from severe myoclonus.

Imaging

MRI findings in sialidoses are normal in the early stages, while cerebellar, pontine, and cerebral atrophy can appear during disease progression (Palmeri *et al.*, 2000).

Myoclonus and associated neurophysiological features

In the earliest description of classic PME resulting from type I sialidosis, the authors reported findings similar to those for Unverricht-Lundborg syndrome, with the exception of photosensitivity that is typically present in Unverricht-Lundborg but not in sialidosis (Engel *et al.*, 1977). As for other types of PME, the subsequent description revealed some degree of phenotypic variability both in terms of the severity of myoclonus and the associated signs of cortical hyperexcitability. In general, the cortical origin of the myoclonus is confirmed by the results of simple back-averaging techniques showing a sharp transient preceding the myoclonus (Franceschetti *et al.*, 1980; Tobimatsu *et al.*, 1985). Since, in patients with sialidosis, myoclonus is often subtle but highly rhythmic and the EEG correlate consists of a discharge of fast activity, the EEG-EMG coherence analysis appears to be a more reliable method to unequivocally reveal a consistent temporal relationship between the EEG spikes and myoclonic jerks through fast cortico-muscular transfer (Panzica *et al.*, 2003). A study comparing between patients with both type I and II sialidosis and patients with Unverricht-Lundborg disease suggested that this strong rhythmicity and the higher cortico-muscular coherence in sialidoses might account for the particularly severe motor impairment observed in sialidosis patients (Canafoglia *et al.*, 2011). The EEG background is usually almost normal in patients with type I sialidosis, but polyspike-waves (often associated with spontaneous jerks) are present on the EEG of patients with infantile type II sialidosis.

In some of the reported patients, the presence of high-amplitude somatosensory evoked potentials and enhanced long-loop reflexes (LLR or C-reflex) further confirms the marked neocortical hyperexcitability, which is responsible for ćortical reflex' and action myoclonus.

The strongly rhythmic recurrence of the jerks reflects on the characteristics of the so-called long-loop reflexes evoked by median nerve stimulation, which include multiple components resulting from recurrent jerks (Canafoglia *et al.*, 2011). Fig. 1 shows the neurophysiological features of the myoclonus in 3 patients with sialidosis.

Differential diagnosis

Sialidosis type II, presenting in infancy or early childhood with dysmorphic features and skeletal abnormalities, should be differentiated from other storage diseases sharing similar features.

Sialidosis type I, presenting with cortical myoclonus as the main symptom, should be differentiated from other forms of progressive myoclonus epilepsy.

Management

Pharmacological treatment is similar to that for other PMEs (see Nirenberg & Frucht [2005] for a review). Valproate can be considered as the first-line drug, but the treatment of severe myoclonus usually requires 2 or 3 additional drugs, including benzodiazepines, levetiracetam, zonisamide or topiramate.

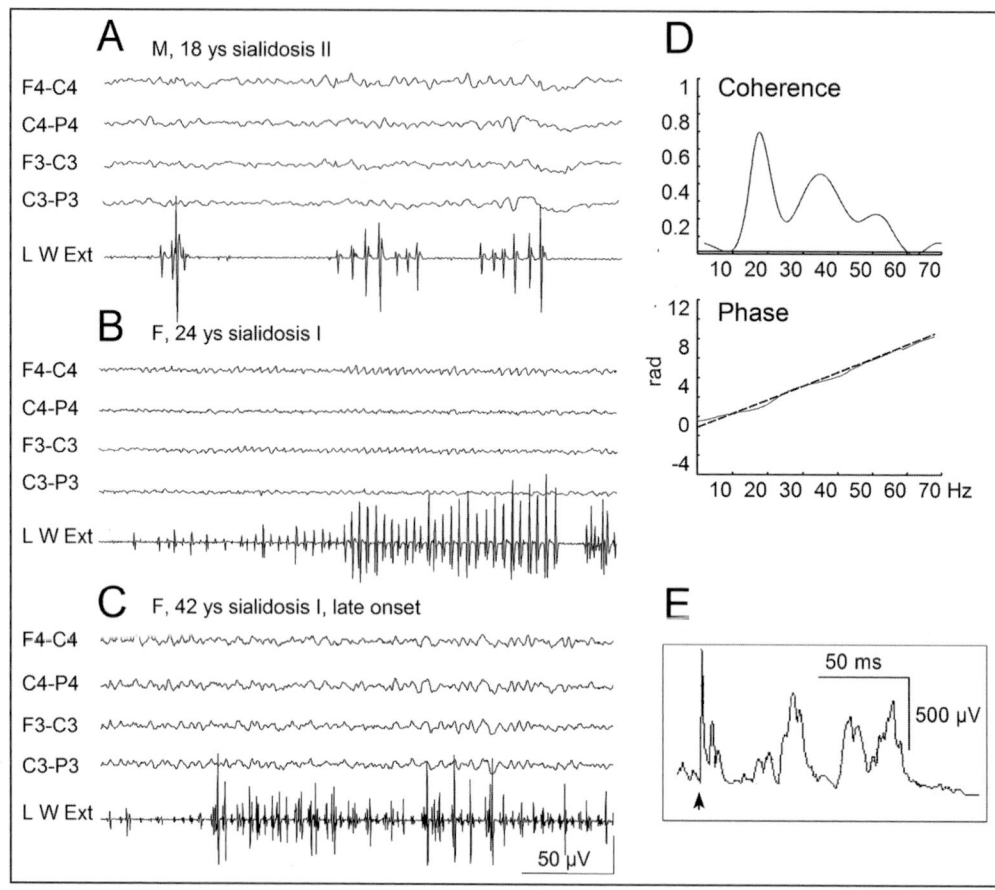

Fig. 1. (A, B, C) EEG-EMG recordings performed in 3 patients with sialidosis type II or I. Even if the jerks show a rhythmic course in the all patients, the less severely affected patient with a late onset (C) shows a combination of brief rhythmic sequences and isolated jerks. The panel D shows the coherence and phase function evaluated on EEG-EMG traces in patient B, with an extremely high coherence value and a linear course of the phase indicating a cortical origin of the myoclonic jerks. The panel E shows the multiphasic long-loop response to median nerve stimulation.

The diversity of clinical phenotypes appears to depend on the type of mutation and the percentage of normal sialidase activity that may protect against most severe forms of the disease. Hence, enzyme replacement therapy is a possible approach to treatment. To date, the effect of enzyme replacement therapy has been evaluated in mouse models. In mice, restored neuraminidase activity persisted for some days, resulting in a significant reduction in lysosomal storage, however, the injected enzyme could not cross the blood-brain barrier. Furthermore, the injected recombinant protein may have induced severe anaphylactic responses (Wang et al., 2005).

Conflicts of interest: none.

References

Allegranza, A., Tredici, G., Marmiroli, P., et al. (1989): Pathological study in an adult. *Clin. Neuropathol.* **8**, 266–271.

Bonten, E., van der Spoel, A., Fornerod, M., Grosveld, G. & d'Azzo (1996): A characterization of human lysosomal neuraminidase defines the molecular basis of the metabolic storage disorder sialidosis. *Genes Dev.* **10**, 3156–3169.

Bonten, E.J., Arts, W.F., Beck, M., et al. (2000): Novel mutations in lysosomal neuraminidase identify functional domains and determine clinical severity in sialidosis. *Hum. Mol. Genet.* **9**, 2715–2725.

Canafoglia, L., Franceschetti, S., Uziel, G., et al. (2011): Characterization of severe actionmyoclonus in sialidoses. *Epilepsy Res.* **94**, 86–93.

Canafoglia, L., Robbiano, A., Pareyson, D., et al. (2014): Expanding sialidosis spectrum by genome-wide screening: *NEU1* mutations in adult-onset myoclonus. *Neurology* **82**, 2003–2006.

Cantz, M., Gehler, J., Spranger, J. & Mucolipidosis, I. (1977): Increased sialic acid content and deficiency of an alpha-N-acetylneuraminidase in cultured fibroblasts. *Biochem. Biophys. Res. Commun.* **74**(2), 732–738.

Engel, J. Jr, Rapin, I. & Giblin, D.R. (1977): Electrophysiological studies in two patients with cherry red spot-myoclonus syndrome. *Epilepsia* **18**, 73–77.

Franceschetti, S., Uziel, G., Di Donato, S., Caimi, L. & Avanzini, G. (1980): Cherry-red spot-myoclonus syndrome and alpha-neuraminidase deficiency: neurophysiological, pharmacological and biochemical study in an adult. *J. Neurol. Neurosurg. Psychiatry* **43**, 934–940.

Kivlin, J.D., Sanborn, G.E. & Myers, G.G. (1985): The cherry-red spot in Tay-Sachs and other storage diseases. *Ann. Neurol.* **17**, 356–360.

Lowden, J.A. & O'Brien, J.S. (1979): Sialidosis: a review of human neuraminidase deficiency. *Am. J. Hum. Genet.* **31**, 1–18.

Lukong, K.E., Landry, K., Elsliger M.A., et al. (2001): Mutations in sialidosis impair sialidase binding to the lysosomal multienzyme complex. *J. Biol. Chem.* **276**, 17286–17290.

Nirenberg, M.J. & Frucht, S.J. (2005): Myoclonus. *Curr. Treat. Options Neurol.* **7**, 221–230.

Palmeri, S., Villanova, M., Malandrini, A., et al. (2000): Type I sialidoses: a clinical, biochemical and neuroradiological study. *Eur. Neurol.* **43**, 88–94.

Panzica, F., Canafoglia, L., Franceschetti, S., et al. (2003): Movement-activated myoclonus in genetically defined progressive myoclonic epilepsies: EEG-EMG relationship estimated using autoregressive models. *Clin. Neuro. Physiol.* **114**, 1041–1052.

Pattison, S., Pankarican, M., Rupar, C.A., Graham, F.L. & Igdoura S.A. (2004): Five novel mutations in the lysosomal sialidase gene (NEU1) in type II sialidosis patients and assessment of their impact on enzyme activity and intracellular targeting using adenovirus-mediated expression. *Hum. Mutat.* **23**, 32–39.

Pshezhetsky, A.V., Richard, C., Michaud, L., et al. (1997): Cloning, expression and chromosomal mapping of human lysosomal sialidase and characterization of mutations in sialidosis. *Nat. Genet.* **15**, 316–320.

Rapin, I., Goldfischer, S., Katzman, R., Engel, J. & O'Brien, J.S. (1978): The cherry-red spot-myoclonus syndrome. *Ann. Neurol.* **3**, 234–242.

Schene, I.F., Ayuso, V.K., de Sain-van der Velden, M., et al. (2015): Pitfalls in diagnosing neuraminidase deficiency: psychosomatics and normal sialic acid excretion. *JIMD Rep.* In press.

Spranger, J., Cantz, M. & Mucolipidosis, I. (1978): The cherry red-spot-myoclonus syndrome and neuraminidase deficiency. *Birth Defects Orig. Artic. Ser.* **14**, 105–112.

Thomas, P.K., Abrams, J.D., Swallow, D. & Stewart G. (1979): Sialidosis type1, cherry red spot-myoclonus syndrome with sialidase deficiency and altered electrophoretic mobilities of some enzymes known to be glycoproteins. 1. Clinical findings. *J. Neurol. Neurosurg. Psychiatry* **42**, 873–880.

Tobimatsu, S., Fukui, R., Shibasaki, H., Kato, M. & Kuroiwa, Y. (1985): Electrophysiological studies of myoclonus in sialidosis type 2. *Electroencephalogr. Clin. Neuro. Physiol.* **60**, 16–22.

Wang, D., Bonten, E.J., Yogalingam, G., Mann, L. & d'Azzo, A. (2005): Short-term, high dose enzyme replacement therapy in sialidosis mice. *Mol. Genet. Metab.* **85**, 181–189.

Yogalingam, G., Bonten, E.J., van de Vlekkert, D., et al. (2008): Neuraminidase 1 is a negative regulator of lysosomal exocytosis. *Dev. Cell* **15**, 74–86.

Chapter 8

Myoclonic epilepsy in mitochondrial disorders

Costanza Lamperti[1] and Massimo Zeviani[1,2]

[1] *Unit of Molecular Neurogenetics, Fondazione I.R.C.C.S. Istituto Neurologico Carlo Besta, via Celoria 11, 20133 Milan, Italy*
[2] *MRC-Mitochondrial Biology Unit, Cambridge, United Kingdom*
mdz21@mrc-mbu.cam.ac.uk

Summary

Mitochondrial disorders are a group of clinical entities associated with abnormalities of the mitochondrial respiratory chain (MRC), which carries out the oxidative phosphorylation (OXPHOS) of ADP into ATP. As the MRC is the result of genetic complementation between two separate genomes, nuclear and mitochondrial, OXPHOS failure can derive from mutations in either nuclear-encoded or mitochondrial-encoded, genes. Epilepsy is a relatively common feature of mitochondrial disease, especially in early-onset encephalopathies of infants and children. However, the two most common entities associated with epilepsy include MERRF, for Myoclonic Epilepsy with Ragged Red Fibers, and AHS, or Alpers-Huttenlocher syndrome, also known as hepatopathic poliodystrophy. Whilst MERRF is a maternally inherited condition caused by mtDNA mutations, particularly the 8344A>G substitution in the gene encoding mt-tRNA^{Lys}, AHS is typically caused by recessive mutations in *POLG*, encoding the catalytic subunit of polymerase gamma, the only mtDNA polymerase in humans. AHS is the most severe, early-onset, invariably fatal syndrome within a disease spectrum, which also includes other epileptogenic entities, all due to *POLG* mutations and including Spino-cerebellar Ataxia and Epilepsy (SCAE). This review reports the main clinical, neuroimaging, biochemical, and molecular features of epilepsy-related mitochondrial syndrome, particularly MERRF and AHS.

Introduction

The term 'mitochondrial disorders' is, to a large extent, applied to the clinical syndromes associated with abnormalities of the common final pathway of mitochondrial energy metabolism, *i.e.* oxidative phosphorylation (OXPHOS). OXPHOS takes place in the inner mitochondrial membrane involving 5 enzymatic complexes which form the mitochondrial respiratory chain (MRC). From a genetic perspective, the MRC is unique since it is encoded by 2 complementary separate genetic systems: the nuclear and the mitochondrial genomes. Because of this dual genetic control, OXPHOS disorders may be due to mutations in mitochondrial deoxyribonucleic acid (mtDNA) or nuclear DNA genes encoding either structural components of the MRC complexes or factors controlling their expression, assembly, function and turnover (Smeitink *et al.*, 2001). Mitochondria contain the only extra-nuclear source of DNA in animal cells (Nass, 1966). MtDNA is a circular, double stranded, 16,569 base-pair molecule of DNA which encodes 37 genes, including 13 polypeptides essential for the formation and function of 4 of the 5 MRC complexes, namely complex I, III, IV and V, two ribosomal RNAs (12S and 16S rRNA), and 22 transfer RNAs (tRNA) (Anderson et al., 1981). All other OXPHOS-related proteins, including most of the MRC subunits, MRC assembly factors, factors necessary for mtDNA maintenance and expression, etc., are synthesized in the cytosol and are specifically targeted, sorted and imported to their final mitochondrial location (Mokranjac & Neupert, 2005). The mitochondrial genome has unique features that distinguish it from the nuclear genome; for instance, in sexuate organisms, mtDNA is strictly maternally inherited and present in several hundred to several thousand copies within a single cell, the number varying amongst different cell types, mostly based on the energy demand of each tissue and organ (Taylor & Turnbull, 2005). The mtDNA genes have no introns, hardly any non-coding intervening regions, and for most cases the termination codons are completed by post-transcriptional polyadenylation (Anderson et al., 1981). The genetic code of mtDNA differs between many species, including humans, such that genomes between species may be reciprocally untranslatable; this partly explains why mtDNA is translated *in situ* by protein synthesis machinery that is completely independent from that operating in the cytosol for the translation of nuclear genes. In human mtDNA, the displacement loop (D-loop) is the only major non-coding region of the molecule which is formed by the displacement of the two DNA strands by a third DNA strand, the so-called 7S DNA.

An important contribution to the elucidation of the molecular basis of mitochondrial disorders has come from the discovery of an impressive, ever-expanding number of pathogenic mutations in mtDNA. In cases in which a mtDNA mutation is not found, mitochondrial disease is defined by the detection of a specific biochemical defect in OXPHOS, or the observation of typical morphological clues, or a combination of the two. In many instances, pathogenic mtDNA mutations can coexist alongside non-mutated mtDNA in the same cell, tissue and organism, a condition known as heteroplasmy (Larsson & Clayton, 1995; Hayashi et al., 1991). The percentage of pathogenic heteroplasmy dictates the phenotype, according to a 'threshold effect', *i.e.* a critical amount below which mutations do not manifest any clinical or biochemical phenotype. This threshold level varies from tissue to tissue and depends on the intrinsic pathogenicity of each mutation but, in general, ranges from 50-60 per cent (Shoubridge, 1994; Moraes et al., 1992; Mita et al., 1990; Hayashi et al., 1991; DiMauro, et al., 1985; Rosing et al., 1985; Traff et al., 1995; Parikh et al., 2008) for the most severe mutations, to more than 90 per cent for the mildest mutations. A paradigmatic example is the m.8993T>G mutation associated with NARP (neuropathy, ataxia, retinitis pigmentosa) syndrome (DiMauro, et al., 1985). The relationship between the mutation load and clinical severity was first documented by Tatuch et al., who showed that around 70 per cent heteroplasmy in skeletal muscle results in adult-onset of a slowly progressive syndrome corresponding to the acronymic features of NARP, whereas higher degrees of heteroplasmy (around 90 per cent) cause severe, early-onset, maternally inherited Leigh syndrome (MILS) (Rosing et al., 1985). MtDNA disease has an extremely variable phenotype and can present at any age (Traff et al., 1995). The clinical features usually affect tissues characterized by high metabolic demand, such as the central nervous system, the skeletal muscle, or the heart. However, other tissues are frequently involved, such as the β cells in the pancreas (leading to diabetes), the hair cells of the cochlea (causing deafness), or the renal tubules (leading to kidney dysfunction).

While epilepsy is a recurrent manifestation of mitochondrial disease, its exact prevalence is not known. In contrast, 35-60 per cent of individuals with refractory seizures display biochemical evidence of mitochondrial dysfunction (Parikh et al., 2008). A few studies have systematically examined the epileptic manifestations of mitochondrial disease (Khurana et al., 2008;

El Sabbagh *et al.*, 2010; Lee *et al.*, 2008). Although seizures may be the presenting symptom at onset (Canafoglia *et al.*, 2001; Hayashi *et al.*, 1991), in more than 80 per cent of cases, the first seizure is preceded by some other symptoms (El Sabbagh *et al.*, 2010), including, for example, failure to thrive, developmental delay, ataxia, or evidence of multi-organ involvement. In children with respiratory chain disorders, different seizure types can occur in as many as 60 per cent of cases (El Sabbagh *et al.*, 2010). Whilst clinical identification of mitochondrial epilepsy may be difficult, one of the most common forms is myoclonic epilepsy, either as typical MERRF syndrome (myoclonic epilepsy with ragged red fibres) or within the context of other, complex epileptic manifestations.

Clinical manifestations

In 1921, Ramsay Hunt described 6 patients with a disorder characterized by ataxia, myoclonus, and epilepsy, which he called *'dyssynergia cerebellaris myoclonica'* (Hunt, 1921). Over 50 years then passed before Tsairis *et al.* linked this entity to mitochondrial abnormalities in the skeletal muscle in one family, hallmarked by the presence of ragged-red fibres (Tsairis *et al.*, 1973). This family was described in great detail, leading to the term 'classic MERRF' in 1989 (Lombes *et al.*, 1989). MERRF was one of the 3 major, multisystem syndromes first classified as 'mitochondrial encephalomyopathy' (DiMauro *et al.*, 1985). MERRF has 2 other historical distinctions: (i) it was the first well-defined human disease in which maternal inheritance was clearly demonstrated, thus suggesting a mitochondrial DNA defect (mtDNA) (Rosing *et al.*, 1985); and (ii) the first mitochondrial encephalomyopathy in which a molecular mtDNA defect was actually identified. It is also one of the most common and clinically better defined mitochondrial syndromes. MERRF is, in fact, a multi-system disorder, hallmarked by myoclonus, episodes of generalized epilepsy, progressive ataxia, and ragged-red fibres (RRF) with partial deficiency of cytochrome c oxidase (COX) (19-20-21) (Fig. 1A, B). Although the onset is usually in childhood, early development is normal and adult onset is not uncommon. Besides the defining criteria, common clinical manifestations include hearing loss, peripheral neuropathy, cognitive decay and eventually dementia, short stature, exercise intolerance, and optic atrophy and ataxia. Less common clinical signs (seen in < 50 per cent of the patients) include cardiomyopathy, pigmentary retinopathy, pyramidal signs, ophthalmoparesis, and the appearance of multiple lipomas, particularly in the neck and upper trunk (Fig. 1C). As is usually the case with mitochondrial encephalomyopathies, maternal family members may be symptomatic, oligosymptomatic, or asymptomatic. While several heteroplasmic point mutations, mostly affecting the gene encoding mt-tRNA^{Lys}, are responsible for MERRF, by far the most frequent MERRF mutation is the m.8344A>G substitution in the T-ψ-C loop of mt-tRNA^{Lys} (Fig. 1D). A few unusual clinical presentations, characterized by overlapping symptoms between MERRF and MELAS (mitochondrial encephalomyopathy with lactic acidosis and stroke-like episodes), have been reported either as isolated cases or, more often, in pedigrees in which typical MERRF patients were also present. Several studies have reported in detail the wide spectrum of clinical presentations associated with the m.8334A>G mutation (Berkovic *et al.*, 1991; Hammans *et al.*, 1993; Silvestri *et al.*, 1993; Howell *et al.*, 1996; Mancuso *et al.*, 2013), but certain features and variants deserve special attention. For instance, peripheral neuropathy is not uncommon in MERRF, being usually sensory-motor and contributing to the onset and progression of gait ataxia. At least one case has been reported to be characterized by predominant motor symptoms, thus phenocopying Charcot-Marie-Tooth disease (Howell *et al.*, 1996).

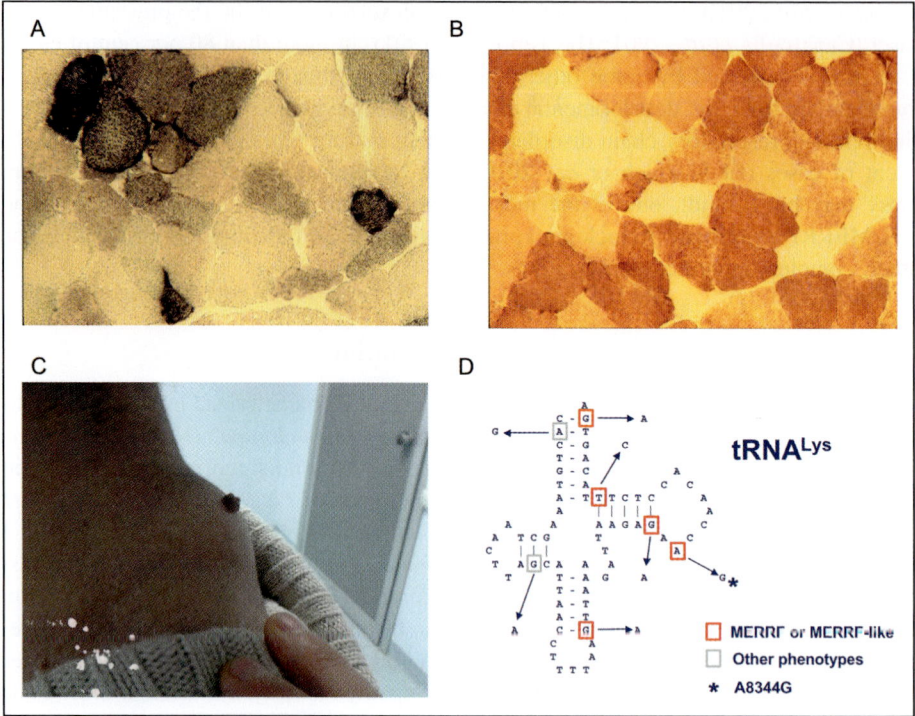

Fig. 1. Muscle biopsy of a MERRF patient presenting with COX deficient (A) and intense SDH-positive (B) RRF. (C) Neck lipoma in a 67-year-old MERRF patient. (D) Lys tRNA highlighting the most frequent mutations associated with MERRF or MERRF-Like syndrome.

In 1975, long before the molecular defects of MERRF became known, Karl Ekbom (Ekbom, 1975) described multiple lipomas in association with hereditary ataxia, photomyoclonus and skeletal deformities in a family in which the 8344A>G mutation was later documented (Traff et al., 1995; Berkovic et al., 1991). These tumours, varying in size from small subcutaneous nodules to disfiguring masses, are usually located in the nape of the neck and the shoulder area. They have been reported in numerous patients with the 8344A>G mutation (Larsson et al., 1992; Holme et al., 1993; Calabresi et al., 1994; Naumann et al., 1995; Austin et al., 1998). Maternal inheritance was evident in a large family (Rosing et al., 1985) which was again confirmed to harbour the m.8344A>G substitution in the mt-tRNALys gene (Shoffner et al., 1990). Not only was this the first molecular defect to be reported for a mitochondrial encephalomyopathy, but also the first to be identified for a specific form of epilepsy. The m.8344A>G mutation is present in about 90 per cent of MERRF patients. Two additional mutations have been associated with MERRF, both affecting the mt-tRNA^{Lys} gene. The first mutation, m.8356T>C, was discovered simultaneously in an American family with typical MERRF (Silvestri et al., 1992), and in an Italian family in which typical MERRF symptoms coexisted with stroke-like episodes and migraines, thus justifying the definition as a 'MERRF/MELAS' overlap syndrome (Zeviani et al., 1993). A common clinical feature of both families was hyperthyroidism, which is rather unusual in mitochondrial diseases and may, therefore, be related to this specific mutation. A third family with the same mutation was later reported in Japan; the proband had typical MERRF, but a maternal aunt had stroke-like episodes, another example of MERRF/MELAS overlap (Sano et al., 1996).

The second mutation, m.8363G>A, was first identified in two unrelated American families with maternally inherited cardiomyopathy, which was severe enough to cause early death in several members of one family (Santorelli et al., 1996). Although cardiomyopathy dominated the clinical picture, additional signs included encephalomyopathy, neurosensory hearing loss, progressive external ophthalmoparesis, intellectual disability, limb weakness, and peripheral neuropathy, variably affecting members of both families. Interestingly, cerebellar symptoms were frequent, including ataxia, dysmetria, slurred speech, and gait instability. Interestingly, one proband had 'horse collar' lipomas. The same mutation was later identified in 2 unrelated Japanese patients with typical MERRF, one of whom also presented cardiomyopathy (Ozawa et al., 1997). Recently a new mutation, m.3291T>C, has been associated with MERRF/MELAS syndrome in a 19-year-old Chinese man (Liu et al., 2014).

The m.8344A>G mutation is virtually always heteroplasmic, and the mutation threshold for typical MERRF is usually high or very high (i.e. affecting about 60-90 per cent of total mtDNA), which suggests that this mutation is relatively benign (Shoffner et al., 1990). As mentioned earlier, the 3 mutations associated with MERRF all affect highly conserved nucleotides in the mt-tRNA^{Lys} gene. The m.8344A>G and the m.8356T>C mutations are located in the T-ψ-C loop, while the m.8363G>A mutation is located in the aminoacyl acceptor stem of the putative cloverleaf (secondary) structure of the mt-tRNA^{Lys} transcript (Santorelli et al., 1996). A single patient with typical MERRF symptoms, i.e. myoclonus, seizures, ataxia, and RRF, but, in addition, peripheral neuropathy, dementia, and neuroradiological evidence of mild cerebral and severe cerebellar atrophy, had no mutation in the tRNA^{Lys} gene, but rather multiple mtDNA deletions in muscle, suggesting impairment in a nuclear gene product controlling mtDNA integrity, such as POLG.

Laboratory tests

Patients with typical MERRF have elevated blood lactate and pyruvate at rest, both increasing abnormally upon moderate exercise. CSF protein levels are often increased, but rarely exceed 100 mg per cent. Electromyography and nerve conduction studies are usually compatible with a predominantly myopathic pattern, except when motor peripheral neuropathy is clearly present. Electroencephalography is typically characterized by generalized spike and wave discharges with background slowing, but focal epileptiform discharges may also be seen (Fig. 2).

A CT or MRI scan may show brain atrophy and basal ganglia calcifications. Phosphorus magnetic resonance spectroscopy of the gastrocnemius muscle in 8 patients (only 3 of whom showed signs of myopathy) revealed mitochondrial dysfunction in all, as evidenced by increased relative intracellular inorganic phosphate (Pi) concentration and decreased phosphocreatine to Pi ratio (Rahman, 2012). However, no mitochondrial dysfunction was seen in the brain using the same technique.

By definition, the muscle biopsy shows RRF using modified Gomori trichrome stain in typical patients (Wolf et al., 2009). These fibres also react intensely to the succinate dehydrogenase (SDH)-specific stain, a more sensitive indicator of excessive mitochondrial proliferation. Both RRF and some non-RRF fail to stain histochemically to COX. Muscle biopsies from MERRF patients can also show strongly SDH-reactive blood vessels (SSVs), similar to those characteristically seen in the muscles of patients with MELAS (Harding, 1990), again emphasizing the concept that the 2 disease entities may overlap to some extent. However, in contrast to MELAS SSVs, which stain positive for COX, MERRF SSVs are uniformly COX-negative

(Lamantea *et al.*, 2002). MRC activities in muscle extracts usually show defects in mtDNA-dependent complexes, particularly COX (Lombes *et al.*, 1989; Silvestri *et al.*, 1993). Neuronal loss and gliosis predominate in the brains of MERRF patients, preferentially involving the cerebellum, the brainstem, and the spinal cord. In the cerebellum, neuronal loss is particularly severe in the dentate nucleus, an observation originally made by Ramsay Hunt, who described 'primary atrophy of the dentate system' in patients with *'dyssynergia cerebellaris myoclonica'* (Hunt, 1921). The inferior olivary nucleus of the medulla oblongata is the most severely affected structure in the brainstem, followed by the red nucleus and the substantia nigra in the mesencephalon. In the spinal cord, severe cell loss has been observed in the thoracic nucleus of Clarke, while milder involvement has been detected in the anterior and posterior horns of the spinal cord. Demyelination preferentially affects the superior cerebellar peduncles and the posterior columns and lateral spinocerebellar tracts of the spinal cord, while the pyramidal system is usually spared or mildly affected.

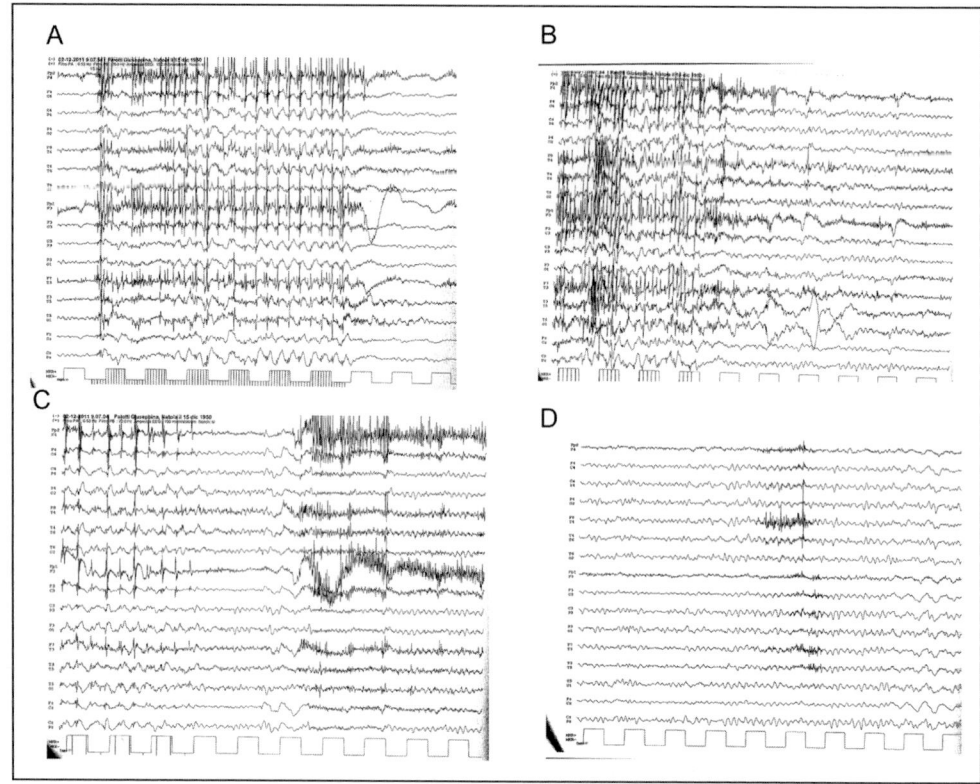

Fig. 2. EEG in adult patients with MERRF. (A, B) Generalized spike and waves, as well as myoclonus, during SLI. (C, D) Paroxysmal activity in the temporal region in both hemispheres with right prevalence.

Private mtDNA mutations and myoclonic epilepsy

Although MERRF is one of the most common mitochondrial encephalomyopathies, a substantial fraction of paediatric patients with myoclonic epilepsy and MRC defects fails to show MERRF mutations (El Sabbagh *et al.*, 2010). In this group, severe myoclonus may be preceded by other seizure types, such as erratic myoclonus, focal motor seizures, myoclonic absences, sor tonic seizures, but becomes predominant during the disease course. Occasionally, the disease may evolve into recurrent myoclonic *status epilepticus*. In the report by El Shabbagh *et al.* on 56 paediatric patients (El Sabbagh *et al.*, 2010), only one showed photosensitivity, with spikes induced by intermittent light stimulation. Brain MRI showed hyper-intense signals on T2/FLAIR (fluid-attenuated inversion recovery) sequences of the basal ganglia ($n = 8$) and/or dentate nuclei ($n = 3$), and cerebellar atrophy ($n = 5$). The basal ganglia were involved irrespective of the age at onset, while cerebellar involvement was present only in patients with early-onset epilepsy, *i.e.* within the first decade of life. Myoclonic seizures were drug-resistant. Six patients died from global neurological failure leading to comatose *status*. Biochemically, 8 patients had complex I deficiency, 3 complex V, 2 complex IV, 1 complex II, and 4 showed multiple defects. In 45 per cent of the cases, a mtDNA mutation was identified; in *MT-ATP6* ($n = 3$), *MT-ND3* ($n = 2$), *MT-TK* ($n = 1$), *MT-ND5* ($n = 1$), and *MT-TL1* ($n = 1$). mtDNA depletion in muscles is only rarely associated with progressive myoclonic epilepsy (Rahman, 2012).

Alpers-Huttenlocher syndrome

The second most common form of mitochondrial myoclonic epilepsy is Alpers-Huttenlocher syndrome (AHS) (OMIM #203700). AHS is clinically characterized by psychomotor retardation, intractable epilepsy, and liver failure. The onset is in infancy or early childhood, often with seizures and/or hypotonia. *Status epilepticus* is common and most patients die from refractory seizures and liver failure before the age of 3 (Luoma *et al.*, 2004). Liver dysfunction can be present at the onset of the neurological symptomatology, or may manifest following treatment with sodium valproate for the control of seizures. Individuals with AHS typically present with focal myoclonic and complex seizures. *Epilepsia partialis continua* is also frequently seen and may lead to fatal *status epilepticus*. The electroencephalogram at onset may point towards the diagnosis, particularly when characterized by unilateral occipital, rhythmic, high-amplitude slow activity with superimposed (poly)spikes, frequently evolving into generalized discharges (Wolf *et al.*, 2009). Other clinical features include global developmental delay and regression, progressive microcephaly, cortical visual impairment with abnormal visual-evoked potentials, and, importantly, evidence of progressive liver failure, heralded by elevated levels of liver enzymes in the blood and hepatomegaly, followed by overt liver cirrhosis. Brain MRI may be normal in the initial stage of disease, or show non-specific changes, such as progressive cerebral atrophy. AHS was firstly diagnosed as a neuropathological entity defined by the presence of extensive necrotizing poliodystrophy; histological features include spongiosis, neuronal loss and astrocytosis affecting the cerebral cortex, particularly the calcarine cortex, which explains the cortical visual loss in this condition (Luoma *et al.*, 2004). Liver histology in AHS may reveal steatosis, hepatocyte loss, bile duct proliferation and fibrosis, evolving into frank cirrhosis (Harding, 1990). By and large, AHS is associated with a few recessive mutations in the *POLG* gene, encoding the catalytic, large subunit of mtDNA polymerase (polymerase gamma). More than 150 mutations have been reported in the *POLG* gene, constituting a major cause of mitochondrial disease. Mutations in this gene are also the most frequent cause of autosomal dominant progressive external ophthalmoplegia (ad-PEO). In adPEO due to *POLG* mutation, distinct features also include severe dysphagia and dysphonia and, occasionally, extra-pyramidal signs, *e.g.* parkinsonism, cerebellar dysfunction, or chorea (Luoma *et al.*, 2004). Recessive mutations of *POLG* may also be responsible for autosomal recessive cases (Lamantea *et al.*, 2002) or apparently sporadic PEO cases characterised by multiple mtDNA deletions (Agostino *et al.*, 2003), with or without additional findings, including parkinsonism, severe peripheral neuropathy, endocrine failure, or psychotic depression (Van Goethem *et al.*, 2003). In addition, recessive *POLG* mutations are responsible for a wide spectrum of syndromes of increasing severity and precocity, including juvenile sensory ataxic neuropathy, dysarthria, ophthalmoplegia, SANDO (Horvath *et al.*, 2006), childhood cerebellar ataxia and epilepsy, SCAE, and possibly infantile AHS, all characterized by exquisite sensitivity of the liver to valproate-associated damage. As mentioned above, liver failure occurs spontaneously in AHS, due to severe, liver-specific mtDNA depletion. The brain lesions in AHS are typically characterized by spongiotic neurodegeneration, particularly in the cortical ribbon and thalami (Davidzon *et al.*, 2005; Van Goethem *et al.*, 2004). The molecular basis of this clinical heterogeneity can be explained, in part, by the structural and functional complexity of the enzyme. Pol-γA, the 145 kDa catalytic subunit encoded by *POLG*, comprises an N-terminal exonuclease domain, with predominantly proofreading functions, and a polymerase domain, which performs the template-directed synthesis of the nascent mtDNA strands. The 2 most prevalent mutations in AHS, but also in SANDO and SCAE, are p.A467T and p.W748S, which are present at a frequency of approximately 1 per cent in the Scandinavian population (Horvath *et al.*, 2006). Rapid molecular diagnosis of AHS syndrome may therefore be achieved by screening these selected 'common' mutations in DNA extracted from blood; however, in several cases, sequence analysis of all exons and exon-intron boundaries is required to identify causative *POLG1* mutations. Liver biopsy of AHS patients shows severe mtDNA depletion while multiple mtDNA deletions are the molecular hallmark in muscle for adPEO or arPEO patients.

Recently, the combination of early encephalopathy, epilepsy, hepatopathy, and sensory axonal neuropathy was found in patients with recessive mutations in the mtDNA helicase, Twinkle (*PEO1*), which co-functions with Pol-γ in mtDNA replication (Saneto & Naviaux, 2010; Lonnqvist *et al.*, 2009). As is the case for POLG-associated AHS, patients with recessive mutations in Twinkle also display mtDNA depletion in the liver.

Therapy

There is no specific therapy for MERRF or other mitochondrial encephalomyopathies associated with myoclonic epilepsy. Patients are empirically treated with 'cocktails' of vitamins and cofactors, including idebenone at high dosage (150 mg x3 daily) and L-carnitine (1 g daily) (Farge *et al.*, 2007). Myoclonus can be controlled with clonazepam (0.5-1 mg 3 times a day) or zonisamide. As with all mitochondrial diseases, valproate has to be used with caution and always in combination with L-carnitine because of its well-documented inhibition of carnitine uptake (DiMauro *et al.*, 2000). Hepatic impairment in AHS, SANDO or SCAE may be precipitated by valproate, leading to fulminant liver failure. These conditions, therefore, represent an absolute contraindication for the use of valproate to control seizures (Tein *et al.*, 1993). Lactic acidosis can be controlled by bicarbonate which, however, has only a transient buffering effect and may exacerbate the cerebral symptoms. Levetiracetam is the first choice of treatment for myoclonus in MERRF and lamotrigine may exert a neuroprotective effect (Lagrue *et al.*, 2007).

Conflicts of interest: none.

References

Agostino, A., Valletta, L., Chinnery, P.F., et al. (2003): Mutations of ANT1, Twinkle, and POLG1 in sporadic progressive external ophthalmoplegia (PEO). *Neurology* **60**, 1354–1356.

Anderson, S., Bankier, A.T., Barrell, B.G., et al. (1981): Sequence and organization of the human mitochondrial genome. *Nature* **290**, 457–465.

Austin, S.A., Vriesendorp, F.J., Thandroyen, F.T., Hecht, J.T., Jones, O.T. & Johns, D.R. (1998): Expanding phenotype of the 8334 transfer tRNA lysine mitochondrial DNA mutation. *Neurology* **51**, 1447–1450.

Berkovic, S., Shoubridge, E., Andermann, F., & Carpenter, S. (1991): Clinical spectrum of mitochondrial, DNA, mutations at base pair 8344. *Lancet* **338**, 457.

Calabresi, P.A., Silvestri, G., DiMauro, S. & Griggs, R.C. (1994): Ekbom's syndrome: lipomas, ataxia, and neuropathy with MERRF. *Muscle & Nerve* **17**, 943–945.

Canafoglia, L., Franceschetti, S., Antozzi, C., et al. (2001): Epileptic phenotypes associated with mitochondrial disorders. *Neurology* **56**, 1340–1346.

Davidzon, G., Mancuso, M., Ferraris, S., et al. (2005): POLG mutations and Alpers syndrome. *Ann. Neurol.* **57**, 921–923.

DiMauro, S., Bonilla, E., Zeviani, M., Nakagawa, M. & DeVivo, D.C. (1985): Mitochondrial myopathies. *Ann. Neurol.* **17**, 521–538.

DiMauro, S., Hirano, M. & Schon, E.A. (2000): Mitochondrial encephalomyopathies: therapeutic approaches. *Neurol. Sci.* **21**, S901–S908.

Ekbom, K. (1975): Hereditary ataxia, photomyoclonus, skeletal deformities and lipoma. *Acta Neurol. Scandinav.* **51**, 393–404.

El Sabbagh, S., Lebre, A.S., Bahi-Buisson, N., et al. (2010): Epileptic phenotypes in children with respiratory chain disorders. *Epilepsia* **51**, 1225–1235.

Farge, G., Pham, X.H., Holmlund, T., et al. (2007): The accessory subunit B of DNA polymerase gamma is required required for mitochondrial replisome function. *Nucleic Acids Res.* **35**, 902–911.

Hammans, S.R., Sweeney, M.G., Brockington, M., et al. (1993): The mitochondrial DNA transfer RNALys A->G(8344): mutation and the syndrome of myoclonic epilepsy with ragged red fibers (MERRF). *Brain* **116**, 617–632.

Harding, B.N. (1990): Progressive neuronal degeneration of childhood with liver disease (Alpers-Huttenlocher syndrome): a personal review. *J. Child Neurol.* **5**, 273–287.

Hayashi, J., Ohta, S., Kikuchi, A., et al. (1991): Introduction of disease related mitochondrial DNA deletions into HeLa Cells lacking mitochondrial DNA results in mitochondrial dysfunction. *Proc. Natl. Acad. Sci.* **88**, 10614–10618.

Holme, E., Larsson, N.G., Oldfors, A., Tulinius, M., Sahlin, P. & Stenman, G. (1993): Multiple symmetric lipomas with high levels of mtDNA with the tRNALys A>G(8344): mutation as the only manifestation of disease in a carrier of myoclonus epilepsy and ragged-red fibers (MERRF) syndrome. *Am. J. Hum. Genet.* **52**, 551–556.

Horvath, R., Hudson, G., Ferrari, G., et al. (2006): Phenotypic spectrum associated with mutations of the mitochondrial polymerase gamma gene. *Brain* **129**, 1674–1684.

Howell, N., Kubacka, I., Smith, R., Frerman, F., Parks, J.K. & Parker, W.D. (1996): Association of the mitochondrial 8344 MERRF mutation with maternally inherited spinocerebellar degeneration and Leigh disease. *Neurology* **46**, 219–222.

Hunt, J.R. (1921): Dyssynergia cerebellaris myoclonica - primary atrophy of the dentate system: a contribution to the pathology and symptomatology of the cerebellum. *Brain* **44**, 490-538.

Khurana, D.S., Salganicoff, L., Melvin, J.J., et al. (2008): Epilepsy and respiratory chain defects in children with mitochondrial encephalopathies. *Neuropediatrics* **39**, 8–13.

Lagrue, E., Chalon, S., Bodard, S., Saliba, E., Gressens, P. & Castelnau, P. (2007): Lamotrigine is neuroprotective in the energy deficiency model of MPTP intoxicated mice. *Pediatr. Res.* **62**, 14–19.

Lamantea, E., Tiranti, V., Bordoni, A., et al. (2002): Mutations of mitochondrial DNA polymerase gamma A are a frequent cause of autosomal dominant or recessive progressive external ophthalmoplegia. *Ann. Neurol.* **52**, 211–219.

Larsson, N.G. & Clayton, D.A. (1995): Molecular genetic aspects of human mitochondrial disorders. *Ann. Rev. Genet.* **29**, 151–178.

Larsson, N.G., Tulinius, M.H., Holme, E., et al. (1992): Segregation and manifestations of the mtDNA tRNALys A->G(8344): mutation of myoclonus epilepsy and ragged-red fibers (MERRF) syndrome. *Am. J. Hum. Genet.* **51**, 1201–1212.

Lee, Y.M., Kang, H.C., Lee, J.S., et al. (2008): Mitochondrial respiratory chain defects: underlying etiology in various epileptic conditions. *Epilepsia* **49**, 685–690.

Liu, K., Zhao, H., Ji, K. & Yan, C. (2014): CMERRF/MELAS overlap syndrome due to the m.3291 T >C., mutation. *C. Metab. Brain Dis.* **29**, 139–144.

Lombes, A., Mendell, J.R., Nakase, H., et al. (1989): Myoclonic epilepsy and ragged-red fibers with cytochrome oxidase deficiency: neuropathology, biochemistry, and molecular genetics. *Ann. Neurol.* **26**, 20-33.

Lonnqvist, T., Paetau, A., Valanne, L., et al. (2009): Recessive twinkle mutations cause severe epileptic encephalopathy. *Brain* **132**, 1553–1562.

Luoma, P., Melberg, A., Rinne, J.O., et al. (2004): Parkinsonism, premature menopause, and mitochondrial DNA polymerase gamma mutations: clinical and molecular genetic study. *Lancet* **364**, 875–882.

Mancuso, M., Orsucci, D., Angelini, C., Bertini, E., et al. (2013): Phenotypic heterogeneity of the 8344A>G mtDNA 'MERRF' mutation. *Neurology* **80**, 2049–2054.

Mita, S., Rizzuto, R., Moraes, C.T., et al. (1990): Recombination via flanking direct repeats is a major cause of large-scale deletions of human mitochondrial DNA. *Nucleic Acids Res.* **18**, 561–567.

Mokranjac, D. & Neupert, W. (2005): Protein import into mitochondria. *Biochem. Soc. Trans.* **33**, 1019–1023.

Moraes, C.T., Ricci, E., Petruzzella, V., et al. (1992): Molecular analysis of the muscle pathology associated with mitochondrial DNA deletions. *Nat. Genet.* **1**, 359–367.

Nass, M.M. (1966): The circularity of mitochondrial DNA. *Proc. Natl. Acad. Sci.* **56**, 1215–1222.

Naumann, M., Reiners, K., Gold, R., et al. (1995): Mitochondrial dysfunction in adult-onset myopathies with structural abnormalities. *Acta Neuropath.* **89**, 152–157.

Ozawa, M., Nishino, I., Horai, S., Nonaka, I. & Goto Y-I. (1997): Myoclonus epilepsy associated with ragged-red fibers: a G-to-A mutation at nucleotide pair 8363 in mitochondrial tRNA(Lys) in two families. *Muscle & Nerve* **20**, 271–278.

Parikh, S., Cohen, B.H., Gupta, A., Lachhwani, D.K., Wyllie, E. & Kotagal, P. (2008): Metabolic testing in the pediatric epilepsy unit. *Pediatr. Neurol.* **38**, 191–195.

Rahman, S. (2012): Mitochondrial disease and epilepsy. *Dev. Med. Child Neurol.* **54**, 397–406.

Rosing, H.S., Hopkins, L.C., Wallace, D.C., Epstein, C.M. & Weidenheim, K. (1985): Maternally inherited mitochondrial myopathy and myoclonic epilepsy. *Ann. Neurol.* **17**, 228–237.

Saneto, R.P. & Naviaux, R.K. (2010): Polymerase gamma disease through the ages. *Dev. Disabil. Res. Rev.* **16**, 163–174.

Sano, M., Ozawa, M., Shiota, S., Momose, Y., Uchigata, M. & Goto, Y. (1996): The T-C(8356) mitochondrial DNA mutation in a Japanese family. *J. Neurol.* **243**, 441–444.

Santorelli, F.M., Mak S-C., El-Schahawi, M., et al. (1996): Maternally inherited cardiomyopathy and hearing loss associated with a novel mutation in the mitochondrial DNA tRNA(Lys) gene (G8363 A). *Am. J. Hum. Genet.* **58**, 933–939.

Shoffner, J.M., Lott, M.T., Lezza, A., Seibel, P., Ballinger, S.W. & Wallace, D.C. (1990): Myoclonic epilepsy and ragged-red fiber disease (MERRF) is associated with a mitochondrial DNA tRNA(Lys) mutation. *Cell* **61**, 931–937.

Shoubridge, E.A. (1994): Mitochondrial DNA diseases: histological and cellular studies. *J. Bioenerg. Biomembr.* **26**, 301–310.

Silvestri, G., Moraes, C.T., Shanske, S., Oh, S.J. & DiMauro, S.A. (1992): New mtDNA mutation in the tRNA(Lys) gene associated with myoclonic epilepsy and ragged-red fibers (MERRF). *Am. J. Hum. Genet.* **51**, 1213–1217.

Silvestri, G., Ciafaloni, E., Santorelli, F., et al. (1993): Clinical features associated with the A→G transition at nucleotide 8344 of mtDNA ('MERRF mutation'). *Neurology* **43**, 1200-1206.

Smeitink, J., van den Heuvel, L. & DiMauro, S. (2001): The genetics and pathology of oxidative phosphorylation. *Nat. Rev. Genet.* **2**, 342–352.

Taylor, R.W. & Turnbull, D.M. (2005): Mitochondrial DNA mutations in human disease. *Nat. Rev. Genet.* **6**, 389–402.

Tein, I., DiMauro, S., Xie, Z-W., De Vivo, D.C. (1993): Valproic acid impairs carnitine uptake in cultured human skin fibroblasts. An in vitro model for pathogenesis of valproic acid-associated carnitine deficiency. *Pediat. Res.* **34**, 281–287.

Traff, J., Holme, E., Nilsson, B.Y. (1995): Ekbom's syndrome of photomyoclonus, cerebellar ataxia and cervical lipoma is associated with tRNA(Lys) A8344 G mutation in mitochondrial DNA *Acta Neurol. Scand.* **92**, 394–397.

Tsairis, P., Engel, W.K., Kark, P. (1973): Familial myoclonic epilepsy syndrome associated with skeletal muscle mitochondrial abnormalities. *Neurology* **23**, 408.

Van Goethem, G., Martin, J.J., Dermaut, B., et al. (2003): POLG mutations presenting with sensory and ataxic neuropathy in compound heterozygote patients with progressive external ophthalmoplegia. *Neuromuscul. Disord.* **13**, 133–142.

Van Goethem, G., Luoma, P., Rantamaki, M., *et al.* (2004): POLG mutations in neurodegenerative disorders with ataxia but no muscle involvement. *Neurology* **63,** 1251–1257.

Wolf, N.I., Rahman, S., Schmitt, B., *et al.* (2009): Status epilepticus in children with Alpers' disease caused by POLG1 mutations: EEG and MRI features. *Epilepsia* **50,** 1596–1607.

Zeviani, M., Muntoni, F. & Savarese, N., *et al.* (1993): A MERRF/MELAS overlap syndrome associated with a new point mutation in the mitochondrial DNA tRNA(Lys) gene. *Eur. J. Hum Genet.* **1,** 80-87.

Chapter 9

Progressive myoclonic epilepsy associated with neuroserpin inclusion bodies (neuroserpinosis)

Benoit D. Roussel[1,2], David A. Lomas[1] and Damian C. Crowther[3,4]

[1] *Wolfson Institute for Biomedical Research, University College London, London, WC1E 6BN, United Kingdom*
[2] *Inserm U919, Serine Proteases and Pathophysiology of the Neurovascular Unit, GIP CYCERON, University Caen Basse Normandie, Boulevard Becquerel, 14074 Caen, France*
[3] *Department of Genetics, University of Cambridge, Downing Street, Cambridge, CB2 3EH, United Kingdom*
[4] *MedImmune Limited, Aaron Klug Building, Granta Park, Cambridge, CB21 6GH, United Kingdom*
damian.crowther@azneuro.com

Summary

Familial encephalopathy with neuroserpin inclusions bodies (FENIB) has been identified as a cause of pre-senile dementia with frontal symptoms as well as progressive myoclonic epilepsy. In affected individuals, mutated neuroserpin accumulates in neuronal inclusions (Collins bodies). FENIB is due to mutations in the *SERPINI1* gene located on chromosome 3q26. Serine protease inhibitors (serpins) are a large superfamily of proteins that employ a conserved molecular mechanism for the inhibition of a wide range of proteases. Mutations may render serpins prone to polymerisation, *i.e.* ordered aggregation, in the endoplasmic reticulum of the synthetic cell. In the case of neuroserpin (NS), a neuronal protein, this aggregation causes gain-of-function neuronal dysfunction that is thought to underpin the neurological manifestations. NS also inhibits tPA and, in this way, is thought to regulate the sensitivity of neurones to glutamatergic excitatory neurotransmission at the NMDA (N-methyl-D-aspartate) receptor. The epileptic component of FENIB may be due to dysfunction of the NS/tPA pathway.

Introduction

Neuroserpin (NS) is a member of the serine protease inhibitor, or serpin, superfamily and has sequence and structural homologies to the archetype α_1-antitrypsin. At the molecular level, serpins are composed of 9 α-helices, 3 β-sheets (A to C) and an exposed mobile reactive centre loop (RCL). The RCL typically contains 20 residues that act as a pseudo-substrate for the target protease (Elliott *et al.*, 1996; Ryu *et al.*, 1996). The main role of NS is to regulate the plasmin proteolytic pathway, in particular by inhibiting tissue-type plasminogen activator (tPA). In this regard, NS plays physiological roles in the development of the central nervous system (Seeds *et al.*, 1999), in learning and memory and also in such pathological events as stroke (Cole *et al.*, 2007) and epilepsy (Qian *et al.*, 1993).

Numerous mutations in human serpins have been linked to a wide range of diseases; examples include emphysema, angioedema, and dementia with progressive myoclonus epilepsy, resulting from mutations in α_1-antitrypsin, C1-inhibitor, and neuroserpin, respectively. Direct toxicity is invariably a consequence of the intracellular accumulation of serpin aggregates that are termed polymers, and may result in death of the synthetic cell. In the case of neuroserpin, cytotoxicity is seen exclusively in neurons of the central nervous system. There may also be associated loss-of-function effects caused by the deregulated hyperactivity of the target proteases and this may underpin the development of epilepsy in patients carrying neuroserpin variants. To date, only a few families and exceptionally rare non-familial cases of progressive myoclonic epilepsy linked to the *SERPINI1* gene have been described. Age at onset is between 13 and 60 years and the disorder is severe with rapid loss of autonomy and premature death.

Pathophysiology of neuroserpin-related disease

NS was first identified as an axonally-secreted glycoprotein in the conditioned medium of embryonic chick dorsal root ganglia cells (Stoeckli *et al.*, 1989; Osterwalder *et al.*, 1996). In mammals it is expressed in the central and peripheral nervous system, predominantly in neurons (Hastings *et al.*, 1997; Osterwalder *et al.*, 1998) where it can inhibit a number of trypsin-like enzymes, including thrombin and plasmin (Osterwalder *et al.*, 1998), however, subsequent studies indicate that tPA is the main physiological target. Accordingly, the highest levels of NS are found in parts of the nervous system that have the highest expression of tPA mRNA and protein (Krueger *et al.*, 1997).

While not all serpins interact with proteases, those such as neuroserpin, which have retained inhibitory activity, employ a highly conserved molecular mechanism. The sequence of events that results in inhibition begins with the serpin's RCL (labelled in red in Fig. 1M) entering the active site of the cognate protease, initially behaving as a substrate. The enzyme and serpin form a transient intermediate called the Michaelis complex (Ye *et al.*, 2001) which precedes the cleavage of the RCL at a specific position, termed the P1-P1' bond. This leads to the release of the P1 residue and the formation of an ester bond between the C-terminal portion of the serpin and the protease. At this stage, however, further hydrolysis, that would otherwise release cleaved serpin and active protease, is prevented by a profound conformational change in the serpin (Wright & Scarsdale, 1995). This transition from a 'stressed to relaxed' form occurs as the protease-attached remainder of the RCL inserts as a α-strand in the main β-sheet A of the serpin core. This insertion is highly energetically favourable and violently flips the enzyme from the upper to the lower pole of the serpin (Huntington *et al.*, 2000), causing steric denaturation and inactivation of the protease. Permanent destruction of the protease is subsequently achieved by third-party proteolysis of those domains of the target protease that have been rendered unstructured (Huntington *et al.*, 2000). Experimentally, the enzyme-serpin complex is relatively stable with a dissociation rate constant that is an order of magnitude slower than the association rate (Belorgey *et al.*, 2002). However, dissociation of the serpin-enzyme complex does occur, in which case the released neuroserpin is in the inactive, cleaved conformation. In contrast, when tPA is liberated from the complex, it may retain its proteolytic activity (Osterwalder *et al.*, 1998).

Clinical features and genotype-phenotype correlations

Mutations in the neuroserpin gene were first reported to cause an autosomal dominant form of pre-senile dementia (Davis *et al.*, 1999a; 1999b; Yerby *et al.*, 1986), described as familial encephalopathy with neuroserpin inclusion bodies (FENIB), characterized histologically by unique neuronal inclusion bodies and biochemically by polymers of the neuron-specific serpin, neuroserpin. These authors reported 2 unrelated Caucasian families living in the United States, carrying 2 different heterozygous mutations (S49P and S52R). In the larger family, affected individuals presented clinically around the fifth decade of life with cognitive decline, including deficits in attention and concentration, response regulation difficulties, and impaired visuospatial skills. Memory was also impaired, but to a lesser degree than is typically seen in individuals with Alzheimer's disease. After several years of disease progression, most affected individuals were unable to work and eventually required nursing-home care. The second, much smaller family showed an earlier clinical onset, during the second or third decade of life. Affected individuals presented with both epilepsy and progressive cognitive decline and their neurohistology was dominated by eosinophilic, PAS-positive intraneuronal inclusions in the brain. Later on, a small family with 2 affected siblings featuring progressive myoclonus epilepsy and dementia was described (Takao *et al.*, 2000). The affected individuals developed generalized seizures in adulthood and progressed to status epilepticus over several years. In addition, they also developed slow speech, diplopia, nystagmus, dysarthria, and myoclonus in the extremities, with rapidly progressive dementia. Their deceased mother was, reportedly, similarly affected.

Davis *et al.* (2002) reported additional patients with the disorder: a 23-year-old man with an 8-year history of progressive myoclonic epilepsy, dementia, tremor, and dysarthria. The second patient was a 13-year-old girl with progressive myoclonus epilepsy with intractable seizures, myoclonus, and dementia. She died at the age of 19 during status epilepticus. Her father was said to be 'mentally deficient', and a paternal uncle had died from epilepsy at the age of 18.

Gourfinkel-An *et al.* (2007) subsequently described a small French family with progressive myoclonic epilepsy associated with a frontal syndrome starting from the age of 18 with severe myoclonus, generalized tonic-clonic seizures, and absences. The EEG of one of the patients showed diffuse slow waves, spikes, and spike-wave discharges superimposed on a slow background, with photic sensitivity at around 1 Hz. Cerebral MRI revealed cortico-subcortical atrophy. The patient's condition progressively worsened and swallowing difficulties were noticed at an early stage. Additionally, cerebellar symptoms and pyramidal signs were also present. Cognitive deterioration was severe (Mini-Mental Status Examination score: 12/30). Signs of frontal dysfunction were observed (emotional lability, distractibility, and poor performance on sequential motor tests) with sparing of long-term explicit memory. In another affected relative, who died at the age of 33, symptoms were similar and were first noticed when she was 18. Behavioural problems, depression, and frontal dysfunction were noticed. Epilepsy was pharmaco-resistant. Status epilepticus took place twice during the course of the disorder. She became mute and bedridden and died of inhalation pneumonia at the age of 33. In these patients, a heterozygous S52R missense mutation at position 273 in exon 2 was detected, the same as in the two families from the United States.

A few non-familial cases have been also described. Coutelier *et al.* (2008) reported an 11-year-old girl who had had normal development until 8 years of age, when she developed a rapidly-progressive symptomatology, including aggressive behaviour, intellectual decline, psychic seizures, and subtle seizures with eyelid myoclonus. The EEG was suggestive of epilepsy with continuous spike-and-waves during slow-wave sleep. This patient was the first person identified with the G392R mutation in neuroserpin that resulted in severe juvenile phenotype and had accordingly appeared *de novo*. Hagen *et al.* (2011) more recently reported an additional sporadic patient with progressive myoclonus epilepsy and declining mental status starting in adulthood. Generalized seizures occurred early with myoclonus and progressive gait disturbances. Neuroimaging revealed mild atrophy and multiple periventricular white matter lesions, consistent with demyelination. The course was one of progressive decline with death occurring at the age of 34. Genetic analysis revealed a nucleotide substitution, resulting in a proline to leucine amino acid substitution (L47P).

The genotype-phenotype correlations are remarkably strong, with mutations causing increasingly severe clinical features in the following order: S49P, S52R, L47P, H338R, G392E and G392R (Table 1). In general, increasing clinical severity is characterized by earlier onset of the symptom and an increasing contribution from the epileptic component of the syndrome. More specifically, individuals with the S49P mutation have diffuse small intraneuronal inclusions of neuroserpin with an onset of dementia between the ages of 45 and 60 (Davis *et al.*, 1999a; Davis *et al.*, 1999b; Bradshaw *et al.*, 2001). People with the S52R, L47P and H338R variants have larger and more numerous intraneuronal inclusions associated with progressively earlier onset of symptoms, during early adulthood (S52R, L47P) and adolescence (H338R) (Hagen *et al.*, 2011; Miranda *et al.*, 2008). In the most severe cases, caused by the most polymerogenic mutations, namely G392R and G392E, the patients exhibit the earliest onset of symptoms, with profound intellectual decline during childhood associated with severe, uncontrolled epilepsy (Coutelier *et al.*, 2008). While FENIB is a rare disease, with only a few known kindreds worldwide, diagnosis should be considered in patients that present with a frontal-type dementia combined with epilepsy, particularly when eosinophilic inclusions are seen on brain biopsy or at post-mortem.

Table 1. There is a clear correlation between the degree of polymerisation seen in patients with neuroserpin variants and the severity of clinical features. Increasingly polymerogenic variants result in earlier onset and a higher incidence of epilepsy, in addition to dementia.

Mutation	Onset (years)	Clinical findings	Inclusions
S49P	45-63	Dementia and terminal seizures	+
S52R	20-40	Myoclonus, Dementia	++
L47P	20-30	Progressive myoclonus epilepsy	+++
H338R	15	Progressive myoclonus epilepsy	+++
G392E	13	Progressive myoclonus epilepsy, chorea	++++
G392R	8	Epilepsy with slow wave sleep	++++

The pathological polymerization of NS variants results in FENIB

These remarkable genotype-phenotype correlations that are evident in the clinic are mirrored by the biophysical and biochemical properties of the variant NS proteins. Under physiological conditions, the rate of aggregation of the least clinically-aggressive NS mutant, S49P, is more than 10 times higher than that of the wild type protein, whereas the association rate constant for tPA is essentially unchanged (Belorgey *et al.*, 2002). The next most severe mutation, S52R, results in a further tenfold increase in the polymerization rate and the loss of effective tPA inhibition (Belorgey *et al.*, 2004). Thereafter, the aggregation rate becomes so high as to be practically immeasurable. In the classic model of serpin polymerisation, proposed by Carrell and Lomas (2002), the functional changes in NS are all caused by the progressive destabilization of the key structural element, termed β-sheet A, which forms the core of NS (Fig. 1). This structural perturbation favours the incorporation of the RCL from a second NS molecule over the physiological process of intra-molecular RCL insertion that occurs during protease inhibition (Takao *et al.*, 2000). An initial loop-sheet polymerization event yields a NS dimer that retains a patent β-sheet A at one end and a destabilized RCL at the other. Such a dimer is competent to undergo further loop-sheet polymerization to form trimers and eventually higher-order polymers. Recently, Huntington and colleagues have proposed alternative mechanisms for polymerization that require a more significant domain swap between the serpins in a chain (Ekeowa *et al.*, 2010; Huntington & Whisstock, 2010; Belorgey *et al.*, 2011; Singh & Jairajpuri, 2011; Yamasaki *et al.*, 2011). In either case, the NS polymers gradually become entangled in the neuronal endoplasmic reticulum (ER) and form inclusions, known as Collins bodies. This phenomenon of aggregation or 'polymerization' has been described in other serpins such as α_1-antitrypsin where it results in hepatocyte inclusions and liver disease (Elliott *et al.*, 1996; Lomas *et al.*, 1992; Huntington *et al.*, 1999). The observation that FENIB was caused by NS mutations (S49P and H338R) that are structurally homologous to substitutions in α_1-antitrypsin, which also lead to polymerization (S53F and H334D, respectively) (Lomas *et al.*, 1993), argues strongly in favour of a shared molecular mechanism. This was confirmed by the finding that the neuronal inclusion bodies of FENIB were formed by polymers of NS with identical morphology to the polymers of mutant α_1-antitrypsin present in hepatocytes from a child with α_1-antitrypsin deficiency-related cirrhosis (Davis *et al.*, 1999a; Carrell & Lomas, 2002).

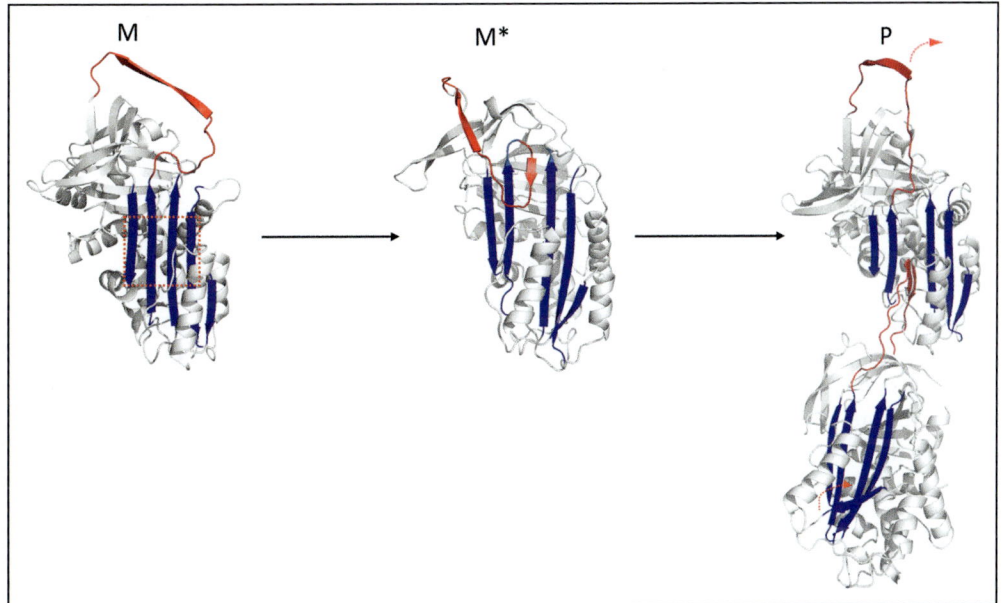

Fig. 1. *Molecular models of serpin conformers. M represents the active protease inhibitor with the reactive loop shown in red and β-sheet A in blue. Mutations that destabilize sheet A (typically in the so-called 'shutter region' signified by the red dashed box) allow the partial insertion of the reactive loop to form a new strand in sheet A (M*). The consequent opening of the sheet allows the reactive loop from another serpin to insert forming a serpin dimer (P). The repeated addition of serpins by loop-sheet polymerisation in this way results in large aggregates.*

Dissecting the pathological mechanisms of the dementing and epileptic components of FENIB

The ER-resident inclusions (Miranda *et al.*, 2004) in the neurones of individuals expressing NS variants are likely to represent the toxic gain-of-function that results in this dominantly-inherited neurodegenerative syndrome. Serpin polymerisation exerts a stress on the cell that differs in important ways from other proteinopathies. In most cases, misfolding of proteins in the ER results in activation of the unfolded protein response (UPR). However, the native-like structure of serpin polymers results in a distinct signalling pathway called the ER overload response (Davies *et al.*, 2009). This ER overload response activates NF-κB by a pathway that is dependent on raised cytoplasmic Ca^{2+} levels. ER-associated degradation or ERAD is involved in the degradation of mutant NS and may be able to degrade the polymers (Ying *et al.*, 2011), whereas autophagy is more important in the bulk turnover of both wild type and mutant NS (Kroeger *et al.*, 2009). In the presence of polymerogenic mutations in serpins, and with increasing age, these mechanisms are overwhelmed and retention of polymers in the ER leads to cell death. This is apparent in the fly model of FENIB where the accumulation of intracellular polymers is associated with locomotor deficits where there was a correlation between the severity of the behavioural deficits and the degree of polymer accumulation (Miranda *et al.*, 2008).

While the intraneuronal accumulation of NS inclusions may underpin the dementia seen in FENIB, there is evidence that other mechanisms may also contribute to the epileptic propensity of these patients. In particular, it is notable that epilepsy is rarely seen when normal levels of tPA inhibitory activity are present, as is the case for wild type and S49P NS. This has been recently highlighted in relation to stroke, where patients thrombolyzed with recombinant tPA present a higher level of seizures (Alvarez *et al.*, 2013). When tPA inhibition is lost (for example, for the S52R and 392 mutants) then epilepsy becomes the major clinical feature (Davis *et al.* 2002; Takao *et al.*, 2000). Notably, neuroserpin is able to dampen neuronal sensitivity to excitotoxic stimuli by regulating tPA activity (Yepes *et al.*, 2000; 2002; Wu *et al.*, 2010). This effect appears to be mediated by the tPA-mediated proteolytic cleavage of the NR1 subunit of the NMDA receptor that increases the functioning of this excitatory glutamate receptor (Fig. 2) (Nicole *et al.*, 2001; Fernandez-Monreal *et al.*, 2004; Samson *et al.*, 2008; Baron *et al.*, 2010).

Excess glutamatergic neurotransmission is also a potent cause of epilepsy (reviewed in Vincent & Mulle [2009]) and increased NMDA signalling in response to dysregulated tPA activity could contribute to FENIB. Indeed, co-injection of neuroserpin with kainate into the hippocampus of the mouse attenuated the spread of consequent epileptic activity when compared to co-injection of kainate with vehicle alone (Yepes *et al.*, 2002). These data suggest a role for tPA in seizure spread in epilepsy and support the use of NS or others tPA inhibitors as a potential therapy.

Conclusion

Familial encephalopathy with neuroserpin inclusion bodies is a recently described neurodegenerative disease that is responsible for progressive myoclonic epilepsy and/or pre-senile dementia. Serpinopathies are unique among conformational diseases because they form native-like aggregates or polymers in the ER of synthetic cells. Serpin variants accumulate as inclusion bodies and thus activate the ER-overload response. It appears that this gain-of-function toxicity is responsible for the neuronal dysfunction and death that underpins dementia in FENIB.

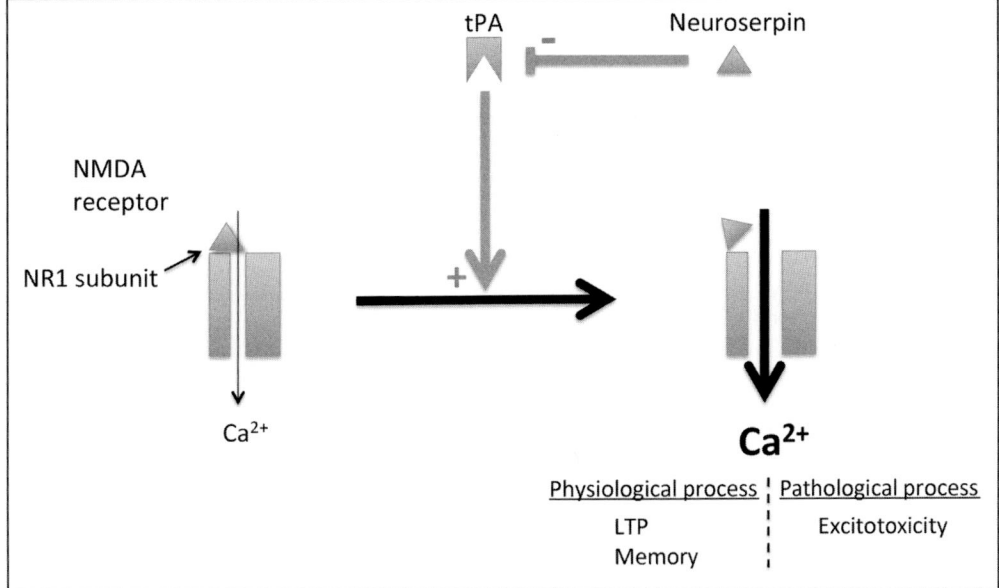

Fig. 2. The NMDA receptor mediates the influx of calcium into neurones in the presence of glutamate. tPA has been shown to cleave the NR1 subunit (triangle) of the receptor and, as a consequence, increases the concentration of intracellular calcium. By inhibiting tPA, neuroserpin is thought to protect neurons from the toxic consequences of excessive NMDA activity, termed 'excitotoxicity'.

The evidence is less clear as to whether similar gain-of-toxicity is the cause of the epilepsy in FENIB or whether this results from dysfunction of the NS/tPA system. The relative importance of these two mechanisms has yet to be clearly elucidated. To date, genetic analysis of the *SERPINI1* gene should be performed in patients with adult-onset PME and early-onset, rapidly progressive cognitive dysfunction or predominantly frontal dementia.

Conflicts of interest: none.

References

Alvarez, V., Rossetti, A.O., Papavasileiou, V. & Michel, P. (2013): Acute seizures in acute ischemic stroke: does thrombolysis have a role to play? *J. Neurol.* **260,** 55–61.

Baron, A., Montagne, A., Cassé, F., et al. (2010): NR2D-containing NMDA receptors mediate tissue plasminogen activator-promoted neuronal excitotoxicity. *Cell Death Differ.* **17,** 860–871.

Belorgey, D., Crowther, D.C., Mahadeva, R. & Lomas, D.A. (2002): Mutant, Neuroserpin (S49P) that causes familial encephalopathy with neuroserpin inclusion bodies is a poor proteinase inhibitor and readily forms polymers in vitro. *J. Biol. Chem.* **277,** 17367–17373.

Belorgey, D., Sharp, L.K., Crowther, D.C., Onda, M., Johansson, J. & Lomas, D.A. (2004): Neuroserpin, Portland (Ser52Arg) is trapped as an inactive intermediate that rapidly forms polymers: implications for the epilepsy seen in the dementia FENIB. *Eur. J. Biochem.* **271,** 3360–3367.

Belorgey, D, Irving, J.A., Ekeowa, U.I., et al. (2011): Characterisation of serpin polymers in vitro and in vivo. *Methods* **53,** 255–266.

Bradshaw, C.B., Davis, R.L., Shrimpton, A.E., et al. (2001): Cognitive deficits associated with a recently reported familial neurodegenerative disease: familial encephalopathy with neuroserpin inclusion bodies. *Arch. Neurol.* **58,** 1429–1434.

Carrell, R.W. & Lomas, D.A. (2002): Alpha1-antitrypsin deficiency-a model for conformational diseases. *N. Engl. J. Med.* **346**, 45–53.

Cole, J.W., Naj A.C., O'Connell, J.R., et al. (2007): Neuroserpin polymorphisms and stroke risk in a biracial population: the stroke prevention in young women study. *BMC Neurol.* **7**, 37.

Coutelier, M., Andries, S., Ghariani, S., et al. (2008): Neuroserpin mutation causes electrical status epilepticus of slow-wave sleep. *Neurology* **71**, 64–66.

Davis, R.L., Shrimpton, A.E., Holohan, P.D., et al. (1999a): Familial dementia caused by polymerization of mutant neuroserpin. *Nature* **401**, 376–379.

Davis, R.L., Holohan, P.D., Shrimpton, A.E., et al. (1999b): Familial encephalopathy with neuroserpin inclusion bodies. *Am. J. Pathol.* **155**, 1901–1913.

Davis, R.L., Shrimpton, A.E., Carrell, R.W., et al. (2002): Association between conformational mutations in neuroserpin and onset and severity of dementia. *Lancet* **359**, 2242–2247.

Davies, M.J., Miranda, E., Roussel, B.D., Kaufman, R.J., Marciniak, S.J., & Lomas D.A. (2009): Neuroserpin polymers activate NF-kappaB by a calcium signaling pathway that is independent of the unfolded protein response. *J. Biol. Chem.* **284**, 18202–18209.

Ekeowa, U.I., Freeke, J., Miranda, E., et al. (2010): Defining the mechanism of polymerization in serpinopathies. *Proc. Natl. Acad. Sci. USA* **107**, 17146–17151.

Elliott, P.R., Lomas, D.A., Carrell, R.W. & Abrahams, J-P. (1996): Inhibitory conformation of the reactive loop of α_1-antitrypsin. *Nature Struc. Biol.* **3**, 676–681.

Fernandez-Monreal, M., López-Atalaya, J.P., Benchenane, K., et al. (2004): Arginine 260 of the amino-terminal domain of NR1 subunit is critical for tissue-type plasminogen activator-mediated enhancement of N-methyl-D-aspartate receptor signaling. *J. Biol. Chem.* **279**, 50850–50856.

Gourfinkel-An, I., Duyckaerts, C., Camuzat, A., et al. (2007): Clinical and neuropathologic study of a French family with a mutation in the neuroserpin gene. *Neurology* **69**, 79–83.

Hagen, M.C., Murrell, J.R., Delisle, M.B., et al. (2011): Encephalopathy with neuroserpin inclusion bodies presenting as progressive myoclonus epilepsy and associated with a novel mutation in the proteinase inhibitor 12 Gene. *Brain Pathol.* **1**, 575–582.

Hastings, G.A., Coleman, T.A., Haudenschild, C.C., et al. (1997): Neuroserpin, a brain-associated inhibitor of tissue plasminogen activator is localized primarily in neurons. Implications for the regulation of motor learning and neuronal survival. *J. Biol. Chem.* **272**, 33062–33067.

Huntington, J.A. & Whisstock, J.C. (2010): Molecular contortionism- on the physical limits of serpin 'loop-sheet' polymers. *Biol. Chem.* **391**, 973–982.

Huntington, J.A., Pannu, N.S., Hazes, B., Read, R.J., Lomas, D.A. & Carrell, R.W. (1999): A 26Å structure of a serpin polymer and implications for conformational disease. *J. Mol. Biol.* **293**, 449–455.

Huntington, J.A., Read, R.J. & Carrell, R.W. (2000): Structure of a serpin-protease complex shows inhibition by deformation. *Nature* **407**, 923–926.

Kroeger, H., Miranda, E., MacLeod, I., et al. (2009): Endoplasmic reticulum-associated degradation (ERAD) and autophagy cooperate to degrade polymerogenic mutant serpins. *J. Biol. Chem.* **284**, 22793–22802.

Krueger, S.R., Ghisu, G.P., Cinelli, P., et al. (1997): Expression of neuroserpin, an inhibitor of tissue plasminogen activator, in the developing and adult nervous system of the mouse. *J. Neurosci.* **17**, 8984–8996.

Lomas, D.A., Evans, D.L., Finch, J.T. & Carrell, R.W. (1992): The mechanism of Z α_1-antitrypsin accumulation in the liver. *Nature* **357**, 605–607.

Lomas, D.A., Finch, J.T., Seyama, K., Nukiwa, T. & Carrell, R.W. (1993): α_1-antitrypsin, S_{iiyama} (Ser^{53}øPhe); further evidence for intracellular loop-sheet polymerisation. *J. Biol. Chem.* **268**, 15333–15335.

Miranda, E., Romisch, K. & Lomas, D.A. (2004): Mutants of neuroserpin that cause dementia accumulate as polymers within the endoplasmic reticulum. *J. Biol. Chem.* **279**, 28283–28291.

Miranda, E., MacLeod, I., Davies, M.J., et al. (2008): The intracellular accumulation of polymeric neuroserpin explains the severity of the dementia FENIB. *Hum. Mol. Genet.* **17**, 1527–1539.

Nicole, O., Docagne, F., Ali C., et al. (2001): The proteolytic activity of tissue-plasminogen activator enhances NMDA receptor-mediated signaling. *Nat. Med.* **7**, 59–64.

Osterwalder, T., Contartese, J., Stoeckli, E.T., Kuhn, T.B. & Sonderegger, P. (1996): Neuroserpin, an axonally secreted serine protease inhibitor. *EMBO J.* **15**, 2944–2953.

Osterwalder, T., Cinelli, P., Baici, A., et al. (1998): The axonally secreted serine proteinase inhibitor, neuroserpin, inhibits plasminogen activators and plasmin but not thrombin. *J. Biol. Chem.* **273**, 2312–2321.

Qian, Z., Gilbert, M.E., Colicos, M.A., Kandel, E.R. & Kuhl, D. (1993): Tissue-plasminogen activator is induced as an immediate-early gene during seizure, kindling and long-term potentiation. *Nature* **361,** 453–457.

Ryu, S.-E., Choi, H.-J., Kwon, K.-S., Lee, K.N. & Yu, M.-H. (1996): The native strains in the hydrophobic core and flexible reactive loop of a serine protease inhibitor: crystal structure of an uncleaved a_1-antitrypsin at 2.7 Å. *Structure* **4,** 1181–1192.

Samson, A.L., Nevin, S.T., Croucher, D., *et al.* (2008): Tissue-type plasminogen activator requires a co-receptor to enhance NMDA receptor function. *J. Neurochem.* **107,** 1091–1101.

Seeds, N.W., Basham, M.E. & Haffke, S.P. (1999): Neuronal migration is retarded in mice lacking the tissue plasminogen activator gene. *Proc. Natl. Acad. Sci. USA* **96,** 14118–14123.

Singh, P. & Jairajpuri, M.A. (2011): Strand 6B deformation and residues exposure towards N-terminal end of helix B during proteinase inhibition by serpins. *Bioinformation* **5,** 315–319.

Stoeckli, E.T., Lemkin, P.F., Kuhn, T.B., Ruegg, M.A., Heller, M. & Sonderegger, P. (1989): Identification of proteins secreted from axons of embryonic dorsal-root-ganglia neurons. *Eur. J. Biochem.* **180,** 249–258.

Takao, M., Benson, M.D., Murrell, J.R., *et al.* (2000): Neuroserpin mutation S52R causes neuroserpin accumulation in neurons and is associated with progressive myoclonus epilepsy. *J. Neuropathol. Exp. Neurol.* **59,** 1070–1086.

Vincent, P. & Mulle, C. (2009): Kainate receptors in epilepsy and excitotoxicity. *Neuroscience* **158,** 309–323.

Wright, H.T. & Scarsdale, J.N. (1995): Structural basis for serpin inhibitor activity. *Proteins* **22,** 210-225.

Wu, J., Echeverry, R., Guzman, J. & Yepes, M. (2010): Neuroserpin protects neurons from ischemia-induced plasmin-mediated cell death independently of tissue-type plasminogen activator inhibition. *Am. J. Pathol.* **177,** 2576–2584.

Yamasaki, M., Sendall, T.J., Pearce, M.C., Whisstock, J.C. & Huntington, J.A. (2011): Molecular basis of alpha1-antitrypsin deficiency revealed by the structure of a domain-swapped trimer. *EMBO Reports* **12,** 1011–1017.

Ye, S., Cech, A.L., Belmares, R., *et al.* (2001): The structure of a Michaelis serpin-protease complex. *Nat. Struct. Biol.* **8,** 979–983.

Yepes, M., Sandkvist, M., Wong, M.K., *et al.* (2000): Neuroserpin reduces cerebral infarct volume and protects neurons from ischemia-induced apoptosis. *Blood* **96,** 569–576.

Yepes, M., Sandkvist, M., Coleman, T.A., *et al.* (2002): Regulation of seizure spreading by neuroserpin and tissue-type plasminogen activator is plasminogen-independent. *J. Clin. Invest.* **109,** 1571–1578.

Yerbi, M.S., Shaw, C.-M. & Watson, J.M.D. (1986): Progressive dementia and epilepsy in a young adult: unusual intraneuronal inclusions. *Neurology* **36,** 68–71.

Ying, Z., Wang, H., Fan, H. & Wang, G. (2011): The endoplasmic reticulum (ER)-associated degradation system regulates aggregation and degradation of mutant neuroserpin. *J. Biol. Chem.* **286,** 20835–20844.

Chapter 10

GOSR2: a progressive myoclonus epilepsy gene

Leanne M. Dibbens[1] and Guido Rubboli[2,3]

[1] *Epilepsy Research Group, School of Pharmacy and Medical Sciences, University of South Australia, and Sansom Institute for Health Research, University of South Australia, Adelaide 5000, South Australia, Australia*
[2] *Danish Epilepsy Center, Filadelfia/University of Copenhagen, Dianalund, Denmark*
[3] *IRCCS, Institute of Neurological Sciences, Bellaria Hospital, Bologna, Italy*
leanne.dibbens@unisa.edu.au
guru@filadelfia.dk

Summary

GOSR2-associated PME is associated with a homozygous mutation in *GOSR2* (c.430G>T, p.Gly144Trp), a Golgi vesicle transport gene. The functional effect of this mutation is a loss of function that results in failure of the GOSR2 protein to localize to the cis-Golgi. The main clinical features of the GOSR2-associated PME are early-onset ataxia, areflexia, action myoclonus and seizures, scoliosis, elevated creatine kinase levels, relative preservation of cognitive function until the late stages of the disease, and relentless disease course. Severe photosensitive myoclonus is a common feature. GOSR2-associated PME is a rare disease with very few cases reported so far and it can be expected that the identification of further patients will contribute to expanding the phenotype and genotype of this condition.

Introduction

In 2011, Corbett *et al.* reported 6 patients with a progressive myoclonus epilepsy (PME) phenotype whose main cardinal features were onset of ataxia in the first years of life, appearance of action myoclonus and seizures later in childhood, and loss of independent ambulation in the second decade. Cognition was not typically affected, although mild memory difficulties occurred for some in the third decade. This condition was found to be associated with a homozygous mutation in *GOSR2* (c.430G>T, p.Gly144Trp), a Golgi vesicle transport gene. This p.Gly144Trp mutation gives rise to a loss of function and results in failure of the GOSR2 protein to localize to the cis-Golgi. Following this, the clinical and neurophysiological characteristics of PME associated with *GOSR2* mutation were further detailed in 12 patients (including the original 6 patients described by Corbett *et al.* [2011]); all patients had the same homozygous mutation (c.430G4T, Gly144Trp) (Boissé Lomax *et al.*, 2013). Interestingly, the birthplaces of all these patients (including the birthplaces of the ancestors of 1 Australian patient) clustered around the North Sea (hence the eponym for this type of PME of 'North Sea progressive myoclonus epilepsy' by Boissé Lomax *et al.* [2013]). This geographic distribution suggests that the identified *GOSR2* mutation may have spread along the North Sea at the time of the Viking conquests in the VIIIth century.

Gene identification

The *GOSR2* gene was identified as a causative gene for PME through the genetic and molecular analyses of a family with one affected child. The proband was an Australian female, born to second-cousin parents of British origin. She, her unaffected brother, and her parents were genotyped using Affymetrix 250K Nsp SNP chips for genome-wide linkage mapping. Homozygosity mapping was performed and a single suggestive linkage region on chromosome 17 was identified, with a maximum possible LOD score of 1.93. Sequence capture followed by next-generation sequencing was carried out and a homozygous variant in *GOSR2* (MIM: 604027), c.430G>T, p.Gly144Trp, (NM_004287.3), was identified as the possible causative mutation. Based on a sequence analysis of a cohort of 73 unrelated individuals with molecularly unsolved PME, 5 additional individuals (from 4 families) were identified who were homozygous for the same *GOSR2* variant, c.430G>T, p.Gly144Trp (Corbett *et al.*, 2011). No consanguinity was reported in any of the families. The c.430G>T *GOSR2* variant was not found in 584 chromosomes from unaffected individuals or in dbSNP132, leading to confirmation that this was the causative mutation. Of the 4 additional families, 1 was of German ancestry and 3 were Dutch. Further analysis of 1 affected individual from each family with both microsatellite markers and Illumina 610 quad SNP chips revealed a founder mutation that was most likely to be of European ancestry (Corbett *et al.*, 2011).

GOSR2 is a member of the Qb-SNARE family of vesicle docking proteins. There are 3 known alternatively spliced isoforms of GOSR2 and all are predicted to be affected by the c.430G>T, p.Gly144Trp mutation. The mutated glycine 144 residue (G144) is within the Qb-SNARE domain of the GOSR2 protein and shows high evolutionary conservation from mammals to yeast. Initial investigations into the pathogenic mechanisms due to the mutation have shown that the GOSR2 p.Gly144Trp mutant protein fails to localize to the cis-Golgi (Corbett *et al.*, 2011).

Clinical features associated with *GOSR2* mutation

The distinct clinical features of PME associated with *GOSR2* mutations are early-onset ataxia (at around 2 years of age), onset of action myoclonus and seizures at around 6 years of age, and scoliosis in adolescence and the absence of cognitive deterioration during evolution, although mild cognitive decline may be observed in the later stages. The clinical history of *Case 1* in the original report by Corbett *et al.* (2011) is paradigmatic in terms of illustrating the characteristics and course of the disease. This patient began to have difficulty walking and was found to be areflexic at the age of 2, but development was otherwise normal. At the age of 7, she had a tremor, and it became clear that action myoclonus and occasional absence seizures were present. At the age of 13, she began having drop attacks as well as major convulsive seizures. The patient required a wheelchair from the age of 14 due to falling attacks and was unable to walk unaided from the age of 16. Notably, the patient had severe scoliosis which required surgical correction. By the age of 22, the patient was confined to bed and she died aged 32 as the result of complications associated with uncontrolled myoclonus. The patient's intellect was preserved until the latter few years of her life, when there was mild cognitive impairment. Autopsy showed mild cerebral atrophy and a lack of gross structural abnormalities. Histological examination revealed subtle, Alzheimer type II gliosis in the basal ganglia region (consistent with metabolic derangement related to her agonal state) and minor loss of Purkinje cells and gliosis in the cerebellar vermis.

The clinical features and evolution of PME caused by mutation of *GOSR2* were detailed in the study by Boissé Lomax *et al.* (2013) who described the original 6 patients with the homozygous *GOSR2* c.430G>T, Gly144Trp mutation (Corbett *et al.*, 2011), as well as 6 new patients (from 11 families) who were molecularly identified with the same mutation. The clinical presentation in the 12 patients was remarkably similar, with features of early-onset ataxia (on average at 2 years of age), followed by myoclonic seizures at the average age of 6.5 years. During the course of the disease, all patients exhibited multiple seizure types, including generalized tonic-clonic seizures, absence seizures, and drop attacks. The patients also uniformly displayed highly photosensitive generalized myoclonus that worsened with action or emotional stress, but was minimal at rest and almost completely absent during relaxation. In some patients, myoclonus and drop attacks were made worse by fever. One patient presented with periods of 'status myoclonicus', characterized by continuous myoclonus lasting for hours up to a day at a time. All patients developed scoliosis by the time they reached adolescence, making this an important diagnostic feature. Additional skeletal deformities were present, including *pes cavus* in 4 patients and syndactyly in 2 patients. Notably, cognition was preserved in the context of severe motor disability until the later stages of the disease. The progression of the disease showed a relentless decline; patients became wheelchair-bound (at a mean age of 13 years) and 4 died during their third or fourth decade of life.

An additional patient with PME caused by mutation in *GOSR2* has been reported by Praschberger *et al.* (2015). This patient was a 61-year-old female presenting with a PME phenotype and was found to be compound heterozygous for two *GOSR2* mutations; the known c.430G>T, Gly144Trp mutation and a novel c.491_493delAGA (p.Lys164del) mutation. She presented with mild ataxia at the age of 2 years, as well as transient episodes of motor deterioration triggered by infection and fever. At the age of 14 years, she started to suffer from action myoclonus and seizures. In her thirties, she was wheelchair-bound. Scoliosis and areflexia were also noted. No cognitive deterioration was observed throughout the course of the disease, although mild cognitive decline was detected after repeated neuropsychological testing. The most relevant distinctive clinical feature of this patient was the milder course of the disease, at variance with the previously reported patients with PME associated with the homozygous *GOSR2* Gly144Trp mutation.

Finally, van Egmond *et al.* (2014) reported the same homozygous c.430G>T, p.Gly144Trp *GOSR2* mutation in 5 Dutch patients with progressive myoclonus ataxia (PMA) (also known as Ramsay Hunt syndrome). These patients showed clinical features that were very similar to those previously described for *GOSR2* mutation-positive PME patients. However, differences include the fact that in the 5 patients with PMA, cognitive function was not seen to decline (however, only 1 patient was in his third decade while the others were younger) and scoliosis was observed in only 3 of the 5 subjects.

Neurophysiological investigations

EEG analysis of *GOSR2* mutation-positive PME patients reveals generalized spike-and-slow-wave discharges with a posterior predominance, often with a slow background. The generalized discharges are highly photosensitive. Focal or multifocal discharges can also be observed (Boissé Lomax *et al.*, 2013) (Fig. 1). Nerve conduction studies have been reported to be consistent with a mild, predominantly axonal peripheral neuropathy, while electromyography was normal in all patients with the exception of 1 in the series reported by Boissé Lomax et al. (2013). Signs of sensory neuronopathy, anterior horn cell involvement, or both, were detected in all patients with absent reflexes reported by van Egmond et al. (2014).

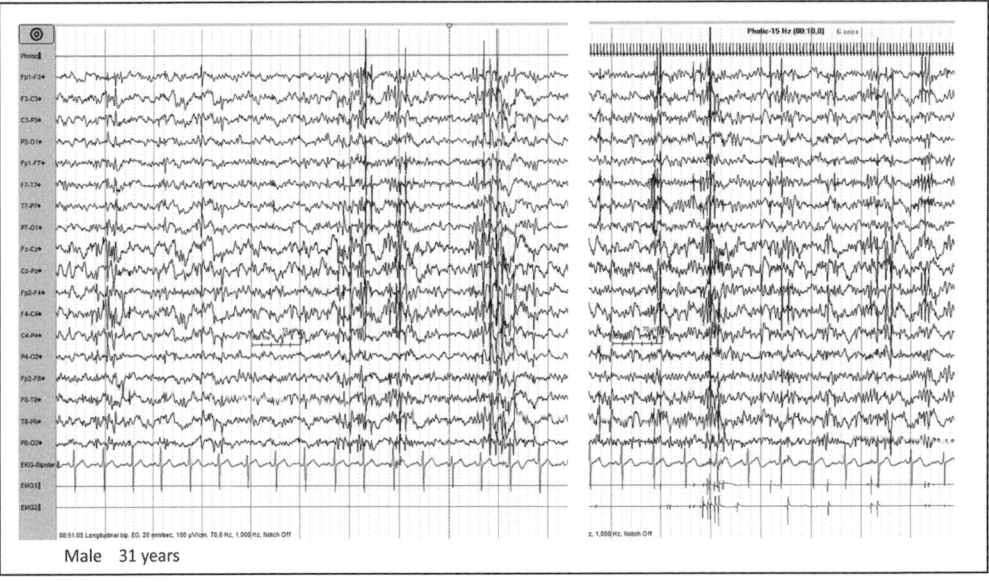

Fig. 1. Polygraphic recording in a 31-year-old male with GOSR2-associated PME. Left panel: the patient is at rest. The tracing shows slowing of background activity, bursts of generalized spike-and-wave discharges, and multifocal spikes in both hemispheres. Myoclonic potentials are not evident at the EMG leads. Right panel: photic stimulation at 15 Hz elicits generalized polyspikes and spike-and-wave discharges, often associated with myoclonic potentials at both EMG leads. EMG1: right deltoid; EMG2: left deltoid.

Multimodal evoked potentials were shown to be unremarkable (Boissé Lomax et al., 2013).

Brain magnetic resonance imaging studies have displayed essentially normal findings or generalized cerebral and cerebellar atrophy (Boissé Lomax et al., 2013; Prachschberger et al., 2015). Elevation of serum creatine kinase levels (median: 734 IU), in the context of normal muscle biopsies, was reported for all patients in the study of Boissé Lomax et al. (2013), but was not a uniform feature in the series described by van Egmond et al. (2014).

Conclusions

GOSR2-associated PME has a relatively homogeneous clinical presentation, characterized by a pattern of early-onset ataxia, areflexia, action myoclonus and seizures, scoliosis, elevated creatine kinase levels, relative preservation of cognitive function until the late stages of the disease, and relentless disease course. Thus far, the same homozygous c.430G>T (p.Gly144Trp) mutation has been detected in all reported patients with GOSR2-mediated PME, with the exception of 1 patient with a milder disease course who was heterozygous for the known c.430G>T (p.Gly144Trp) mutation and a novel c.491_493delAGA (p.Lys164del) *GOSR2* mutation. The identification of additional patients will contribute to further expanding the phenotype and genotype and will add to our knowledge of GOSR2-related disease.

Conflicts of interest: none.

References

Boissé Lomax, L., Bayly, M.A., Hjalgrim, H., *et al.* (2013): 'North Sea' progressive myoclonus epilepsy: phenotype of subjects with *GOSR2* mutation. *Brain* **136,** 1146–1154.

Corbett, M.A., Schwake, M., Bahlo, M., *et al.* (2011): A mutation in the Golgi Qb-SNARE gene *GOSR2* causes progressive myoclonus epilepsy with early ataxia. *Am. J. Hum. Genet.* **88,** 657–663.

Praschberger, R., Balint, B., Mencacci, N.E., *et al.* (2015): Expanding the phenotype and genetic defects associated with the *GOSR2* gene. *Mov. Disord. Clin. Pract.* Published online Wiley InterScience, DOI: 10.1002/mdc3.12190.

van Egmond, M.E., Verschuuren-Bemelmans, C.C., Nibbeling, E.A., *et al.* (2014): Hunt syndrome: clinical characterization of progressive myoclonus ataxia caused by *GOSR2* mutation. *Mov. Disord.* **29,** 139–143.

Chapter 11

KCTD7-related progressive myoclonic epilepsy

Patrick Van Bogaert

Department of Paediatric Neurology, CHU d'Angers and Laboratoire Angevin de Recherche et d'Ingénierie des Systèmes (LARIS), University of Angers, France
patrick.vanbogaert@chu-angers.fr

Summary

Progressive myoclonic epilepsy associated with *KCTD7* mutations has been reported in 19 patients from 12 families. Patients show homozygous mutations in the coding regions of the *KCTD7* gene. The disease starts in infancy. Patients typically show an initial severe epileptic disorder, with abundant epileptiform discharges on EEG and myoclonic seizures in the foreground, associated with cognitive regression and ataxia. Continuous multifocal myoclonus aggravated by action is observed in more than half of the cases. After a few years, the disease tends to stabilize and long peiod of survival can be expected. Some patients remain able to walk independently. The severity of the disease is variable from one patient to another, even within the same family. It is hypothesized that the epileptic disorder may influence the neurological regression observed in patients.

Introduction

In 2007, Van Bogaert *et al.* reported 3 siblings from a consanguineous family with a clinical picture of progressive myoclonic epilepsy (PME) which was associated with a homozygous mutation of the gene encoding potassium channel tetramerization domain-containing protein 7 (*KCTD7*) (Van Bogaert *et al.*, 2007). Since this original family, 16 other patients from 11 new families have been reported (Blumkin *et al.*, 2012; Krabichler *et al.*, 2012; Staropoli *et al.*, 2012; Kousi *et al.*, 2012; Farhan *et al.*, 2014). The disease is inherited as an autosomal recessive trait and its incidence is unknown. In a study in which *KCTD7* was screened in a cohort of more than 100 unconfirmed PME patients after exclusion of neuronal ceroid lipofuscinosis (NCL), 5 positive families were identified, suggesting that *KCTD7* is not an exceptional cause of PME (Kousi *et al.*, 2012). In a pilot study evaluating a panel of 265 genes, including *KCTD7*, in 33 index patients with various epileptic syndromes randomly selected in Germany and Switzerland, 1 patient was shown to have a homozygous mutation for *KCTD7* (Lemke *et al.*, 2012). The present chapter focuses on the clinical characteristics of *KCTD7*-related PME from the 19 published cases reported so far and discusses the pathophysiology and genotype/phenotype correlation of the disease.

Clinical characteristics

The 12 families reported so far (Van Bogaert *et al.*, 2007; Blumkin *et al.*, 2012; Krabichler *et al.*, 2012; Staropoli *et al.*, 2012; Kousi *et al.*, 2012; Farhan *et al.*, 2014) had variable ethnic origin and showed a high rate of consanguinity (5/12). Epileptic seizures were the first signs in all cases. Onset ranged between 5 months and 3 years, after a period of psychomotor development that was described as either normal or slightly delayed. Independent walking was usually acquired. However, 1 reported patient with onset in the second year of life never walked (Kousi *et al.*, 2012). The first seizures were described as either myoclonic or generalized tonic-clonic seizures, and were precipitated by fever in some cases. Myoclonic seizures were reported in the course of the disease in all but 1 patient. In 11 patients, continuous multifocal myoclonus, aggravated by action and posture, was reported either at presentation or during the course of the disease. In 1 patient, myoclonus was associated with opsoclonus, which prompted the authors to consider a diagnosis of opsoclonus-myoclonus syndrome (Blumkin *et al.*, 2012). Other types of seizures (atonic seizures and atypical absences) were also reported. Epilepsy responded poorly to antiepileptic drugs in 2 thirds of patients, the most effective drugs being levetiracetam, valproate and clobazam. All patients had cognitive decline leading to severe dementia. Progressive ataxia was reported in all but 1 patient, and two thirds of them became wheelchair-bound. Pyramidal signs were described in 8 patients and microcephaly in 6 patients.

Concerning complementary examinations, electroencephalograms (EEG) were described to be abnormal, except for those very early during the course of the disease. The most common findings were very frequent multifocal and/or generalized spike-waves associated with an excess of slow activity. In many patients, EEG abnormalities were more prominent in the posterior areas, and intermittent light stimulation evoked generalized or posterior epileptiform discharges. In some patients, the EEG was reported as either hypsarrhythmic or showing continuous spike waves during slow-wave sleep. Action myoclonus was not associated with concomitant epileptiform discharges. One patient had negative focal myoclonus. Fig. 1 illustrates EEG findings from 2 affected siblings from the first family (Van Bogaert *et al.*, 2007).

Cerebral magnetic resonance imaging was either normal or showed non-specific findings (atrophy or posterior white matter hyperintensities). Metabolic work-up of blood and cerebrospinal fluid was not suggestive of mitochondrial dysfunction. Fundoscopy was normal in most patients.

The search for storage material was performed by skin biopsy in 9 patients from 8 different families and was normal except for 1 patient who was reported to have electron-dense storage material in fibroblasts and a lymphoblastoid cell line based on electron microscopy (Staropoli *et al.*, 2012). This finding is noteworthy as it was the only finding of storage material in a patient mutated for *KCTD7*, which prompted the authors to designate *KCTD7* mutations as the cause of a new subtype of NCL that was called 'NCL type 14'. It should be noted that the screening for *KCTD7* mutation performed in a cohort of 22 NCL patients with storage material demonstrated by electron microscopy analysis was negative, suggesting that *KCTD7* is not a common cause of NCL after exclusion of the already known NCL genes (Kousi *et al.*, 2012). Moreover, the patient reported by Starapoli *et al.* (2012), as well as his affected brother, had a very atypical clinical course that differed from other KCTD7 patients. First, these 2 patients were the only reported cases with severe ocular involvement, *i.e.* optic atrophy leading to visual loss. Second, constant clinical deterioration was observed in these 2 patients who died in their mid-teens. This contrasted with the other reported KCTD7 patients who showed clinical stabilization after a period of early regression, most of whom were still alive at the last assessment.

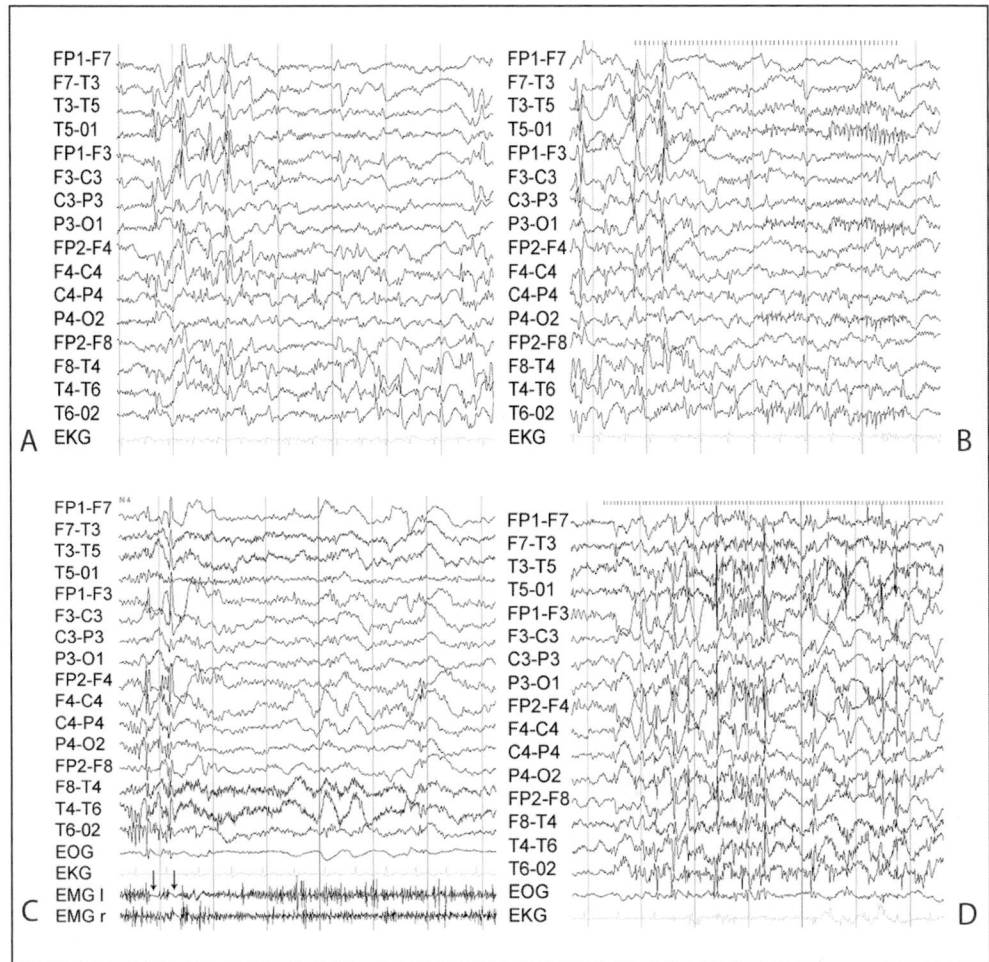

Fig. 1. The EEG of Patients 1 and 2 from the original report by Van Bogaert et al. (2007). (A) EEG of Patient 1 at the age of 5 years, awake and at rest, showing slow dysrythmia and multifocal high-amplitude epileptiform discharges. (B) Intermittent light stimulation (ILS) at 12 Hz inducing occipital spikes in addition to the spike-wave complexes still present at rest. (C) EEG of Patient 2 at the age of 14 years, awake with arms maintained in flexion and forearms in extension. On EMG, performed with surface electrodes placed over the left (l) and right (r) deltoid muscles, two negative myocloni appear as flattening of the EMG discharge (arrows), the first one on the left side and the second on both sides. Myoclonus was preceded by right-sided spike-wave discharges, followed by generalized spike-wave discharges. (D) ILS, at 15 Hz, induced generalized spike-waves, together with clinical bilateral myoclonus; these discharges were followed by rhythmic occipital spikes diffusing into a secondary generalized tonic-clonic seizure.

To our knowledge, the oldest patient (Patient 2 from the original report [Van Bogaert et al., 2007]) is now aged 25 years and is still able to walk independently.

Differential diagnosis

The typical presentation follows a 3-stage evolution that is quite unique among PME: (1) a period of normal development; (2) a period of mental and motor regression with epileptic myoclonic seizures that starts at around 1-2 years of age; and (3) a period of stabilization after a few years. Rare cases with optic atrophy and storage material on skin biopsy may complicate differential diagnosis with the classic late-infantile form of NCL. Clues to resolve this differential diagnosis are summarized in Table 1. The rare presence of associated opsoclonus can evoke opsoclonus-myoclonus syndrome. Finally, in rare patients, ataxia or myoclonus may not be present, which raises the issue of whether such patients have an epileptic syndrome other than PME.

Table 1. Differential diagnosis between *KCTD7*-related PME and late-infantile NCL

	KCTD7-related PME	Late-infantile NCL
Gene defect	KCTD7	*CLN2* gene (*TPP1*)
Age at onset	0.5-3 years	2-3 years
Epileptic seizures	+++ (myoclonic, GTCS, atypical absences)	+++ (myoclonic, GTCS, atypical absences)
Action myoclonus	++	++
Progressive ataxia	+++	+++
Cognitive regression	+++	+++
Optic atrophy	- (*)	+++
Retinitis	-	+++
Atrophy on MRI	+	++
Photosensitivity on EEG	++	+++ (low frequency)
Storage material on EM	- (*)	+++ (curvilinear bodies)
Course	Stabilization (*)	Bedridden at 5-7 years

+++seen in nearly all patients; ++ seen in > 50%; + seen in < 50%; - absent; TPP1: tripeptidyl peptidase 1; GTCS: generalized tonic-clonic seizures; EM: electron microscopy; *except in the family reported by Starapoli *et al.* (2012).

Physiopathology

All 11 different mutations identified so far are within the coding region of *KCTD7*, which is a member of the *KCTD* gene family. This family of proteins shares an N-terminal BTB/POZ domain that demonstrates sequence homology to the T1 domain in voltage-gated potassium channels that allows its tetramerization (Stogios *et al.*, 2005). The KCTD7 protein is extremely conserved across species and, in mice, is expressed in the olfactory bulbs, the CA1 and CA3 hippocampal cells, and the Purkinje cells of the cerebellum (Azizieh *et al.*, 2011). KCTD7 overexpression in transfected primary cultures of murine neurons resulted in hyperpolarization of the resting membrane potential, and decreased their excitability in patch clamp experiments (Azizieh *et al.*, 2011). This is consistent with an epileptogenic effect of a KCTD7 defect. KCTD7 is much smaller than a typical potassium channel subunit, and its computed hydrophobicity profile does not indicate a transmembrane segment. It is hence extremely unlikely that KCTD7 would function as a transmembrane channel for potassium. The demonstration of a direct molecular interaction between KCTD7 and Cullin 3 suggests that the effect on the plasma membrane resting potential is likely to be mediated by Cullin 3 (Azizieh *et al.*, 2011). Although additional experiments are required to understand how the KCTD7 defect causes PME, this may already explain the lack of genotype/phenotype correlation observed in affected patients. Indeed, mutations within the functional BTB/POZ domain (5/11 reported mutations) did not result in a more severe phenotype.

An interesting finding is that the severity of the disease may be highly variable among affected members within the same family (Van Bogaert *et al.*, 2007; Farhan *et al.*, 2014). Since the more severely affected members also had a more severe epileptic disorder, this suggests that the epileptic activity itself played a role in the neurological deterioration observed in patients. From this point of view, *KCTD7*-related epilepsy could be considered as an epileptic encephalopathy, *i.e.* a condition in which epileptic activity may contribute to progressive neurological decline (Berg *et al.*, 2010), such that effective antiepileptic intervention might improve developmental outcome.

Conflicts of interest: none.

References

Azizieh, R., Orduz, D., Van Bogaert, P., *et al.* (2011): Progressive myoclonic epilepsy-associated gene KCTD7 is a regulator of potassium conductance in neurons. *Mol. Neurobiol.* **44,** 111–121.

Berg, A.T., Berkovic, S.F., Brodie, M.J., *et al.* (2010): Revised terminology and concepts for organization of *Seizure*s and epilepsies: report of the ILAE Commission on Classification and Terminology, 2005-3009. *Epilepsia* **51,** 676–685.

Blumkin, L., Kivity, S., Lev, D., *et al.* (2012): A compound heterozygous missense mutation and a large deletion in the KCTD7 gene presenting as an opsoclonus-myoclonus ataxia-like syndrome. *J. Neurol.* **259,** 2590–2598.

Farhan, S.M., Murphy, L.M., Robinson, J.F., *et al.* (2014): Linkage analysis and exome sequencing identify a novel mutation in KCTD7 in patients with progressive myoclonus epilepsy with ataxia. *Epilepsia* **55,** e106–111.

Kousi, M., Anttila, V., Schulz, A., *et al.* (2012): Novel mutations consolidate KCTD7 as a progressive myoclonus epilepsy gene. *J. Med. Genet.* **49,** 391–399.

Krabichler, B., Rostasy, K., Baumann, M., *et al.* (2012): Novel mutation in potassium channel related gene KCTD7 and progressive myoclonic epilepsy. *Ann. Hum. Genet.* **76,** 326–331.

Lemke, J.R., Riesch, E., Scheurenbrand, T., *et al.* (2012): Targeted next generation sequencing as a diagnostic tool in epileptic disorders. *Epilepsia* **53,** 1387–1398.

Staropoli, J.F., Karaa, A., Lim, E.T., *et al.* (2012): A homozygous mutation in KCTD7 links neuronal ceroid lipofuscinosis to the ubiquitin-proteasome system. *Am. J. Hum. Genet.* **91,** 202–208.

Stogios, P.J., Downs, G.S., Jauhal, J.J., Nandra, S.K. & Prive, G.G. (2005): Sequence and structural analysis of BTB domain proteins. *Genome Biol.* **6,** R82.

Van Bogaert, P., Azizieh, R., Desir, J., *et al.* (2007): Mutation of a potassium channel-related gene in progressive myoclonic epilepsy. *Ann. Neurol.* **61,** 579–586.

Chapter 12

Autosomal recessive progressive myoclonus epilepsy due to impaired ceramide synthesis

Edoardo Ferlazzo[1], Pasquale Striano[2], Domenico Italiano[3], Tiziana Calarese[4], Sara Gasparini[1], Nicola Vanni[2], Floriana Fruscione[2], Pierre Genton[5] and Federico Zara[2]

[1] *Regional Epilepsy Center, Reggio Calabria, Italy; Department of Medical and Surgical Sciences, Magna Graecia University, Catanzaro, Italy*
[2] *Department of Neurosciences, 'G. Gaslini' Institute, Genova, Italy*
[3] *Department of Clinical and Experimental Medicine, University of Messina, Italy*
[4] *Division of Child Neurology and Psychiatry, University of Messina, Italy*
[5] *Hôpital Henri-Gastaut, Marseille, France*
strianop@gmail.com
federicozara@ospedale-gaslini.ge.it

Summary

Autosomal recessive progressive myoclonus epilepsy due to impaired ceramide synthesis is an extremely rare condition, so far reported in a single family of Algerian origin presenting an unusual, severe form of progressive myoclonus epilepsy characterized by myoclonus, generalized tonic-clonic seizures and moderate-to-severe cognitive impairment, with probable autosomal recessive inheritance. Disease onset was between 6 and 16 years of age. Based on a genetic study, a homozygous nonsynonymous mutation in CERS1 was identified. This gene encodes for ceramide synthase 1, a transmembrane protein of the endoplasmic reticulum (ER) which catalyzes the biosynthesis of C18 ceramids. The identified mutation was associated with decreased C18 ceramide levels. In addition, downregulation of CERS1 in a neuroblastoma cell line was shown to lead to activation of ER stress response and induction of proapoptotic pathways. This observation demonstrates that impairment of ceramide biosynthesis underlies neurodegeneration in humans.

Introduction

Despite great advances in molecular analytical techniques, aetiology remains undetermined in ~28 per cent of cases of progressive myoclonus epilepsies (PMEs) (Franceschetti *et al.*, 2014). We herein report clinical, neurophysiological, and genetic findings of an Algerian family with a new form of PME with autosomal recessive inheritance, in which 4 out of 6 siblings presented a peculiar clinical picture, characterized by epilepsy, action myoclonus, and moderate-to-severe cognitive impairment.

This family was first observed at the Hôpital Henri-Gastaut in Marseilles (France), in November 2007, by 2 of the authors (EF and PG), and was extensively reported by Ferlazzo *et al.* (2009). Fig. 1 shows the pedigree of the family with the 4 affected siblings (II:2, II:4, II:5, and II:6). The history and the clinical picture of this family appeared unusual and our first impression was that we were faced with a peculiar form of PME. In particular, we were intrigued by the presence of a severe myoclonic syndrome in most (II:2 was wheelchair-bound, and II:4 and II:5 walked with bilateral support) and the persistence of frequent generalized tonic-clonic seizures (GTCS) over the years, the dramatic reduction of action myoclonus following every GTCS, moderate-to-severe intellectual disability, and the unresponsiveness to common antimyoclonic agents (piracetam, levetiracetam and benzodiazepines).

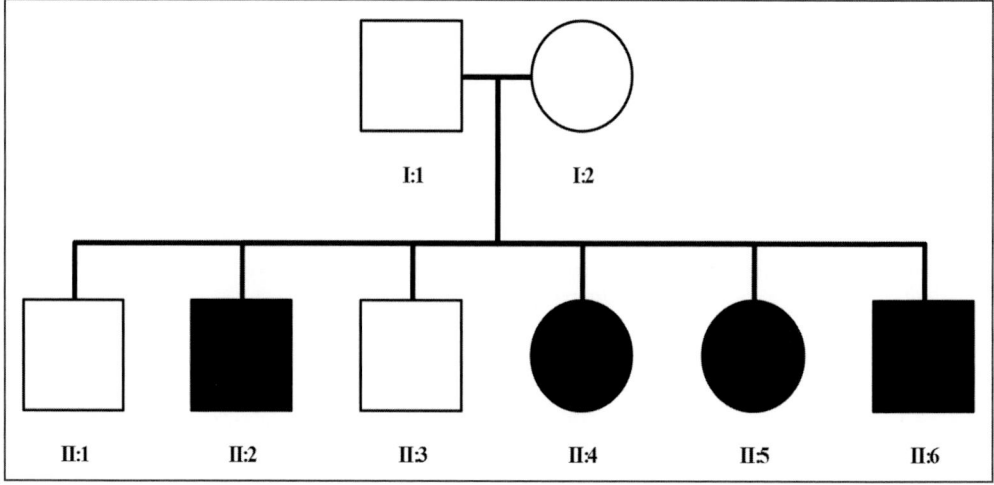

Fig. 1. Family pedigree.

Parents (I:1 and I:2) originated from two small but close Algerian villages and denied consanguinity. All affected siblings underwent neurological examination as well as neurophysiological evaluations, including video-EEG recordings at awakening. Sleep EEG was performed in Patients II:4 and II:6. To evaluate severity of action myoclonus, section 4 of the Unified Myoclonus Rating Scale (UMRS) was completed for all patients (normal score: 0). Serologic screening for coeliac disease was performed for Patients II.2, II:4, and II:6. Patient II:2 underwent extensive studies including: EMG; a peripheral nerve conduction study; somatosensory, brainstem and visual evoked potentials (SSEP, BAEP, VEP); and brain MRI. He also underwent muscle biopsy to analyze the presence of abnormal mitochondria using routine methodology. This patient also underwent armpit skin biopsies in order to investigate Lafora bodies in sweat duct cells; ultrastructural studies of skin and rectal biopsy specimens were performed to search for typical neurolipofuscinosis inclusions. Biochemical assays for ceruloplasmin, hexosaminidases A and B, arylsulfatase, urine sialyloligosaccharides, leucocitary betagalactosidase, neuraminidase and betaglucocerebrosidase, as well as serum and CSF lactate and pyruvate levels, were performed. Molecular analysis for EPM1, EPM2A, EPM2B, MERRF, MELAS and *KCTD7*, were performed according to standard techniques.

Finally, homozygosity mapping was carried out to identify mutations in common using the Web-based tool, HomozygosityMapper. Based on the autosomal recessive pattern of inheritance, we carried out homozygosity mapping of the available family members using the Affymetrix Axiom Genome-Wide Human SNP Array. Genotypes of 567 k single nucleotide polymorphisms were analyzed by HomozygosityMapper software to identify runs of homozygous markers (ROHs) shared by the affected siblings.

Results

Patient II:2

This 29-year-old boy presented his first generalized tonic-clonic seizure (GTCS) at 7 years. Afterwards, GTCS presented at monthly intervals despite trials with different antiepileptic drugs. Onset of myoclonus probably occurred at the same time as the first seizure and worsened over the years; by the age of 20 years, the patient was wheelchair-bound. After each GTCS, myoclonus was reduced over 3-4 days. Lamotrigine worsened myoclonus, and levetiracetam and piracetam were ineffective. Clonazepam and phenobarbital produced a sedative effect. At consultation, the patient was being treated with VPA at 1,250 mg/day. Neurological examination revealed severe action myoclonus (UMRS score: 124). Neuropsychological tests revealed severe cognitive impairment. EEG showed background activity at 4-6 Hz with diffuse or multifocal spike- and polyspike-and-wave discharges (Fig. 2). Intermittent photic stimulation (IPS) was negative. EMG, ENG, BAEP and VEP were normal. SSEP showed giant potentials. Brain MRI showed mild atrophy of the cerebellum and brainstem. Abdominal ultrasound was normal. Fundus oculi and campimetry were normal. Muscle biopsy showed normal morphology and histochemistry without ragged red fibres. No Lafora bodies were observed in skin biopsies. No typical lipofuscin inclusions were present in skin or rectal biopsies. Biochemical assays were normal. Mutation analyses of the cystatin B gene, Lafora genes (laforin and malin), mtDNA for MERRF, MELAS or other mitochondrial diseases, were negative.

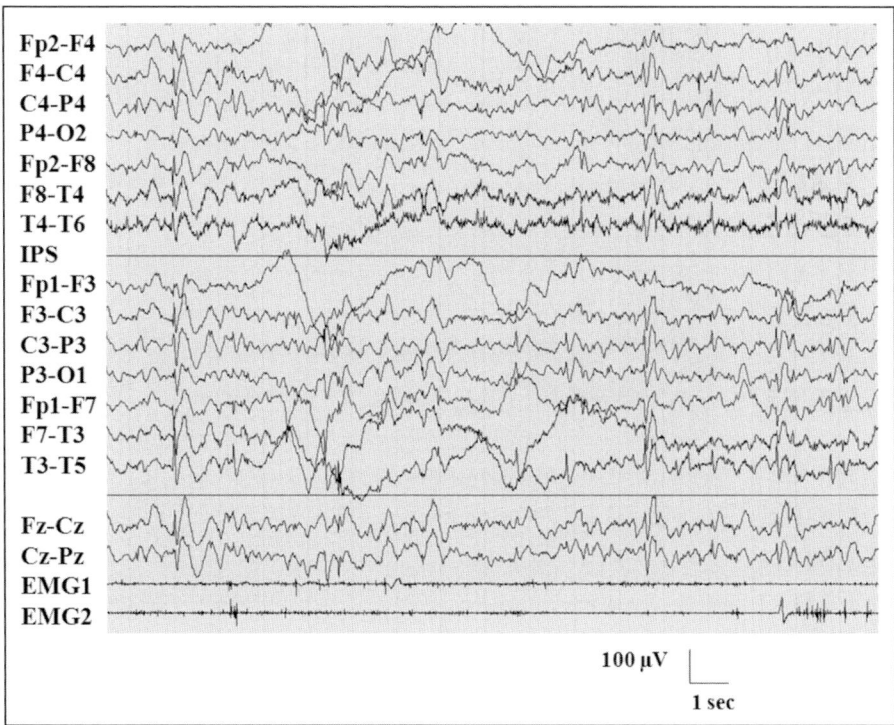

Fig. 2. Patient II:2. EEG showing slow background activity in the theta-delta range and low- and midvoltage spikes, spike- and polyspike-wave discharges, with fast spike components, both diffuse or multifocal, predominant over the centro-parieto-temporal regions. Note myoclonic jerks recorded over both deltoid muscles (EMG1: right deltoid; EMG2: left deltoid).

Patient II:4

This 24-year-old girl had GTCS that started at the age of 8 years and thereafter occurred monthly. Onset of myoclonus was at around 10 years and worsened over the years. The girl started to attend a specialized institution for disabled persons by the age of 13 years. At consultation, she was being treated with VPA at 1,000 mg/day, which was the only drug she was ever given. Neurological examination revealed severe action myoclonus (UMRS score: 106), and she was unable to walk without support. Neuropsychological evaluation showed severe cognitive impairment. Following GTCS, a marked reduction in myoclonus severity was observed over 3 to 4 days. EEG showed slow background activity mixed with low-voltage fast activity, along with diffuse, irregular, spike- and polyspike-and-wave discharges. IPS from 10 to 20 Hz provoked a photoparoxysmal response. Sleep EEG showed spikes and polyspikes over the vertex and the centro-parietal regions during the first and second stages of non-REM sleep (Fig. 3-5).

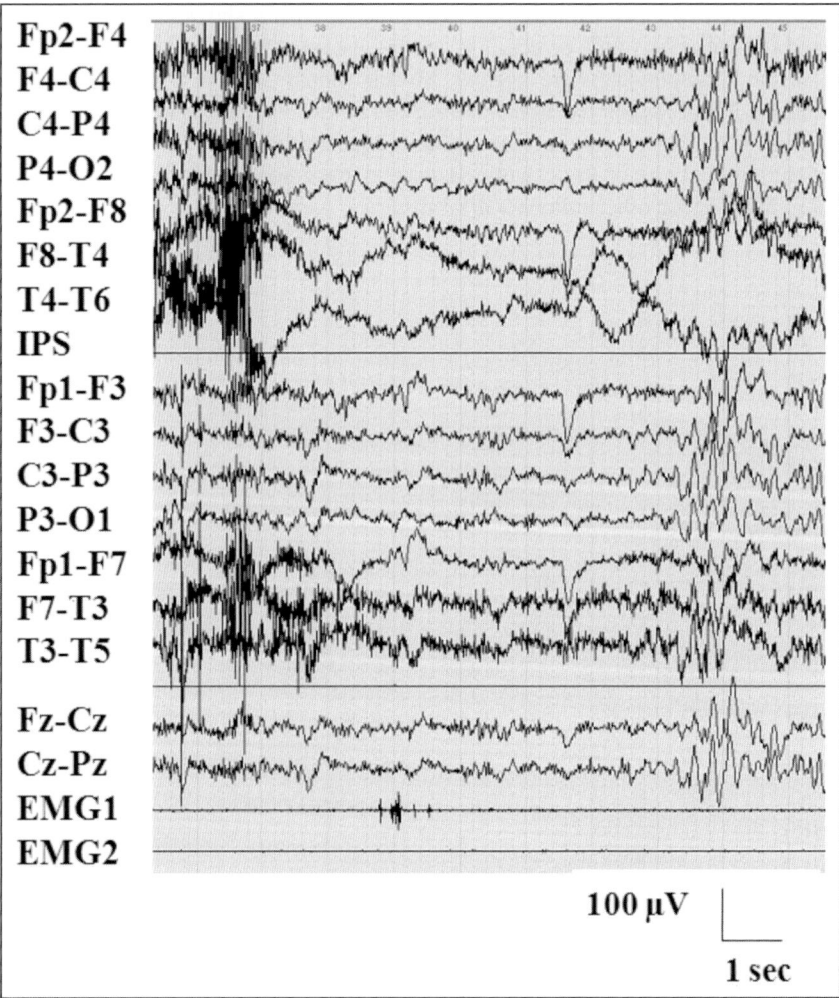

Fig. 3. Patient II:4. EEG showing slow background activity at 6 Hz mixed with low-voltage fast activity, and diffuse, irregular, spike- and polyspike-and-wave discharges at 3-4 Hz. Note myoclonic jerks recorded over the right deltoid (EMG1: right deltoid; EMG2: left deltoid).

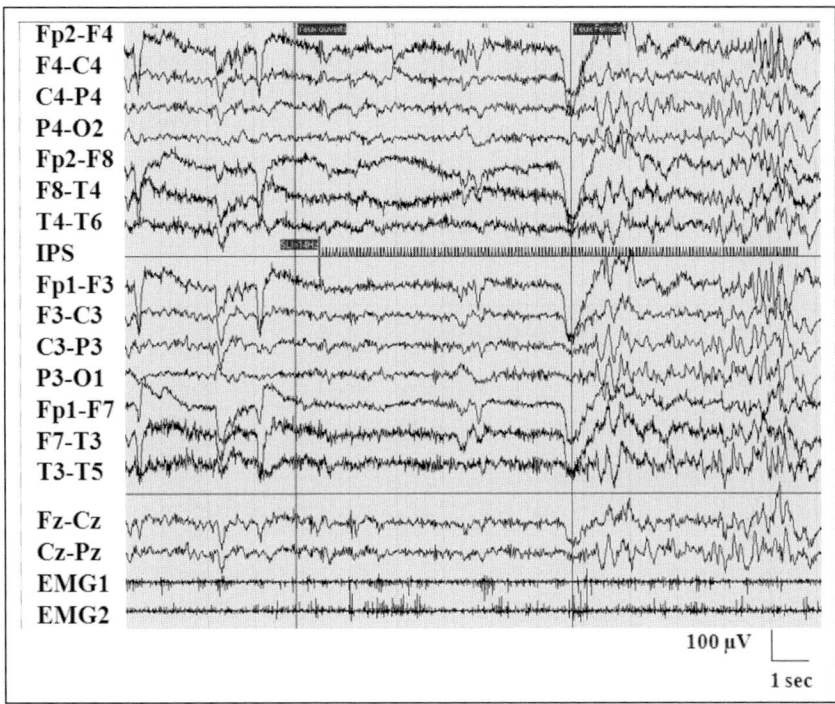

Fig. 4. Patient II:4. The same EEG recording as in Fig. 3. Diffuse, irregular spike- and polyspike-and-wave discharges provoked by IPS at 14 Hz, associated with eye closure.

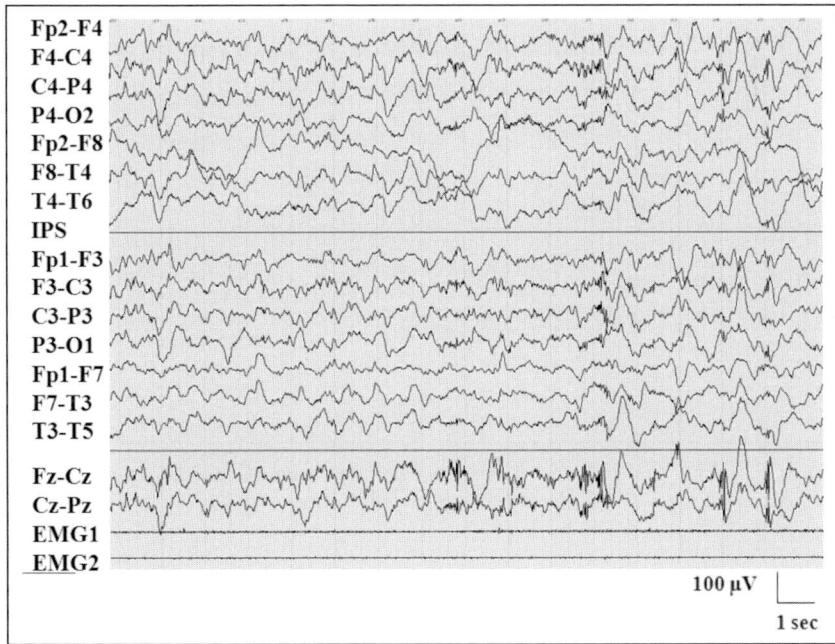

Fig. 5. Patient II:4. During stages N1 and N2 of sleep, low- and mid-voltage spikes, polyspikes and polyspike-wave discharges, with fast spike components, were recorded over the vertex and both centro-parietal regions.

Patient II:5

Myoclonus began at the age of 6 years. GTCS occurred at the age of 7 years and persisted weekly/monthly. At consultation, she was being treated with VPA at 1,250 mg/day. Neurological examination revealed action and stimulus-sensitive myoclonus (UMRS score: 99). A reduction in myoclonus severity was observed after each GTCS, which persisted for 3-4 days. Neuropsychological evaluation showed severe cognitive impairment. EEG showed slow background activity and multifocal fast spikes, polyspikes and polyspike-and-wave discharges (Fig. 6, 7). IPS was ineffective.

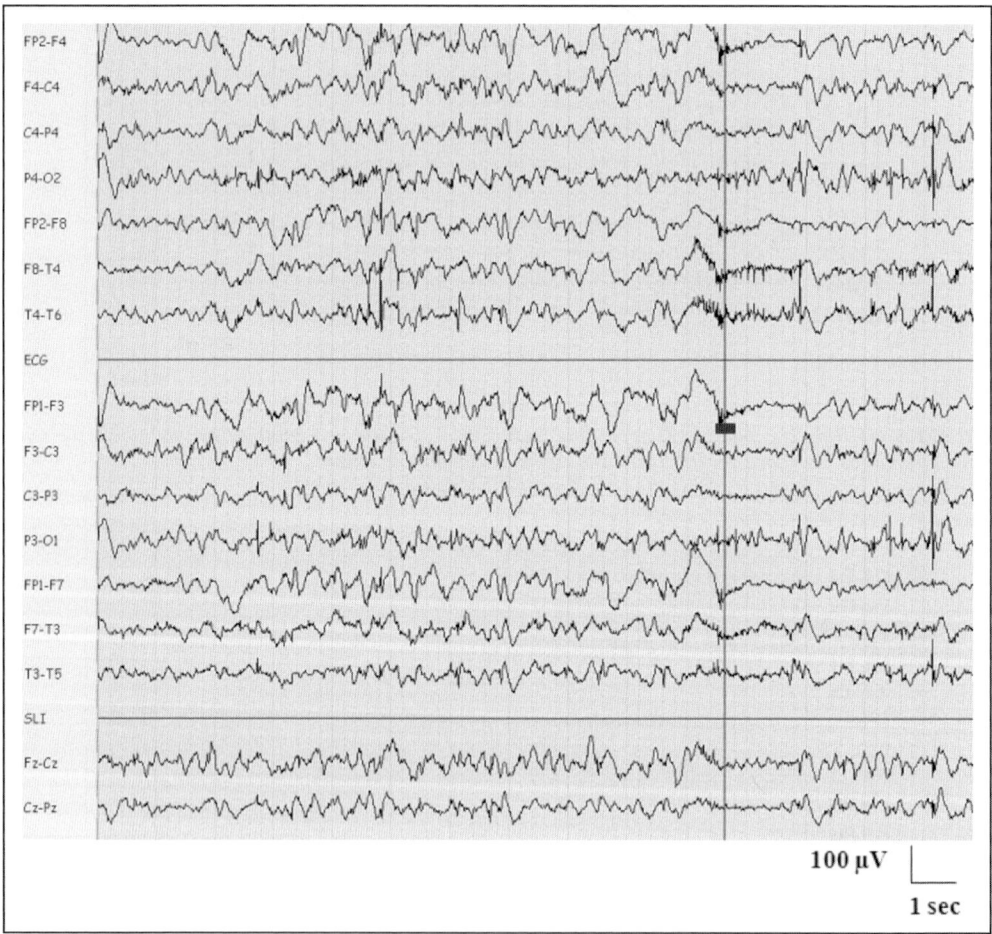

Fig. 6. Patient II:5. EEG showing slow background activity in the theta-delta range mixed with low-voltage fast activity, along with multifocal fast spikes, polyspikes and polyspike-and-wave discharges.

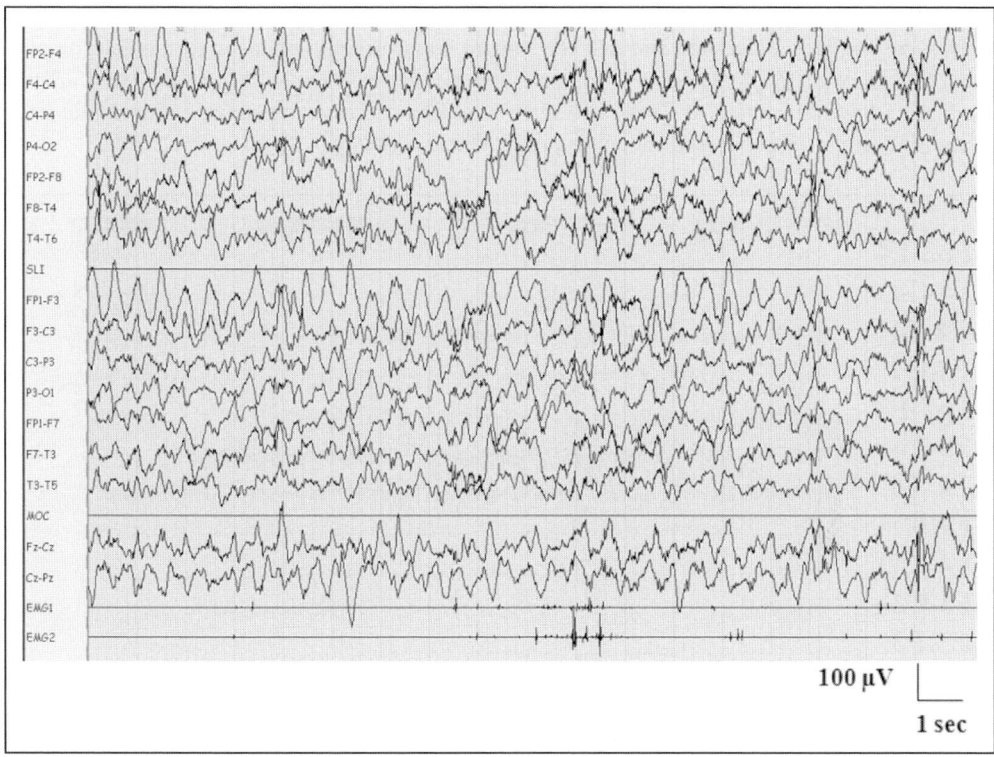

Fig. 7. Patient II:5. EEG recorded after a GTCS showing continuous polymorphic delta activity over both frontal regions. Note myoclonic jerks recorded over both deltoid muscles (EMG1: right deltoid; EMG2: left deltoid).

Patient II:6

This 19-year-old boy presented two GTCS at the age of 16 years (only a few months before consultation) and had never had specialized medical attention. He was described to be completely normal by his father. A very mild action myoclonus was observed according to neurological evaluation (UMRS score: 14). He attended normal school with low performance until age 13, after which he was moved to a specialized school. Neuropsychological evaluation showed moderate cognitive impairment, with visual perception impairment and reduction in spontaneous language. EEG showed slow background activity, as well as diffuse spike- and polyspike-and-wave discharges and multifocal spikes activated by non-REM sleep (Fig. 8). IPS between 6 and 20 Hz provoked a photoparoxysmal response. He was untreated at referral and was prescribed VPA up to 1,000 mg/day.

Homozygosity mapping

Homozygosity mapping revealed a unique unreported non-synonymous coding variant of the *CERS1* gene (c.549 C>G, NM_021267.3; p.H183Q, NP_067090) (Vanni *et al.*, 2014). The mutation affects a critical histidine conserved in all human ceramide synthases and throughout evolution, which proved to be essential for enzymatic activity. Sanger sequencing confirmed the presence of the homozygous mutation in all affected individuals, whereas both parents and 2 unaffected siblings were heterozygous. By transfecting wild-type H183-tagged and mutant

Q183-CerS1 V5-tagged vectors into HeLa cells, we found that the mutant and wild-type proteins were similarly expressed and that the mutant was correctly localized to the ER compartment (Vanni *et al.*, 2014). However, this mutation was shown to severely impair CerS1 activity leading to down-regulation of CerS1 in a neuroblastoma cell line, triggering endoplasmic reticulum (ER) stress response and inducing proapoptotic pathways (Vanni *et al.*, 2014).

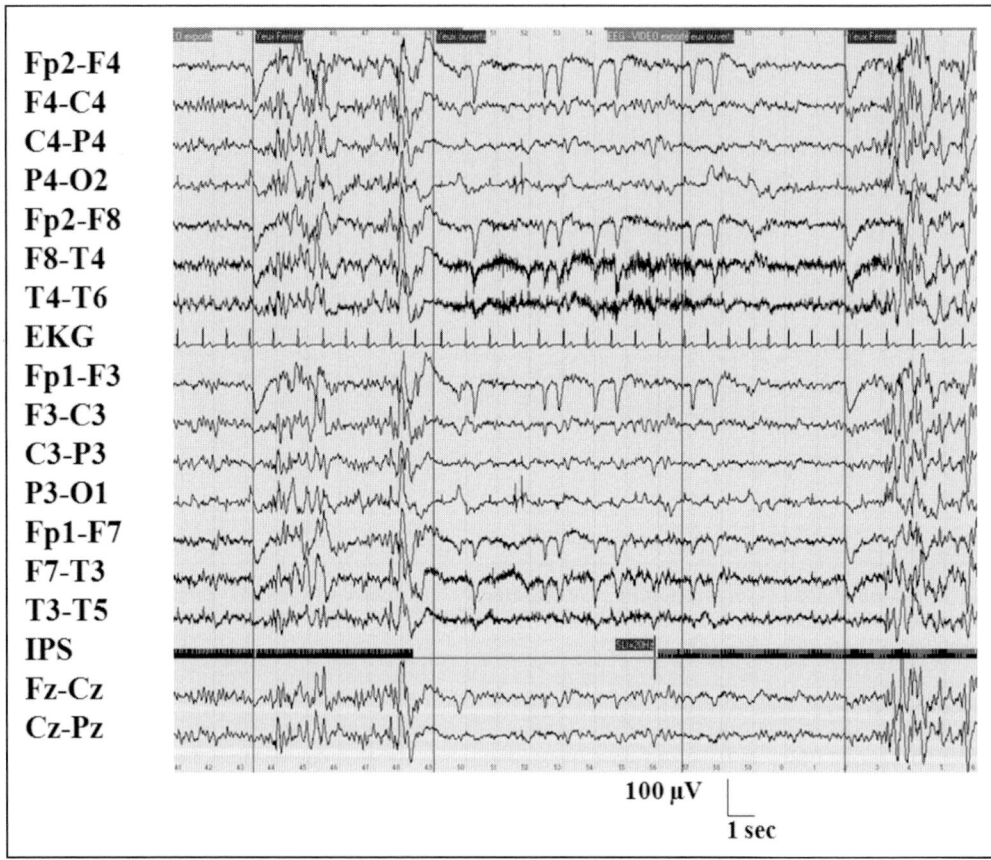

Fig. 8. Patient II:6. *Diffuse, irregular spike- and polyspike-and-wave discharges provoked by IPS at 16 and 20 Hz, associated with eye closure.*

Discussion

We herein describe clinical, neurophysiological and genetic features of a family with a novel neurodegenerative disorder featuring PME. The main characteristics distinguishing our family from Unverricht-Lundborg Disease (ULD), the most common form of PME, are the presence of relevant cognitive impairment and seizure persistency even in the late phase of the disease. However, EEG findings partially overlap with those of ULD (Magaudda *et al.*, 2006). Indeed, normal or mildly slow background activity, generalized spike- and polyspike-and-wave discharges, photoparoxysmal response at IPS between 10 and 25 Hz, bursts of low voltage, and spikes and polyspikes over the central and vertex regions during sleep are usually found in ULD. Moreover, in ULD, generalized epileptiform discharges, both spontaneous or induced by IPS, tend to decrease after 10 to 15 years of disease (Ferlazzo *et al.*, 2007). For the family reported here, generalized epileptic discharges with a fast spike component, as well as a photoparoxysmal response, were observed in 2 out of 4 patients. Moreover, one affected sibling (Patient II:4) showed fast low-voltage spikes and polyspikes over the vertex and both centroparietal regions during sleep. Unlike ULD, background activity was slow in all patients, and epileptic abnormalities persisted in all subjects for many years after disease onset.

A mutation in the *CERS1* gene, leading to the impairment of C18 ceramide biosynthesis, was shown to be the cause of this peculiar form of PME, providing evidence of the involvement of ceramide metabolism in the pathogenesis of these conditions. Moreover, we observed that impairment of CerS1 activity is associated with up-regulation of key ER stress markers, highlighting a possible link between ceramide metabolism, ER stress response, and neurodegeneration.

The significance of impaired ceramide synthesis in the development of PMEs was also shown by Mosbech *et al.*, (2014) who described a novel 27-kb heterozygous deletion in the *CERS2* gene in a PME patient. This was a 30-year-old man presenting febrile and afebrile seizures at 2 years of age. Developmental delay and myoclonus became evident at the age of 13 years, and GTCS and myoclonia increased over the years despite administration of several antiepileptic drugs. At the last follow-up visit, he presented 4-8 GTCS per month and severe myoclonus. Compared to parental controls, levels of *CERS2* mRNA, protein, and activity were reduced by ~50 per cent in fibroblasts isolated from this proband, resulting in significantly reduced levels of ceramides and sphingomyelins containing the very long-chain fatty acids C24:0 and C26:0.

However, *CERS1* and *CERS2* mutations were not found in a recent whole-exome sequencing study of 84 undiagnosed PME patients with unknown aetiology (Muona *et al.*, 2015) and, to date, have not been reported elsewhere (June 2015). Hence, we cannot exclude that the mutation reported here represents a private mutation within this family.

Finally, the interest of these findings extends beyond the field of rare forms of PMEs because ceramide represents a central element in sphingolipid metabolism, since disturbed sphingolipid levels may be found in ceroid lipofuscinosis (CLN1-6 and CLN8), as well as other common neurodegenerative diseases, such as Parkinson disease, Alzheimer disease, amyotrophic lateral sclerosis, and prion diseases.

Conflicts of interest: none.

References

Ferlazzo, E., Magaudda, A., Striano, P., Nguyen, V.H., Serra, S. & Genton, P. (2007): Long-term evolution of EEG in Unverricht-Lundborg disease. *Epilepsy Res.* **73**, 219–227.

Ferlazzo, E., Italiano, D., An, I., *et al.* (2009): Description of a family with a novel progressive myoclonus epilepsy and cognitive impairment. *Mov. Disord.* **24**, 1016–1022.

Franceschetti, S., Michelucci, R., Canafoglia, L., *et al.* (2014): Progressive myoclonic epilepsies: definitive and still undetermined causes. *Neurology* **82**, 405–411.

Magaudda, A., Ferlazzo, E., Nguyen, V.H. & Genton, P. (2006): Unverricht-Lundborg disease, a condition with self-limited progression: long-term follow-up of 20 patients. *Epilepsia* **5**, 860–866.

Mosbech, M-B., Olsen, A.S.B., Neess, D., *et al.* (2014): Reduced ceramide synthase 2 activity causes progressive myoclonic epilepsy. *Ann. Clin. Transl. Neurol.* **1**, 88–98.

Muona, M., Berkovic, S.F., Dibbens, L.M., *et al.* (2015): A recurrent de novo mutation in *KCNC1* causes progressive myoclonus epilepsy. *Nat. Genet.* **47**, 39–46.

Vanni, N., Fruscione, F., Ferlazzo, E., *et al.* (2014): Impairment of ceramide synthesis causes a novel progressive myoclonus epilepsy. *Ann. Neurol.* **76**, 206–212.

Chapter 13

Spinal muscular atrophy associated with progressive myoclonic epilepsy

Haluk Topaloglu[1] and Judith Melki[2]

[1] Hacettepe University, Departments of Paediatric Neurology, Ankara, Turkey
[2] Unité mixte de recherche (UMR)-1169, Inserm and University Paris Sud, 94276, Le Kremlin Bicêtre, France
htopalog@hacettepe.edu.tr
judith.melki@inserm.fr

Summary

A rare syndrome characterized by lower motor neuron disease associated with progressive myoclonic epilepsy, referred to as 'spinal muscular atrophy associated with progressive myoclonic epilepsy' (SMA-PME), has been described in childhood and is inherited as an autosomal recessive trait. SMA-PME is caused by mutation in the *ASAH1* gene encoding acid ceramidase. Ceramide and the metabolites participate in various cellular events as lipid mediators. The catabolism of ceramide in mammals occurs in lysosomes through the activity of ceramidase. Three different ceramidases (acid, neutral and alkaline) have been identified and appear to play distinct roles in sphingolipid metabolism. The enzymatic activity of acid ceramidase is deficient in two rare inherited disorders; Farber disease and SMA-PME. Farber disease is a very rare and severe autosomal recessive condition with a distinct clinical phenotype. The marked difference in disease manifestations may explain why Farber and SMA-PME diseases were not previously suspected to be allelic conditions. The precise molecular mechanism underlying the phenotypic differences remains to be clarified. Recently, a condition with mutation in *CERS1*, the gene encoding ceramide synthase 1, has been identified as a novel form of PME. This finding underlies the essential role of enzymes regulating either the synthesis (CERS1) or degradation (ASAH1) of ceramide, and the link between defects in ceramide metabolism and PME.

Introduction

Progressive myoclonic epilepsy (PME) represents a heterogeneous group of epilepsies characterized by myoclonic and generalized seizures with progressive neurological deterioration (Girard *et al.*, 2013). A rare syndrome characterized by lower motor neuron disease associated with progressive myoclonic epilepsy (SMA-PME) has been described in childhood (Jankovic & Rivera, 1979; Haliloglu *et al.*, 2002). This condition is inherited as an autosomal recessive trait and the disease-causing gene has been recently identified. SMA-PME is caused by mutation in the *ASAH1* gene, which encodes acid ceramidase (Zhou *et al.*, 2012).

A total of 11 affected individuals have been reported thus far, leading to a relatively precise phenotypic characterization (Zhou et al., 2012; Rubboli et al., 2015; Dyment et al., 2014, 2015; Giráldez et al., 2015).

Mutations in the same gene are responsible for Farber disease, a very rare autosomal recessive condition with a distinct clinical phenotype, resulting from marked reduction or complete lack of acid ceramidase activity (Sugita et al., 1972; Levade et al., 2009). The marked difference in disease manifestations may explain why Farber and SMA-PME diseases were previously not suspected to be allelic conditions.

Several therapeutic strategies have been adopted to treat Farber disease, including allogeneic bone marrow transplantation and introduction of wild-type human acid ceramidase cDNA, using recombinant oncoretroviral or lentiviral vectors. The latter approach performed in non-human primates was recently shown to result in increased acid ceramidase activity. This underlines the importance of screening for *ASAH1* or acid ceramidase activity in patients with undiagnosed SMA or PME, for the purposes of diagnosis and future treatment.

Clinical description of SMA-PME

Based on the clinical description of cases reported to date ($n = 11$), SMA-PME is mainly characterized by progressive lower motor neuron degeneration followed by progressive myoclonic epilepsy (Table 1) (Jankovic & Rivera, 1979; Haliloglu et al., 2002; Zhou et al., 2012; Rubboli et al., 2015; Dyment et al., 2014, 2015; Giráldez et al., 2015).

Lower motor neuron disease manifestations

Early development milestones are usually normal, with an ability to walk unaided between 14 to 17 months of age. Progressive symmetric weakness and muscle atrophy of the lower and then the upper limbs are the main clinical features, usually occurring between 2.5 to 6 years of age (Table 1). The patients begin to show slowness of gait and difficulties in standing from the sitting position. The motor deficit is purely peripheral, with a decrease in or absence of deep tendon reflexes. The disease is progressive, leading to the inability to stand up from the floor, the inability to sit unsupported, a lack of head control, difficulty swallowing, fasciculations of the tongue, severe scoliosis, and subsequent respiratory insufficiency. Electromyography (EMG) shows a chronic denervation process while muscle biopsy shows neurogenic atrophy, although there are no changes suggestive of a mitochondrial disorder.

However, in 1 of these 11 patients, atonic and absence seizures and myoclonic jerks were the main and first clinical features. Once the *ASAH1* gene mutations were identified, an EMG was performed, showing evidence of motor neuron disease despite only mild proximal muscle weakness (Dyment et al., 2014, 2015).

Progressive myoclonic epilepsy

Later on, myoclonic epilepsy is observed from 3 to 12 years of age (Table 1). This is characterized by brief myoclonic seizures without loss of consciousness, generalized epileptic seizures and myoclonic jerks, myoclonic seizures, absences with head drop or postural lapses in the upper limbs, atonic seizures, or upper limb myoclonic jerks. The EEG shows subcortical myoclonic epileptiform abnormalities which are sensitive to hyperventilation, paroxysmal activity consisting of frequent, diffuse bursts of sharp waves and polyspike and wave complexes, bursts

Table 1. Literature review

	Zhou et al., 2012 (family D)	Zhou et al., 2012 (family ITA)	Zhou et al., 2012 (family ITB)	Rubboli et al., 2015 (case 1)	Rubboli et al., 2015 (case 2)	Rubboli et al., 2015 (case 3)	Dyment et al., 2014 & 2015	Giráldez et al., 2015
Nb. of affected individuals	3	2	1	1	1	1	1	1
MOTOR DEVELOPMENT								
Ability to walk (m.)	14	Normal	Normal	Normal	17 (abnormal deambulation)	Not reported	Not reported	17 (unsteady gait)
Age of onset of weakness (y.)	5	4 to 5	5	6	2,4	3	?	3
Muscle symptoms	Proximal weakness	Progressive muscle weakness	Progressive muscle weakness	Progressive muscle weakness	Progressive muscle weakness and limb tremor	Mild proximal weakness	Mild proximal muscle weakness	Proximal muscle weakness
EMG	Chronic denervation process	Denervation process	Denervation-reinnervation process	Chronic denervation process	Chronic denervation process	Chronic denervation process	Evidence of motor neuron disease	Chronic denervation process
Muscle biopsy	Neurogenic atrophy	Denervation process	Denervation-reinnervation	Neurogenic damage	Neurogenic damage	Neurogenic damage	nd	Neurogenic atrophy
EPILEPSY								
Age of onset (y.)	7	12	10	8	3	12	10	7
Clinical symptoms	Brief myoclonic seizures without loss of consciousness	Generalized epileptic seizures and myoclonic jerks	Loss of consciousness associated with myoclonic jerks	Brief episodes of impairment of consciousness associated with 'jerks' at the upper limbs	Staring and myoclonic jerks	Myoclonic seizures, absences with head drop or postural lapses at the upper limbs	Absence and atonic seizures; frequent myoclonic jerks	Multiple and brief absences, upper limb myoclonic jerks and/or head nodding episodes
EEG	Subcortical myoclonic epileptiform abnormalities sensitive to hyperventilation	Not reported	Paroxysmal activity consisting in frequent diffuse bursts of sharp waves and poly-spike and wave complexes	Bursts of generalized spike- and polyspike-and-wave complexes associated with myoclonic phenomena	Similar to case 1	Similar to case 1	Generalized polyspike and wave discharges	Frequent interictal bursts of posterior delta activity and ictal generalized spike-wave and polyspike-wave discharges

	Zhou et al., 2012 (family D)	Zhou et al., 2012 (family ITA)	Zhou et al., 2012 (family ITB)	Rubboli et al., 2015 (case 1)	Rubboli et al., 2015 (case 2)	Rubboli et al., 2015 (case 3)	Dyment et al., 2014 & 2015	Giráldez et al., 2015
Brain MRI	Normal	Normal	Normal	Normal	Diffuse supratentorial and subtentorial cortical atrophy	Normal	Normal then mildly increased size of the III and IV ventricles and mild volume loss	Normal
EVOLUTION	Progressive	Progressive	Progressive	Progressive	Progressive	Progressive	Not reported	Progressive
Age of death (y.)	13-17	na	15	19	na	na	na	na
ASAH1 MUTATION								
Nucleotide (NM_177924.3)	c.125C>T; homozygous	c.125C>T; homozygous	c.125C>T; ASAH1 deletion	c.125C>T; homozygous	c.223_224insC; c.125C>T	c.177C>G; c.456A>C	c.850G>T; c.456A>C	c.125C>T; lack of the other allele (deletion?)
Protein	p.Thr42Met	p.Thr42Met	p.Thr42Met	p.Thr42Met	p.Val75Alafs*25; p.Thr42Met	p.Tyr59*; p.Lys152Asn	p.Gly284*; p.Lys152Asn	p.Thr42Met
Acid ceramidase activity (% of normal value)	32%	32%	32%	Not reported	Not reported	Not reported	5.5%	Not reported

Nb.: number; y.: year; m.: month; nd: not done; na: not applicable of generalized spike- and polyspike-and-wave complexes associated with myoclonic phenomena, generalized polyspike-and-wave discharges, or interictal bursts of posterior delta activity and ictal generalized spike-wave and polyspike-wave discharges. Brain MRI is most often normal or displays mild supratentorial and subtentorial cortical atrophy. Myoclonic seizures are most often refractory to antiepileptic drugs.

Other symptoms

Variable degrees of cognitive impairment occur. When reported, cognition is usually mildly impaired. Neither skin, joint abnormalities, or hoarseness of the voice, as observed in Farber disease, has been reported. Ophthalmological examination did not reveal corneal opacities or cherry red spots.

SMA-PME is caused by mutations in *ASAH1*

This condition is inherited as an autosomal recessive trait. Genome-wide linkage analysis combined with exome sequencing in two multiplex families and one sporadic case suffering from childhood SMA-PME revealed mutations in *ASAH1* which were responsible for the disease (Zhou *et al.*, 2012). *ASAH1*, located on chromosome 8, was the only gene to have a mutation that was shared by the unrelated affected individuals. The same missense mutation in exon 2 of *ASAH1* (NM_177924.3; c.125C>T; p.Thr42Met) was found in the affected individuals. The p.Thr42Met missense substitution affected an evolutionarily conserved amino acid among different species and was predicted to be damaging. In 2 families, both parents were heterozygous and affected siblings were homozygous for this missense mutation. In one family, the affected child carried compound heterozygous mutations, the c.125C>T missense mutation on one allele and a deletion of the whole gene on the other. Transient expression of the mutant cDNA in immortalized fibroblasts derived from an individual with Farber disease with very low acid ceramidase activity (less than 3.5 per cent of control value), revealed a mild reduction in acid ceramidase activity when compared to that of the wild type cDNA (about 32 per cent of the control value) (Zhou *et al.*, 2012). To analyze the effect of *ASAH1* loss-of-function *in vivo*, a morpholino antisense oligonucleotide of the *ASAH1* ortholog was used to knock down *ASAH1* in zebrafish embryos. Analysis of this model revealed a marked defect in motor neuron axonal branching associated with a significant increase in apoptosis in the spinal cord (Zhou *et al.*, 2012).

For other SMA-PME patients reported to date, *ASAH1* mutations were identified using sanger or whole-exome sequencing (Rubboli *et al.*, 2015; Dyment *et al.*, 2014, 2015; Giráldez *et al.*, 2015). The same c.125C>T mutation was identified in three additional patients, and other mutations including missense, non-sense, or large deletion of *ASAH1* were identified (Table 1). Although acid ceramidase activity was reported *in vitro* to be mildly reduced as the consequence of the p.Thr42Met mutation (Zhou *et al.*, 2012), acid ceramidase activity in patient fibroblasts carrying the compound *ASAH1* heterozygous mutation (p.Gly284*; p.Lys152Asn) was markedly reduced (5.5 per cent of normal activity), similar to that observed in Farber patients. Surprisingly, this patient did not develop manifestations of Farber disease (Dyment *et al.*, 2014, 2015).

Pathogenesis of SMA-PME is linked to *ASAH1* gene mutations

Ceramide is synthesized in the endoplasmic reticulum and transported by the ceramide-transfer protein, CERT, to the trans-Golgi membrane where it is converted to sphingomyelin by the sphingomyelin synthase-1,2. Ceramide and the metabolites (sphingosine and sphingosine 1-phosphate) participate in various cellular events as lipid mediators. The catabolism of ceramide in mammals occurs in lysosomes through the activity of ceramidase. Three different ceramidases (acid, neutral, and alkaline) have been identified and characterized according to optimum pH and primary structure; these include the acid (ASAH1), neutral (ASAH2), and alkaline ceramidases (ASAH3). The three families of ceramidase appear to play distinct roles in sphingolipid metabolism.

The enzymatic activity of acid ceramidase is deficient in two rare inherited disorders, Farber disease and SMA-PME. Importantly, in addition to the role of acid ceramidase in ceramide catabolism, the enzyme may have other functions depending on its subcellular location and the local pH. The other putative functions of ASAH1 may account for the clinical spectrum of the disease associated with *ASAH1* mutation. Refined characterization of acid ceramidase activity in the subcellular domain should contribute to a better understanding of the genotype-phenotype correlation.

Ceramides are the precursors to complex sphingolipids, which are important for normal functioning of both the developing and mature brain. Recently, a mutation in *CERS1*, the gene encoding ceramide synthase 1, has been identified as a novel cause of PME (Vanni *et al.*, 2014). This data underlies the essential role of enzymes in terms of regulating the synthesis (CERS1) or degradation (ASAH1) of ceramide and the link between ceramide metabolism defects and PME.

Molecular basis of Farber *versus* SMA-PME diseases

Farber disease is a rare and severe autosomal recessive lysosomal storage disorder (Levade *et al.*, 2009) which, like SMA-PME, is linked to the disease gene, *ASAH1*. It is characterized by a marked deficiency in acid ceramidase activity (Sugita *et al.*, 1972). Farber disease is characterized by a severe early onset (from 2 weeks to 4 months of age) of a unique triad of clinical manifestations including painful and progressively deformed joints, subcutaneous nodules, and progressive hoarseness as the result of laryngeal involvement. The illness advances rapidly, with progressive neurological deterioration, leading to death at a mean age of 1.45 years. At late stages of disease progression, 13 per cent of Farber disease patients display hypotonia and muscular atrophy with reduced or absent deep tendon reflexes and signs of denervation, as observed on EMG. These data strongly suggest that while a dramatic reduction in acid ceramidase activity leads to Farber disease, a milder reduction in enzymatic activity leads to a later onset of symptoms restricted to spinal cord motor neurons and subsequently other areas of the CNS responsible for PME. However, as reported recently (Dyment *et al.*, 2014, 2015), one patient presenting with features of PME, with mild motor weakness, had a marked reduction in acid ceramidase activity, similar to that observed in Farber patients, but did not present any manifestations of Farber disease, suggesting that additional factors are likely to be involved in the different phenotypic expression.

Animal models and therapeutic research strategies

Previously, homozygous *ASAH1* knockout mouse embryos were shown not to live beyond the four-cell stage, indicating that acid ceramidase plays an essential role during development (Eliyahu *et al.*, 2007). Recently, a knock-in mouse model was created by introducing a single-nucleotide mutation, identified in human Farber patients, into the murine *ASAH1* gene (Pro362Arg) (Alayoubi *et al.*, 2013). Homozygous mutant mice displayed Farber disease manifestations and died within 7-13 weeks. Treating mutant mice during the neonatal period with a single injection of lentivector expressing human acid ceramidase diminishes the severity of the disease. It would be of great interest to determine whether, using this model, partial correction of acid ceramidase deficiency could prevent both Farber and SMA-PME disease manifestations or only the Farber phenotype, which should reinforce the hypothesis that the clinical expression of the disease correlates with residual acid ceramidase activity. This model should contribute to a better understanding of the pathogenesis of Farber and SMA-PME diseases and represents a valuable tool towards developing therapeutic strategies.

While bone marrow transplantation has been reported to be effective in relieving joint contractures and subcutaneous nodules in a patient with Farber disease (Yeager *et al.*, 2000), the affected individual developed progressive muscle weakness and features consistent with the occurrence of lower motor neuron involvement, the main clinical features found in SMA-PME individuals. More recently, a preclinical gene therapy study for Farber disease involving a lentiviral vector was performed in non-human primates. Acid ceramidase activity was detected above normal levels in various cell types, including bone marrow cells, spleen and liver 1 year after lentiviral vector transduction (Walia *et al.*, 2011).

Genetic counselling

The identification of the *ASAH1* gene mutations found in SMA-PME patients has greatly improved diagnostic testing and family-planning options of SMA-PME family members. Because the risk of recurrence of the disease in the sibling of an affected child is high (1/4), information should be given to parents early after diagnosis. Explanations regarding molecular pathology, risk evaluation, and prenatal testing possibilities should be given to the parents and their relatives within the context of a genetic counselling visit.

Conclusion

Mutations in *ASAH1*, which encodes acid ceramidase, are the major cause of SMA-PME. Based on an overview of patients reported to date, the main clinical characteristic features are onset, most often within the first 6 years of age, characterized by lower motor neuron disease leading to progressive muscle weakness, followed by the occurrence of clinical and EEG characteristics of myoclonic epilepsies, and a progressive course. This data underlies the link between ceramide metabolism defects and PME. Taking into account ongoing therapeutic research for Farber disease, a disease allelic to SMA-PME, screening for *ASAH1* or acid ceramidase activity should be proposed for the diagnosis and future treatment of patients with PME or SMA.

Conflicts of interest: none.

Acknowledgments: This work was supported by Inserm, the Association française contre les myopathies, Paris-Sud and Hacettepe Universities.

References

Alayoubi, A.M., Wang, J.C., Au, B.C., *et al.* (2013): Systemic ceramide accumulation leads to severe and varied pathological consequences. *EMBO Mol. Med.* **5,** 827–842.

Dyment, D.A., Sell, E., Vanstone, M.R. *et al.* (2014): Evidence for clinical, genetic and biochemical variability in spinal muscular atrophy with progressive myoclonic epilepsy. *Clin. Genet.* **86,** 558–563.

Dyment, D.A., Tétreault, M., Beaulieu, C.L., *et al.* (2015): Whole-exome sequencing broadens the phenotypic spectrum of rare pediatric epilepsy: a retrospective study. *Clin. Genet.* **88,** 34–40.

Eliyahu, E., Park, J.H., Shtraizent, N., He, X. & Schuchman, E.H. (2007): Acid ceramidase is a novel factor required for early embryo survival. *FASEB J.* **21,** 1403–1409.

Giráldez, B.G., Guerrero-López, R., Ortega-Moreno, L., *et al.* (2015): Uniparental disomy as a cause of spinal muscular atrophy and progressive myoclonic epilepsy: phenotypic homogeneity due to the homozygous c.125 C>T mutation in ASAH1. *Neuromuscul. Disord.* **25,** 222–224.

Girard, J.M., Turnbull, J., Ramachandran, N. & Minassian, B.A. (2013): Progressive myoclonus epilepsy. *Handb. Clin. Neurol.* **113,** 1731–1736.

Haliloglu, G., Chattopadhyay, A., Skorodis, L., *et al.* (2002): Spinal muscular atrophy with progressive myoclonic epilepsy: report of new cases and review of the literature. *Neuropediatrics* **33,** 314–319.

Jankovic, J. & Rivera, V.M. (1979): Hereditary myoclonus and progressive distal muscular atrophy. *Ann. Neurol.* **6,** 227–231.

Levade, T., Sandhoff, K., Schulze, H. & Medin, J.A. (2009): Acid ceramidase deficiency: Farber lipogranulomatosis. In: *Scriver's OMMBID (Online Metabolic and Molecular Bases of Inherited Disease)*, eds. D. Valle, A.L. Beaudet, B. Vogelstein, K.W. Kinzler, S.E. Antonarakis & A. Ballabio A. McGraw-Hill.

Rubboli, G., Veggiotti, P., Pini, A., *et al.* (2015): Spinal muscular atrophy associated with progressive myoclonic epilepsy: a rare condition caused by mutations in *ASAH1*. *Epilepsia* **56,** 692–698.

Sugita, M., Dulaney, J.T. & Moser, H.W. (1972): Ceramidase deficiency in Farber's disease (lipogranulomatosis). *Science* **178,** 1100-1102.

Vanni, N., Fruscione, F., Ferlazzo, E., *et al.* (2014): Impairment of ceramide synthesis causes a novel progressive myoclonus epilepsy. *Ann. Neurol.* **76,** 206–212.

Walia, J.S., Neschadim, A., Lopez-Perez, O., *et al.* (2011): Autologous transplantation of lentivector/acid ceramidase-transduced hematopoietic cells in nonhuman primates. *Hum. Gene Ther.* **22,** 679–687.

Yeager, A.M., Uhas, K.A., Coles, C.D., Davis, P.C., Krause, W.L. & Moser, H.W. (2000): Bone marrow transplantation for infantile ceramidase deficiency (Farber disease). *Bone Marrow Transplant.* **26,** 357–363.

Zhou, J., Tawk, M., Tiziano, F.D., *et al.* (2012): Spinal muscular atrophy associated with progressive myoclonic epilepsy is caused by mutations in *ASAH1*. *Am. J. Hum. Genet.* **91,** 5–14.

Chapter 14

Myoclonus epilepsy and ataxia due to potassium channel mutation (MEAK) is caused by heterozygous *KCNC1* mutations

Fábio A. Nascimento and Danielle M. Andrade

*Division of Neurology, Department of Medicine,
University of Toronto- Adult Epilepsy Genetics Program, University of Toronto, Toronto Western Hospital, Krembil Neurosciences Program, 5W-445, 399 Bathurst Street, Toronto, ON, M5T 2S8, Canada*
Danielle.andrade@uhn.ca

Summary

Progressive myoclonus epilepsy (PME) is a distinct group of seizure disorders characterized by gradual neurological decline with ataxia, myoclonus and recurring seizures. There are several forms of PME, among which the most recently described is MEAK - myoclonus epilepsy and ataxia due to potassium channel mutation. This particular subtype is caused by a recurrent *de novo* heterozygous mutation (c.959G>A, p.Arg320His) in the *KCNC1* gene, which maps to chromosome 11 and encodes for the Kv3.1 protein (a subunit of the Kv3 subfamily of voltage-gated potassium channels). Loss of Kv3 function disrupts the firing properties of fast-spiking neurons, affects neurotransmitter release and induces cell death. Specifically regarding Kv3.1 malfunctioning, the most affected neurons include inhibitory GABAergic interneurons and cerebellar neurons. Impairment of the former cells is believed to contribute to myoclonus and seizures, whereas dysfunction of the latter to ataxia and tremor. Phenotypically, MEAK patients generally have a normal early development. At the age of 6 to 14 years, they present with myoclonus, which tends to progressively worsen with time. Tonic-clonic seizures may or may not be present, and some patients develop mild cognitive impairment following seizure onset. Typical electro-encephalographic features comprise generalized epileptiform discharges and, in some cases, photosensitivity. Brain imaging is either normal or shows cerebellar atrophy. The identification of MEAK has both expanded the phenotypic and genotypic spectra of PME and established an emerging role for *de novo* mutations in PME.

Introduction

The term 'progressive myoclonus epilepsy' (PME) provides us with a broad, but reliable, characterization for this distinct subgroup of seizure disorders. 'Progressive' depicts the gradual neurological decline seen in patients affected with a PME. 'Myoclonus' and 'epilepsy' summarize the other two cardinal clinical features observed in these individuals

(Berkovic et al., 1986). Aetiologically, most PMEs are the result of genetic abnormalities. The vast majority are inherited in an autosomal recessive fashion, although some cases exhibit autosomal dominant or mitochondrial inheritance.

Despite the impressive range of specific forms of PME, their phenotypes are fairly similar, which makes accurate clinical diagnosis very challenging, especially in the early stages. However, significant heterogeneity exists in terms of the genetic causes of the subtypes of progressive myoclonus epilepsies.

As is the case with countless other diseases in the realm of neurology, a proportion of PME cases still have no identified genetic basis. In this context, a cohort of 84 unconfirmed, unrelated PME patients was extensively investigated in a recent multicentre study. With a view to trying to elucidate their molecular diagnoses, all cases underwent whole-exome sequencing, and Sanger sequencing was performed for a secondary cohort of 28. The most remarkable finding was the identification of a recurrent heterozygous *de novo* mutation in the *KCNC1* gene, which encodes for a subunit of a specific potassium channel. The new PME subtype was named 'myoclonus epilepsy and ataxia due to potassium channel mutation' (MEAK) (Muona et al., 2015). Notably, prior to this study, *KCNC1* had never been associated with any human disease. In addition, this group of researchers importantly demonstrated that *de novo* mutations play a significant role in the genesis of progressive myoclonus epilepsies.

This chapter aims to review the most recent PME subtype described: MEAK. We begin by introducing the micro-world of potassium channels, since an understanding of this is of fundamental importance. We then focus on how *KCNC1* was identified to be associated with MEAK and discuss how the effects of such a mutation are translated into clinical signs and symptoms. Finally, the phenotypes of all the reported individuals with MEAK are discussed.

Potassium ion channels

Potassium ion channels are ubiquitous membrane proteins responsible for a range of cellular functions, including maintenance of membrane potential, regulation of cell volume, and electrical excitability modulation. The latter is particularly important for the membrane physiology of excitable cells, such as neurons. According to their functional properties, potassium channels can be categorized into several groups, such as *voltage-gated potassium channels*, calcium-activated potassium channels, and sodium-activated potassium channels, among others. Furthermore, each of these groups can be subdivided into families and subfamilies, based on molecular similarity (Sansom et al., 2002).

Voltage-gated potassium channels (Kv channels) play an essential role in the generation and propagation of electrical impulses in the nervous system. By enabling the selective flow of potassium ions through neuronal membranes (upon changes in transmembrane potentials), Kv channels help set the resting potential and degree of excitability of the membrane (repolarization), influence action potential waveforms and firing patterns, and modulate synaptic activity (Ried et al., 1993). Voltage-gated potassium channels are classified into four subfamilies: Kv1, Kv2, Kv3, and Kv4.

Kv3 channels, in particular, are known for their high activation threshold and fast activation and deactivation properties (Rudy & McBain, 2001). Kv3 channels are crucial components of the circuitry of neurons that are able to fire action potentials at high frequencies or follow high frequency inputs (Wang et al., 2007). The Kv3 subfamily is composed of 4 subunits, Kv3.1, Kv3.2, Kv3.3, and Kv3.4, which are encoded by 4 genes, *KCNC1* to *KCNC4*, respectively.

These 4 subunits assemble as either homomers or heteromers to form voltage-gated tetrameric potassium ion channels. Each of the 4 subunits consists of 6 transmembrane segments (S1-S6) with a re-entrant P-loop region. The transmembrane segments S1-S4 are referred to as the voltage-sensing domain, of which the primary voltage-sensing unit is S4. The segments S5-P-S6 represent the ion-conducting pore domain. Upon membrane de- or hyper-polarization, which is sensed by positively charged arginine residues at the S4 segment, the S4 segment undergoes the largest reorientation, leading to channel opening and generation of transient gating currents (Aggarwal & MacKinnon, 1996; Chanda & Bezanilla, 2008).

Within the *KCNC* gene family, *KCNC3* has been previously reported as a human disease associated gene. *KCNC3* mutations have been recognized as a cause of spinocerebellar ataxia type 13 (*SCA13*) (Herman-Bert et al., 2000; Middlebrooks et al., 2013). Only very recently, *KCNC1* mutations have been identified as a cause of human disease: myoclonus epilepsy and ataxia due to potassium channel mutation (MEAK).

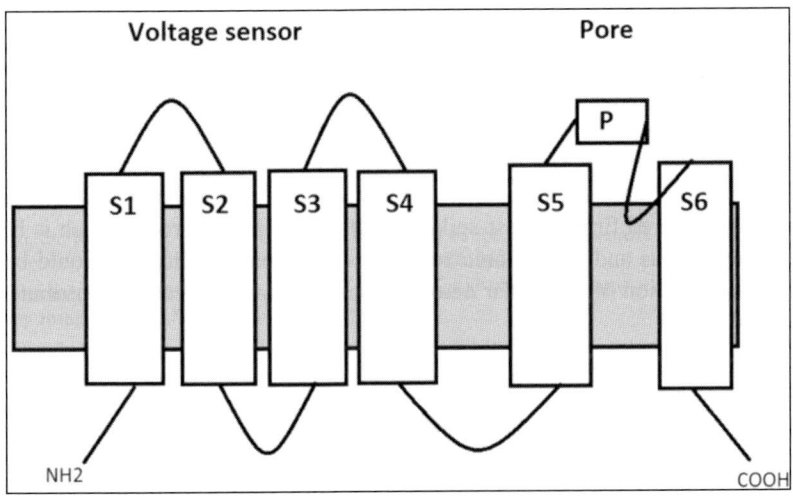

Fig. 1. Transmembrane topology of a Kv channel subunit.

Discovering *KCNC1* mutations in myoclonus epilepsy and ataxia (MEAK)

Eighty-four clinically confirmed cases of PME without clear genetic aetiology from multiple centres (including Europe, North America, Asia, and Australia), were investigated using whole-exome sequencing. A recurrent heterozygous missense mutation, c.959G>A (p.Arg320His), in *KCNC1* was identified in 11 unrelated patients (13.1 per cent). Sanger sequencing confirmed the mutation in 2 new cases, as well as in an affected sister and 2 affected children of 1 of the original 11 cases. In total, 16 cases, 13 of them unrelated, had the same *KCNC1* mutation. The parents of all patients with the *KCNC1* mutation were unaffected. Segregation analysis, where DNA was available for both parents, revealed that in each case the mutation occurred *de novo*. The family with 4 MEAK cases was further evaluated to rule out parental mosaicism (Muona et al., 2015). Based on a recently published mutation model (Samocha et al., 2014), the rate of this specific mutation was estimated at 1.75×10^{-7} mutations per person, representing an occurrence in 1 out of every 5,700,000 conceptions.

Chapter 15

Autosomal dominant cortical tremor, myoclonus and epilepsy

Pasquale Striano and Federico Zara

Department of Neurosciences, 'G. Gaslini' Institute, University of Genoa, Genoa, Italy
strianop@gmail.com
federicozara@ospedale-gaslini.ge.it

Summary

The term 'cortical tremor' was first introduced by Ikeda and colleagues to indicate a postural and action-induced shivering movement of the hands which mimics essential tremor, but presents with the electrophysiological findings of cortical reflex myoclonus. The association between autosomal dominant cortical tremor, myoclonus and epilepsy (ADCME) was first recognized in Japanese families and is now increasingly reported worldwide, although it is described using different acronyms (BAFME, FAME, FEME, FCTE and others). The disease usually takes a benign course, although drug-resistant partial seizures or slight intellectual disability occur in some cases. Moreover, a worsening of cortical tremor and myoclonus is common in advanced age. Although not yet recognized by the International League Against Epilepsy (ILAE), this is a well-delineated epilepsy syndrome with remarkable features that clearly distinguishes it from other myoclonic epilepsies. Moreover, genetic studies of these families show heterogeneity and different susceptible chromosomal loci have been identified.

Introduction

In 1990, Ikeda *et al.* described an action and postural tremor originating from the cerebral cortex, which was thus defined as a cortical tremor. Due to its electrophysiological features, this involuntary movement was considered to be a variant of cortical reflex myoclonus (Ikeda *et al.*, 1990). Uyama and colleagues reported 54 patients in 7 families, estimating a prevalence of approximately 1:35,000 based on their observation in Kumamoto Prefecture (Uyama *et al.*, 2005).

Cortical tremor was recognized to occur in families often in association with generalized tonic-clonic seizures, and this observation led to the definition of a peculiar autosomal dominant (AD) trait named 'benign adult familial myoclonic epilepsy' (BAFME). BAFME was first described in Japanese families and the genetic locus mapped to chromosome 8q24. However, several European families fulfilling the diagnostic criteria for BAFME have been described and in these families, linkage to chromosome 8q24 has been excluded (reviewed in Striano & Zara [2010]). These findings suggest a worldwide distribution and genetic heterogeneity for this condition. Guerrini *et al.* (2001) described a family who also presented drug-resistant focal seizures and mild intellectual disability in three affected individuals and considered this phenotype as a peculiar syndrome named 'AD cortical myoclonus and epilepsy' (ADCME). The mapping of a gene on chromosome 2p11.1-q12.2 reinforced the hypothesis that ADCME was an independent (genetically distinct from BAFME) clinical entity. A founder effect may possibly explain the high frequency of families originating from the same topographic areas of Japan and southern Italy (Uyama *et al.*, 2005; Madia *et al.*, 2008). An in-frame insertion/deletion in the α_2-adrenergic receptor subtype B gene (*ADRA2B*), encoding the α2-adrenergic receptor subtype B, has been reported in two apparently unrelated ADCME pedigrees of Italian origin (De Fusco *et al.*, 2014). This mutation alters several conserved residues of the third intracellular (3i) loop and alters the binding with the scaffolding protein called spinophilin upon neurotransmitter activation, thus increasing epinephrine-stimulated calcium signalling.

Additional loci have also been mapped to 5p15.31-p15 and 3q26.32-q28 in single families of French (Depienne *et al.*, 2010) and Thai (Yeetong *et al.*, 2013) origin. Stogmann *et al.* (2013) recently described a consanguineous Egyptian family presenting focal epilepsy, neuropsychiatric features, borderline cognitive level, and myoclonus, resembling BAFME, but inherited in an autosomal recessive manner. A homozygous deletion (c.503_503delG) leading to a frameshift in the coding region of *CNTN2* and segregating in the 5 affected family members was identified. The *CNTN2* gene (mapped at 1q32.1) encodes for contactin 2, a glycosylphosphatidylinositol-anchored neuronal membrane protein, which is necessary to maintain voltage-gated potassium channels at the juxtaparanodal region. Finally, a unique south Indian community, including 241 patients with ADCME belonging to 48 families has been described. The 48 families are domiciled in 2 southern districts of Tamilnadu, India, which belongs to the Nadar community, and their origin is confined to these southern districts, with reported unique genetic characteristics. This is the largest single report of ADCME worldwide (Mahadevan *et al.*, 2016).

The pathophysiological and biochemical bases of this condition also remain largely speculative. Both clinical and electrophysiological features of the syndrome suggest a cortical hyperexcitability, which may be the result of decreased cortical inhibition by the cerebellum via its cerebello-thalamo-cortical projections (Striano *et al.*, 2005). Sporadic post-mortem histological studies have shown evidence of cerebellar pathology (Uyama *et al.*, 2005).

Clinical features

Age at onset is highly variable (ranging from 11 to 50 years) but the disease usually starts with a slight hand 'tremor' within the second decade of life and progresses to rare tonic-clonic seizures and myoclonus by the third or fourth decade of life. Prevalence is unknown, but this condition is likely to be under-recognized. The dominant clinical picture is characterized by cortical tremor, myoclonus and epilepsy. Cortical tremor is an action and postural fine shivering movement consisting of continuous, arrhythmic, mainly distal, fine twitches in the hands. There is no significant progression over time, but a worsening of the disturbance may be observed over the age of 70. The cortical tremor is enhanced by emotion or fatigue and may be easily misdiagnosed as essential tremor, but may be distinguished from the latter clinically (Fig. 1A). To definitively distinguish between cortical tremor and benign essential tremor requires a neurophysiological demonstration of cortical origin (Striano *et al.*, 2005). In addition to cortical tremor, most patients present distal segmental, arrhythmic, erratic myoclonic jerks in the upper limbs which are exacerbated by posture and action. The involvement of more proximal, as well

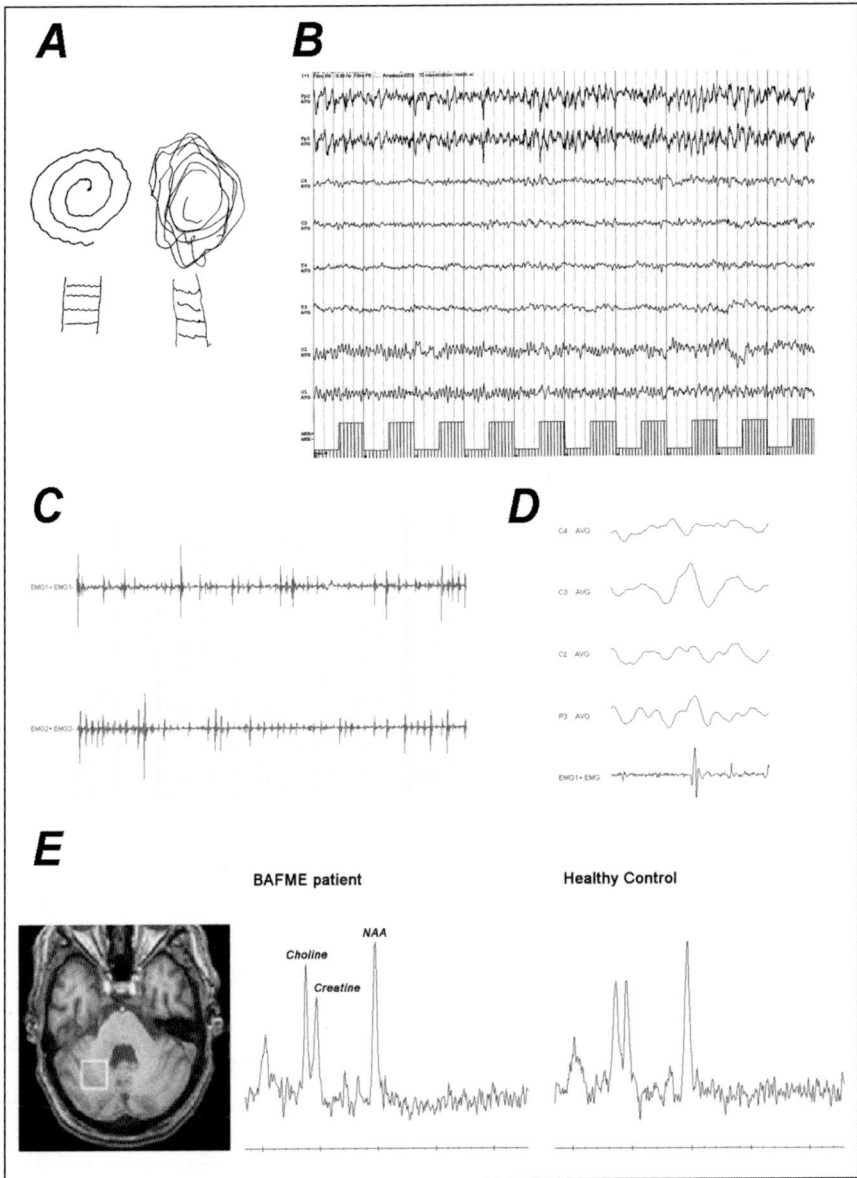

Fig. 1. Electroclinical and MRI features of familial cortical tremor, myoclonus and epilepsy. (A) free-hand drawing (Archimedes' spiral and ladder) showing the differences between essential (left) and cortical (right) tremors. The cortical tremor is fairly irregular, and sudden, brisk jerks cause disruption to the drawing. (B) EEG of a patient during photic stimulation with eyes closed, showing the photomyoclonic response consisting of increasing, mainly anteriorly, myogenic potentials related to each flash stimuli. (C) EMG recording of bursts between agonist and antagonist muscles (EMG1: right wrist extensor; EMG2: right wrist flexor) with extended arms; irregular, high-frequency, short EMG bursts without the regular alternating pattern typically found in tremors. (D) Jerk-locked averaging analysis shows a positive-negative potential, recognizable over the left centroparietal electrodes, preceding myoclonus by about 30 ms (right wrist extensor muscle; number of triggers = 100). (E) 1H-MR Spectroscopy using a PRESS sequence (TR 1,500 ms; TE 144 ms) showing abnormal spectral peak areas at 3.22 ppm, corresponding to choline (location of the $8\,cm^3$ voxel: right cerebellar hemisphere). Reproduced from Striano and Zara (2010), with permission.

as facial, muscles, particularly the eyelids, is also possible. The onset of myoclonus is difficult to clearly establish but usually starts at around the same age as that for cortical tremor (Striano & Zara, 2010).

Most patients experience generalized tonic-clonic seizures starting later than the tremor. The age at first seizure ranges widely between 12 and 67 years, with a peak around the age of 30. Seizures are generally rare (up to 5-10 episodes over the person's lifetime) and are not preceded by any warning. However, in some cases, they may be heralded by progressively increasing myoclonic jerks. Precipitating factors, such as sleep deprivation, emotional stress, and photic stimulation are often reported (Striano et al., 2005; Uyama et al., 2005). In rare cases, patients may also present with drug-resistant complex partial seizures and focal EEG abnormalities (Guerrini et al., 2001).

Patients usually present normal cognitive levels. However, mild-to-moderate intellectual disability may be present in some cases, particularly at a more advanced age (Fig. 2) (Striano et al., 2005; Coppola et al., 2011). Night blindness, with a reduced b-wave response on electroretinography, has been reported in three patients from Japan and migraine attacks have been reported as a predominant feature in a Turkish family (reviewed by Striano et al. [2005] and Uyama et al. [2005]).

Instrumental diagnostic procedures

Detailed electrophysiological investigations are essential to confirm the cortical origin of myoclonus. However, some of these electrophysiological features may be masked by antiepileptic treatments. The EEG background activity is usually normal or slightly slow in the slower alpha band. Generalized paroxysmal abnormalities and photoparoxysmal responses are frequently found in patients without therapy (Striano et al., 2005; Uyama et al., 2005). Furthermore, a photomyogenic response (i.e. a muscular, mainly anterior response, synchronous with photic stimulation) may be present (Fig. 1B). Focal paroxysmal activity can occur in some patients, in addition to generalized EEG abnormalities (Guerrini et al., 2001; Striano & Zara, 2010).

Polymyographic recording helps to differentiate between tremor and myoclonus. The electromyographic (EMG) pattern is consistent with irregular, arrhythmic or semi-rhythmic, high-frequency (around 10/s) myoclonic jerks. EMG bursts last about 50 ms and are usually synchronous between agonist and antagonist muscles, but do not regularly alternate between agonist/antagonist muscles, as in essential tremor (Fig. 1C). Jerk-locked averaging analysis commonly discloses a positive-negative, biphasic, premyoclonic spike or a more complex pattern of wavelets related to myoclonus on the contralateral sensorimotor regions (Fig. 1D). The evaluation of somatosensory evoked potentials and long-loop reflex I may show an enlargement of cortical components (P25-N33 amplitude larger than 8.5-15 µV) and enhanced long-latency (40 ms) C-reflex response evoked by stimulation of the peripheral nerve. A reduction in the resting motor threshold intensity and post-motor evoked potential silent period has been reported in a few patients evaluated by transcranial magnetic stimulation, indicating that central motor inhibitory mechanisms are impaired in these cases (Guerrini et al., 2001). MRI examination is usually normal although minor, non-specific abnormalities (such as mild enlargement of the subarachnoid spaces of the lateral ventricles) are sometimes reported. An MRI spectroscopy study revealed an elevated choline/creatine ratio in the cerebellum cortex of patients compared with controls (Fig. 1E) (Striano et al., 2009).

Chapter 15 Autosomal dominant cortical tremor, myoclonus and epilepsy

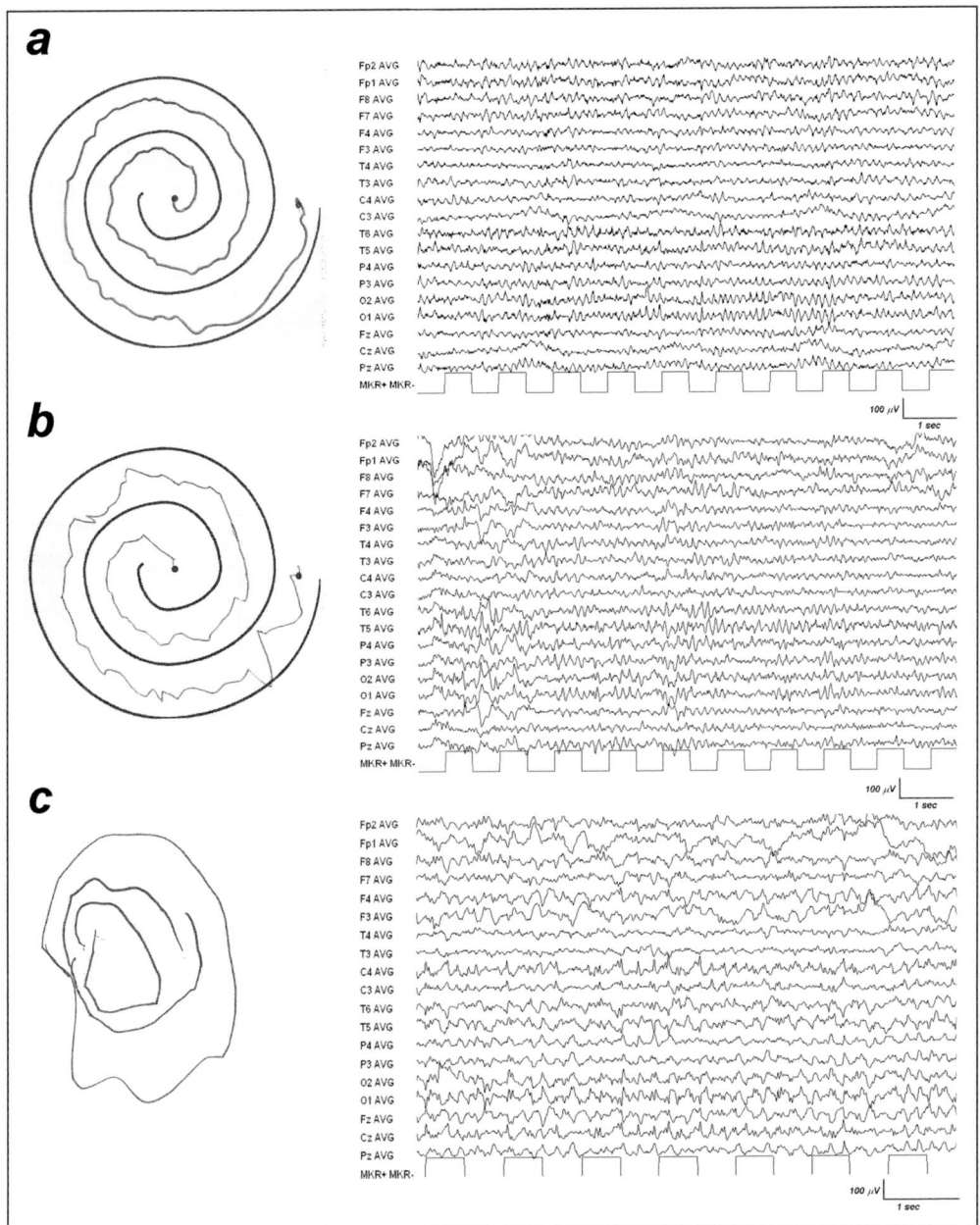

Fig. 2. Free-hand drawing, Archimede's spiral hands (left) and basal EEG of patient C/3 obtained at the age of 59 (A), 70 (B), and 80 years (C), showing worsening of myoclonus and progressive slowing of EEG background activity. Reproduced from Coppola et al. (2011), with permission.

Differential diagnosis

Cortical tremor may be easily misinterpreted as essential tremor and seizures may be overlooked or considered to be coincidental, or interpreted as a side effect of valproate treatment (Striano *et al.*, 2005). The clinical observation and demonstration of cortical reflex myoclonus by means of electrophysiological investigation enables confirmation of the diagnosis. ADCME must be differentiated from epilepsy syndromes with prominent myoclonus features. In particular, patients may easily be misdiagnosed with juvenile myoclonic epilepsy (JME) because of the occurrence of myoclonic jerks and generalized tonic-clonic seizures. However, JME clinically differs with regards to the absence of cortical tremor and predominant proximal myoclonic seizures which typically occur upon awakening. The absence of ataxia and dementia, adult onset, and the usually benign outcome of epilepsy differentiate ADCME from progressive myoclonic epilepsies (Striano & Zara, 2010).

Treatment and evolution

Cortical tremor is not responsive to alcohol or l-dopa/carbidopa but improves with antiepileptic drugs (Ikeda *et al.*, 1990; Striano *et al.*, 2005; Uyama *et al.*, 2005). Valproate, levetiracetam and benzodiazepines produce the greatest benefit against cortical tremors and myoclonus, combining both antiepileptic and antimyoclonic activity. In some cases, epilepsy may be difficult to treat.

As for other idiopathic generalized epilepsies, some antiepileptic drugs may precipitate myoclonic status. In these cases, a correct diagnosis and prompt discontinuation of the drug may reverse a potentially severe, life-threatening condition (Striano *et al.*, 2007). In advanced age, worsening of the myoclonus is possible, as well as difficulty in walking and mild ataxia (Striano & Zara, 2010; Coppola *et al.*, 2011).

Conflicts of interest: none.

References

Coppola, A., Santulli, L., Del Gaudio, L., *et al.* (2011): Natural history and long-term evolution in families with autosomal dominant cortical tremor, myoclonus, and epilepsy. *Epilepsia* **52**, 1245–1250.

De Fusco, M., Vago, R., Striano, P., *et al.* (2014): The α2 B adrenergic receptor is mutant in cortical myoclonus and epilepsy. *Ann. Neurol.* **75**, 77–87.

Depienne, C., Magnin E., Bouteiller D., *et al.* (2010): Familial cortical myoclonic tremor with epilepsy: the third locus (FCMTE3) maps to 5p. *Neurology* **74**, 2000–2003.

Guerrini, R., Bonanni, P., Patrignani, A., *et al.* (2001): Autosomal dominant cortical myoclonus and epilepsy (ADCME) with complex partial seizures and generalized seizures. A newly recognized epilepsy syndrome with linkage to chromosome 2 p11.1-q12.2. *Brain* **124**, 2459–2475.

Ikeda, A., Kakigi, R., Funai, N., Neshige, R., Kuroda, Y. & Shibasaki, H. (1990): Cortical tremor: a variant of cortical reflex myoclonus. *Neurology* **40**, 1561–1565.

Madia, F., Striano, P., Di Bonaventura, C., *et al.* (2008): Benign adult familial myoclonic epilepsy (BAFME): evidence of an extended founder haplotype on chromosome 2 p11.1-q12.2 in five Italian families. *Neurogenetics* **9**, 139–142.

Mahadevan, R., Viswanathan, N., Shanmugam, G., Sankaralingam, S., Essaki, B. & Chelladurai, R.P. (2016): Autosomal dominant cortical tremor, myoclonus, and epilepsy (ADCME) in a unique south Indian community. *Epilepsia* **57**, e56–9.

Stogmann, E., Reinthaler, E., Eltawil, S., *et al.* (2013): Autosomal recessive cortical myoclonic tremor and epilepsy: association with a mutation in the potassium channel associated gene *CNTN2*. *Brain* **136**, 1155–1160.

Striano, P. & Zara, F. (2010): Autosomal dominant cortical myoclonus and epilepsy. In: *Atlas of Epilepsy, Part 11,* eds. C.P. Panayiotopoulos. pp. 1051–1054. London, Springer Ltd.

Striano, P., Zara, F. & Striano, S. (2005): Autosomal dominant cortical tremor, myoclonus and epilepsy: many syndromes, one phenotype. *Acta Neurol. Scand.* **111,** 211–217.

Striano, P., Coppola, A., Madia, F., *et al.* (2007): Life-threatening status epilepticus following gabapentin administration in a patient with benign adult familial myoclonic epilepsy. *Epilepsia* **48,** 1995–1998.

Striano, P., Caranci, F., Di Benedetto, R., Tortora, F., Zara, F. & Striano, S. (2009): 1H MR spectroscopy indicates prominent cerebellar dysfunction in benign adult familial myoclonic epilepsy. *Epilepsia* **50,** 1491–1497.

Uyama, M.D., Fu, Y.H. & Ptacek, L. (2005): Familial adult myoclonic epilepsy (FAME). In: *Advances in Neurology. Myoclonic epilepsies.* eds. A.V. Delgado-Escueta, R. Guerrini, M.T. Medina, P. Genton, M. Bureau, C. Dravet, Vol. 95. Ch. 22. pp. 281–288. Lippincott Williams & Wilkins.

Yeetong, P., Ausavarat, S., Bhidayasiri, R., *et al.* (2013): A newly identified locus for benign adult familial myoclonic epilepsy on chromosome 3 q26.32–3 q28. *Eur. J. Hum. Genet.* **21,** 225–228.

Chapter 16

Myoclonus and seizures in PMEs: pharmacology and therapeutic trials

Roberto Michelucci[1], Elena Pasini[1], Patrizia Riguzzi[1], Eva Andermann[2], Reetta Kälviäinen[3] and Pierre Genton[4]

[1] *IRCCS Institute of Neurological Sciences of Bologna, Unit of Neurology, Bellaria Hospital, via Altura 3, 40139 Bologna, Italy*
[2] *Montreal Neurological Hospital & Institute, Neurology & Neurosurgery and Human Genetics, McGill University, 3801 University St., Room 127, Montreal, Quebec H3A 2B4, Canada*
[3] *Kuopio Epilepsy Center, Department of Neurology, Kuopio University Hospital, Puijonlaaksontie 2, P.O. Box 1777, Kuopio, 70210, Finland*
[4] *Centre Saint-Paul - Hôpital Henri-Gastaut, 300 Bd De Sainte Marguerite, 13009 Marseille, France*
roberto.michelucci@ausl.bo.it

Summary

Generalized motor seizures, usually tonic-clonic, tonic-vibratory, myoclonic or clonic, and stimulus-sensitive/action myoclonus are typical features of progressive myoclonus epilepsies (PMEs). Despite the introduction of many anticonvulsants, the treatment of these symptoms, particularly myoclonus, remains challenging, due to the incomplete and often transitory effects of most drugs. Moreover, treatment is only symptomatic, since therapy targeting the underlying aetiology for these genetic conditions is in its infancy. Traditional antiepileptic drugs for the treatment of PMEs are valproate, clonazepam, and phenobarbital (or primidone). These drugs may improve the overall performance of PME patients by decreasing their generalized seizures and, to a lesser extent, their myoclonic jerks. Newer drugs which have been shown to be effective include piracetam, levetiracetam, topiramate, zonisamide, and possibly perampanel for Lafora disease. The potential of other drugs (such as L-triptophan and N-acetylcysteine) and procedures (such as vagal and deep brain stimulation) has also been discussed. The available data on the efficacy of drugs are mainly based on small series or anecdotal reports. Two prospective, randomized, double blind studies investigating the novel SV2A ligand, brivaracetam, in genetically confirmed Unverricht-Lundborg patients have been performed with disappointing results. When treating PMEs, particular care should be paid to avoid drugs known to aggravate myoclonus or myoclonic seizures, such as phenytoin, carbamazepine, oxcarbazepine, lamotrigine, vigabatrin, tiagabine, gabapentin, and pregabalin. The emergency treatment of motor status, which often complicates the course of PMEs, consists of intravenous administration of benzodiazepines, valproate, or levetiracetam.

Introduction

Progressive myoclonus epilepsies (PMEs) are a group of uncommon diseases characterized by the association between myoclonus, epileptic seizures, and neurological deterioration, particularly ataxia and dementia (Marseille Consensus Group, 1990). A large number of rare specific genetic disorders may cause PME, but 5 principal causes are responsible for most cases of PME worldwide: Unverricht-Lundborg disease (ULD), Lafora disease (LD), mitochondrial encephalomyopathies (ME) with the phenotype of myoclonic epilepsy with ragged red fibres (MERRF), and sialidosis and neuronal ceroid lipofuscinoses (NCL). In order to establish a precise diagnosis, the clinical and neurophysiological characteristics of each PME are crucial to guide the clinician to the correct diagnostic algorithm, which may include complex and sometimes invasive procedures (Berkovic et al., 1986; Shahwan et al., 2005). Despite extensive investigations, a number of PMEs remain undiagnosed (Franceschetti et al., 2014); however, these unsolved cases are decreasing over time as a result of recent genetic advances (including wide-genome/exome sequencing), which have led to the discovery of new major causative genes, such as *SCARB2* (Dibbens et al., 2009) and *KCNC1* (Muona et al., 2015).

Myoclonus, the main symptom of PMEs, is typically fragmentary and multifocal, involving the musculature of the face and distal limbs. Bilateral massive myoclonic jerks, which tend to involve proximal limb muscles, may also occur, sometimes causing the patient to fall to the ground. Myoclonus may be spontaneous or, more often, induced or exacerbated by a variety of stimuli (such as light, sound, touch, and emotional strain), as well as movement or posture. Action myoclonus, in which muscular jerking is induced by movement or attempts at movement, is the most frequent and disabling form, commonly seen in almost all conditions underlying PME. A mixture of positive and negative myoclonus is the rule in patients with PME, especially LD. The generators for myoclonus in PME remain controversial, but neurophysiological studies suggest that cortical reflex myoclonus is the most common type, while reticular reflex myoclonus is less frequent (Tassinari et al., 1998b). Myoclonus is often difficult to control in these conditions and is usually a significant cause of disability in daily life.

PMEs are characterized by a wide range of epileptic seizures (Michelucci et al., 2002). Generalized tonic-clonic seizures are usually reported at the onset of LD and ULD and may, therefore, suggest the alternative diagnosis of idiopathic generalized epilepsies. They may occur without any warning or after a long build-up of myoclonias. Polygraphic recording may reveal these generalized motor seizures to be tonic-vibratory seizures (as in LD) or true myoclonic or clonic seizures (as in ULD). Absences or focal seizures (such as occipital seizures in LD) have also been encountered.

Other symptoms, which appear at various times during the course of the illness, include ataxia, cognitive dysfunction (sometimes leading to dementia), pyramidal signs, and a variety of other neurological and extraneurological signs (particularly in mitochondrial diseases).

Overall, the treatment of PMEs remains palliative, since there is no specific treatment for most genetic disorders underlying a PME syndrome (Uthman & Reichl, 2002; Shahawan et al., 2005). Despite a variety of anticonvulsants on the market, effective treatment remains challenging due to the fact that although these drugs may control major convulsive seizures, myoclonus does not really respond to the use of classic antiepileptic drugs (AEDs). Moreover a pathogenetic variety exists among the subtypes of PME, which means that medications which benefit one patient may be less effective in patients with another particular type of PME. Another problem is that clinical trials are difficult to perform due to the small number of patients, the progression of the clinical condition, and the choice of reliable efficacy endpoints. Hence, available data on the efficacy of newer antiepileptic medications in PME are primarily anecdotal or observational, based on individual responses in very small groups of patients.

In the present review, we summarize the results of the treatment of PMEs using a number of drugs (including AEDs) and procedures. The issues of designing and performing controlled clinical trials, as well as the emergency treatment, for patients with PMEs are also addressed.

Pharmacological treatment

Traditional AEDs used to treat PMEs are valproate, clonazepam, and phenobarbital (or primidone, a parent compound). These drugs may improve the overall performance of PME patients by decreasing their generalized seizures and, to a lesser extent, their myoclonic jerks. Other drugs which have shown to be effective include piracetam, levetiracetam, topiramate, zonisamide, brivaracetam, and perampanel (at least for LD). The overall therapy of PMEs is summarized in Table 1.

Table 1. Treatment of PMEs.
(A combination of multiple drugs is commonly needed).

First-line AEDs	Second-line AEDs	Third-line strategies	Emergency treatment
Valproate	Zonisamide	5-hydroxy-L-tryptophan	Benzodiazepines i.v.[1]
Clonazepam	Levetiracetam	Lamotrigine	Levetiracetam i.v.
	Topiramate	N-acetylcystein	Valproate i.v.
	Piracetam	VNS or DBS	Phenytoin i.v.[2]
	Phenobarbital	Experimental drugs	
		Brivaracetam	
		Perampanel[3]	

[1] Diazepam, lorazepam, clonazepam, midazolam.
[2] Phenytoin may be successfully used to treat motor status epilepticus in late-stage PMEs (Miyahara et al., 2009).
[3] Used thus far for Lafora disease.

Valproate

Valproate (at doses ranging from 15 mg/kg to 60 mg/kg) is the treatment of choice for PMEs. It may be used as monotherapy in mild cases or combined with other drugs in more serious cases. Its usefulness was clearly demonstrated by Iivanainen & Himberg (1982) in a prospective study conducted with 26 Finnish adults with severe forms of PME, likely to be related to ULD. These patients were severely disabled at the onset of the study (due to stimulus-sensitive myoclonus and ataxia) and were receiving chronic treatment with different combinations of AEDs, including carbamazepine, phenytoin, phenobarbital, primidone, and diazepam. These drugs were discontinued and treatment with valproate and clonazepam was commenced simultaneously, with rapid titration to optimal doses (1,500 to 1,800 mg for valproate and 6 to 10 mg for clonazepam). If the patients still had generalized tonic-clonic seizures, 50 to 100 mg of phenobarbital was added. The patients showed a dramatic improvement, particularly in locomotor ability, which continued in the 19 patients who were followed for 6 years. According to Iivanainen & Himberg (1982), these favourable results contributed to improving the prognosis of Baltic' PME and were also due, at least in part, to the discontinuation of phenytoin.

Despite its widespread use for all types of PME, valproate should be given with caution for mitochondrial disorders, due to its inhibitory effect on complex IV (cytocrome c oxidase) activity in the respiratory chain (Lam et al., 1997) and carnitine uptake (Tein et al., 1993). If used, therefore, supplementation with L-carnitine is recommended (Tein et al., 1993).

Clonazepam

The efficacy of clonazepam for the treatment of myoclonus and myoclonic seizures in different clinical contexts is well established (Nanda et al., 1977; Obeid & Panayiotopoulos, 1989; Tassinari et al., 1998a). The role of clonazepam in PMEs was highlighted in the study of Iivanainen & Himberg (1982), as described in the above section. Clonazepam is used as add-on therapy, at doses ranging from 3 to 16 mg/day for adults and 0.2 mg/kg/day for children. Due to the possible development of tolerance in some patients after 1 to 6 months of treatment, the dosage may need to be adjusted. Since it is commonly used in combination with other drugs for PMEs, the sedative effects of clonazepam may increase with the concomitant administration of phenobarbital. The effect of other, commonly used benzodiazepines, such as diazepam or clobazam, has not been assessed. However, these drugs may be used alternatively, especially when tolerance to clonazepam has developed.

Phenobarbital

Phenobarbital is a major AED with a wide efficacy spectrum. In PMEs, it may be used as an add-on treatment, at doses ranging from 30 to 200 mg/day (adults) and 3 to 8 mg/kg/day (children), particularly for the control of generalized tonic-clonic seizures (Iivanainen & Himberg, 1982). Particular attention should be paid to the inhibitory effect of valproate on phenobarbital elimination, resulting in phenobarbital accumulation and increased somnolence. Toxic signs may also be precipitated by elevated blood ammonia levels, because the magnitude of valproic acid-induced hyperammonaemia is increased in patients comedicated with phenobarbital (Michelucci et al., 2009). Primidone, which is at least partially metabolized into phenobarbital, has also been used with positive results in patients with myoclonus (Obeso, 1995).

Piracetam

Piracetam, a pyrrolidone derivative with a potent antimyoclonic effect and good tolerability profile, has long been used for the treatment of PMEs. Koskiniemi et al. (1998) reported a significant reduction in myoclonic jerks, and improvement in gait, in a double-blind, placebo-controlled trial in 20 patients with ULD, especially with the highest dose used (24 g/day). In this study, a linear dose-effect relationship of piracetam was established. High piracetam doses (up to 45 g/day) were also used by Genton et al. (1999) to obtain a stable and long-lasting improvement in 12 patients with PME. Other reports have also stressed the positive antimyoclonic effects of 20 g/day for advanced forms of PMEs (Fedi et al., 2001). The major drawback of these higher doses is the number of tablets taken and their bulk, sometimes making adherence to treatment difficult. Piracetam is well tolerated and the side effects (usually consisting of gastrointestinal discomfort) are rare, transitory, and mild even at high doses and can be avoided by slow titration (Ikeda et al., 1996).

Levetiracetam

Levetiracetam, a potent AED with a wide spectrum and a unique mechanism of action (mediated by binding to presynaptic vescicular protein, SV2A), was developed within the class of pyrrolidone derivatives and belongs to the same family of piracetam. For PMEs, levetiracetam has been evaluated in several series and appears to be effective for both myoclonus and generalized seizures (Genton & Gelisse, 2000; Frucht et al., 2001; Kinrions et al., 2003; Crest et al., 2004; Magaudda et al., 2004; Lim & Ahmed, 2005; Mancuso et al., 2006; Papacostas et al., 2007). Overall, of 23 patients with ULD treated with levetiracetam in open label trials at doses ranging from 1,000 to 4,000 mg, 15 (65 per cent) showed some clinical improvement while 8 (35 per cent) were unchanged. Seven patients (30 per cent) showed a dramatic improvement, which tended to subside, however, with long-term treatment. Levetiracetam is usually well tolerated in this group of patients and does not interact with concomitant drugs used for PMEs.

Topiramate

Topiramate, a sulfamate-substituted monosaccharide molecule, is a widely recognized broad-spectrum AED which is particularly effective for the treatment of refractory focal seizures, as well as primary or secondary generalized seizures. There are scattered reports in the literature showing that topiramate, when used for PMEs, may cause a marked decrease in myoclonus and myoclonic seizure frequency, and an improvement in daily functioning (Uldall & Bucholt, 1999). These effects do not appear to be specific to any given PME, but have been particularly studied in LD (Aykutlu et al., 2005; Demir et al., 2013). In one study, however, topiramate efficacy tended to decrease over time and the drug was discontinued in 2 out of 5 patients because of a rapid increase in cognitive impairment and vomiting (Aykutlu et al., 2005).

Zonisamide

Zonisamide, a sulfonamide derivative chemically distinct from any of the previously established AEDs, is indicated for the treatment of refractory partial epilepsy, but is also useful for a variety of generalized epilepsies, including epileptic encephalopathies, such as Lennox-Gastaut and West syndrome.

A number of case reports and small studies have suggested that zonisamide may be effective for treating patients with PME. More specifically, almost all patients with ULD who were treated with zonisamide as add-on therapy showed a dramatic reduction in myoclonus and a marked improvement in generalized tonic-clonic seizures and daily functioning, although this effect may subside over time (Henry et al., 1988; Kyllerman & Ben-Menachem, 1998; Yoshimura et al., 2001). Tassinari et al. (1999) investigated the efficacy and tolerability of zonisamide in the treatment of severely disabling action myoclonus. In the 4 patients with PME (2 with ULD and 2 cryptogenic), the authors observed a dramatic improvement, as documented by video-polygraphic recording of the patients before and at various times after the start of zonisamide therapy. Vossler et al. (2008) used add-on zonisamide (up to 6 mg/kg/die) in 30 patients with a variety of PME syndromes refractory to common AEDs. They found a ≥ 50 per cent decrease in myoclonic seizure frequency, measured over a 24-hour period, in 38 per cent of patients. About half of the patients experienced side effects consisting of anorexia, asthenia, and somnolence. Italiano et al. (2011) carried out a pilot, open-label trial of add-on zonisamide (up to 6 mg/kg/day) in 12 patients with EPM1 and studied the effect on myoclonus by means of the Unified Myoclonus Rating Scale, obtained for each subject before and after zonisamide add-on treatment. The authors observed a significant reduction in myoclonus severity following the introduction of zonisamide, associated with a good tolerability profile.

Lamotrigine

Lamotrigine, a triazine derivative developed from a series of folate antagonists, is a useful medication for a wide variety of epilepsies, including partial and generalized conditions. Its plasma levels are markedly increased by valproate co-administration, an interaction which largely explains the significant increase in lamotrigine potency after the addition of valproate.

The clinical experience with the use of lamotrigine for the treatment of myoclonus has given conflicting results. Wallace (1998) reviewed the effect of lamotrigine on different myoclonic syndromes and concluded that lamotrigine could be useful for the control of myoclonus for a variety of conditions, including PMEs. It was noted to be particularly efficacious for the treatment of seizures (of any type) of infantile and juvenile neuronal ceroid lipofuscinosis (Aberg et al., 1999). More recently, lamotrigine was revealed to improve disabling myoclonus in a patient with a mtDNA A3243G mutation (Costello & Sims, 2009).

In juvenile myoclonic epilepsy, however, lamotrigine was reported to exacerbate myoclonus in some cases and, in severe myoclonic epilepsy, was also shown to be dangerous (Guerrini et al., 1998). Genton et al. (2006) retrospectively analyzed the effect of add-on lamotrigine in 5 patients with ULD and observed either an aggravation of myoclonic jerks or a lack of improvement. The authors concluded that lamotrigine is not a sensible treatment option for ULD.

Brivaracetam

Following the discovery of the mechanism of action of levetiracetam, which involves a specific binding site on the presynaptically located synaptic vesicle protein, SV2A, great efforts were made to identify molecules which had structural analogy to levetiracetam and showed high binding constants to SV2A. Brivaracetam, a novel molecule with a 10-fold higher affinity for the SV2A binding site than levetiracetam, was proposed as a drug with high potential efficacy for myoclonus, as suggested by preclinical studies in an established rat model of cardiac arrest post-hypoxic myoclonus (Tai & Truong, 2007) and a phase IIa trial in which its efficacy in the photoparoxysmal response model was analyzed for photosensitive epilepsies (Kasteleijn-Nolst Trenité et al., 2007). In this study, brivaracetam, administered at a daily dose of 80 mg, eliminated the photoparoxysmal responses in 14/18 patients for a period of time exceeding the half-life of the drug.

In 2005, brivaracetam received orphan drug designation by the European Medicines Agency for development in PME and from the US Food and Drug Administration for the treatment of symptomatic myoclonus. Two prospective, multicentre, randomized, double-blind, placebo-controlled, parallel-group studies of brivaracetam as adjunctive treatment in 50 and 56 patients, respectively, with genetically ascertained ULD have recently been completed (N01187, N01236) (Kälviäinen et al., 2016). In the first study, dosages of 50 and 150 mg/day were tested and in the second study, dosages of 5 and 150 mg/day were applied. These patients suffered from moderate-to-severe action myoclonus and were stratified for concomitant use of levetiracetam or piracetam. Both studies failed to reach the primary goal of reducing the severity of action myoclonus, as measured by the Unified Myoclonus rating scale. However, a favourable trend was observed with brivaracetam at a dose of 50 mg/day in the 12-week maintenance period, and a significant improvement in quality of life (measured by QOLIE-31-P) was found with brivaracetam at daily doses of 50 and 150 mg. Moreover, 87 per cent of patients who completed the studies entered the long-term follow-up study. Overall, brivaracetam was well tolerated in this patient population, as evidenced by the high retention rate and the fact that it did not aggravate seizures or myoclonus. The most frequently reported adverse events were dizziness, headaches, and somnolence.

Although these controlled studies did not appear to support significant efficacy of brivaracetam for the treatment of ULD, a number of factors could have biased the results, including the severity and long duration of the disease, the small scale of the patient population, a high inter- and intra-patient variability, and, perhaps most importantly, the fact that many patients were already on high doses of levetiracetam and/or piracetam, which also act on the SV2A vesicles. A considerable number of patients continued to use brivaracetam after the controlled phase of the trial, for over 6 years, which appears to indicate that this compound has some benefits.

Other drugs and procedures

Perampanel, one of the newer AEDs, is a selective non-competitive antagonist of the AMPA-type glutamate receptors and was recently licensed as adjunctive therapy for the treatment of refractory focal-onset seizures (Krauss *et al.*, 2012; French *et al.*, 2012). Two reports document its efficacy when used as add-on therapy for the treatment of LD. The first case was a 21-year-old female patient who was administered perampanel at a dose of 8-10 mg, in addition to a regimen that included clonazepam, levetiracetam, piracetam, valproate, zonisamide, a ketogenic diet, and VNS. This therapeutic change resulted in seizure remission for more than 3 months and led to a reduction in the number of epileptiform discharges on EEG (Schorlemmer *et al.*, 2013). The second case was a 15-year-old girl who experienced a dramatic decrease in her seizure frequency, as well as improvement in neurological and cognitive function following initiation of treatment with 10 mg perampanel, administered as monotherapy. Perampanel was therefore proposed as the first potentially efficacious treatment for LD (Dirani *et al.*, 2014).

In line with the serotoninergic hypothesis of myoclonus, which suggests that serotonergic hypofunction is involved in the genesis of myoclonus in PMEs and other myoclonic disorders, 5-hydroxy-L-tryptophan, a precursor of serotonin, was used for the treatment of PMEs. In 1980, Koskiniemi *et al.* performed a double-blind, placebo-controlled, cross-over study with 2 g L-tryptophan in 7 patients with ULD and found a significant improvement in 6 patients, mostly concerning ambulation, myoclonic jerks, and general condition. With long-term L-tryptophan treatment, however, the effect disappeared or was even reversed in 3 of the 7 patients after 3 to 4 weeks. Similar positive short-term results were obtained in a further group of 11 Finnish patients with ULD who received up to 100 mg/kg of L-tryptophan plus carbidopa (in order to prevent metabolism outside of the brain) over a 6-week period (Leino *et al.*, 1981). In contrast, Pranzatelli *et al.* (1995) reported no significant change in myoclonus or ataxia evaluation score in a double-blind, cross-over study with L-5HTP in 8 patients with a variety of PME. Overall, this drug does not appear to have a place in the modern treatment of ULD.

N-acetylcysteine is a sulfhydryl antioxidant that increases cellular glutathione and the activity levels of several antioxidant enzymes. Hurd *et al.* (1996) reported marked beneficial effects on mobility, speech, and seizures in at least 2 of 4 severely affected siblings with ULD treated with N-acetylcysteine in combination with other antioxidants (riboflavin, vitamin E, selenium, and zinc).

Antioxidant vitamins and cofactors, including coenzyme Q_{10} and L-carnitine, are empirically used to treat mitochondrial disorders (Shahwan et al., 2005; Di Mauro & Mancuso, 2007). Baclofen, a muscle relaxant normally used to treat spasticity by inhibiting both monosynaptic and polysynaptic reflexes at the spinal level, has shown promising results in a few PME cases with prominent spasticity and polymyoclonus (Awaad & Fish, 1995). Ropirinole, a dopamine agonist commonly used to treat Parkinson's disease, was shown to improve myoclonus, writing, and muscular balance in a single patient with ULD (Karvonen et al., 2010). Ethosuximide is active against negative myoclonus, which is often found in PMEs, in association with positive myoclonus.

Alcohol was proven to have some beneficial effects in patients with myoclonus by decreasing myoclonic jerks and improving speech and gait (Genton & Guerrini, 1990). This compound, however, can be used only occasionally to improve the quality of a patient's social life; in contrast, regular use can induce the development of tolerance or even dependence.

A high-fat and low-carbohydrate diet (with a ratio of fat to carbohydrate of 3:1 or 4:1), also known as a ketogenic diet, has been shown to be useful for a variety of severe, drug-resistant epilepsies, including infantile myoclonic seizures. An Italian study of 5 patients with LD, a condition which causes a specific glycogen metabolism disorder, showed that a ketogenic diet, though well tolerated, was unable to stop disease progression (Cardinali et al., 2006). It is now hypothesized that potential targets of new molecules for LD could involve the inhibition or modulation of glycogen synthesis (Pedersen et al., 2013).

Different stimulation procedures have also occasionally been employed for patients with PMEs. Vagal nerve stimulation was implanted in an adult patient with a ULD-type PME, who was followed for 1 year, and the procedure resulted in a marked reduction in seizures (more than 90 per cent) and a significant improvement in cerebellar function, as demonstrated on neurological examination (Smith et al., 2000). Chronic high-frequency deep brain stimulation (DBS) of the subthalamic nucleus has been used in an adult patient with an undiagnosed form of PME who was disabled due to frequent seizures, despite vagal nerve stimulation and a complex antiepileptic regimen (Vesper et al., 2007). After a 12-month follow-up, the seizures were reduced in intensity and frequency by 50 per cent. More recently, 5 adult patients with PME underwent chronic high-frequency DBS (Wille et al., 2011). Electrodes were implanted in the substantia nigra pars reticulata (SNr)/subthalamic nucleus (STN) region in the first patient and additionally in the ventral intermediate nucleus (VIM) bilaterally in the next four cases. After a mean follow-up of 24 months, a reduction in myoclonic seizures was observed in all patients, ranging between 30 and 100 per cent, as quantified by a standardized video protocol. All patients reported clinically relevant improvements of various capabilities, such as free standing, walking, and improved fine motor skills. The best clinical effects were seen with SNr/STN DBS in all patients.

Drugs and circumstances to avoid

Interestingly, rather than being beneficial, some AEDs have the potential to exacerbate myoclonic seizures and should be used with caution in patients with PME (Table 2). More specifically, sodium channel blockers (carbamazepine, oxcarbazepine, and phenytoin) and GABAergic drugs (vigabatrin and tiagabine), as well as gabapentin and pregabalin, should, in general, be avoided as they may aggravate myoclonus and myoclonic seizures (Medina et al., 2005).

Table 2. Antiepileptic drugs and effects on myoclonus in PME

Antimyoclonic	Potentially aggravating	To be used with caution	Not documented
Valproate	Phenytoin	Lamotrigine	Lacosamide
Clonazepam	Carbamazepine	Valproate for MERRF	Felbamate
Phenobarbital/Primidone	Oxcarbazepine		Rufinamide
Piracetam	Vigabatrin		Ethosuximide
Levetiracetam	Gabapentin		Eslicarbazepine
Topiramate	Pregabalin		
Zonisamide	Tiagabine		

Phenytoin has also been found to aggravate neurological symptoms and cerebellar ataxia in ULD and its widespread use in the past has been proposed as an explanation for the poor prognosis of ULD described in the early series reports (Iivanainen & Himberg, 1982; Elridge et al., 1983).

Emergency treatment of PMEs

In situations where myoclonic jerks are exacerbated, leading to a series of jerks or status myoclonicus, loud noises and bright lights should be avoided and the patient should be treated in a quiet room, as calmly as possible. Emergency treatment includes the intravenous use of benziodiazepines (diazepam, lorazepam, clonazepam, and midazolam), valproate, and levetiracetam (Fernandez-Baca Vaca et al., 2012). Phenytoin, although usually contraindicated for PMEs, has proven to be useful in selected cases of refractory status epilepticus, particularly when this occurs in the late stages of a variety of PMEs or in the presence of focal status (Riguzzi et al., 1997; Kälviäinen et al., 2008; Miyahara et al., 2009).

Conclusions

The treatment of PME disorders essentially continues to involve the management of seizures and myoclonus, together with palliative, supportive, and rehabilitative measures. The treatment of myoclonus and seizures in PME can prove to be difficult and both tend to be refractory to conventional medications. Available data on the efficacy of drugs are primarily anecdotal or observational based on small groups of patients. It is difficult to conduct controlled clinical trials in these patients because the incidence of these disorders is exceedingly rare; however, collaborative trials involving many specialized centres could be designed to bring together a sufficient number of patients with a genetically verified diagnosis. Following the availability of brivaracetam, a potentially effective antimyoclonic agent, 2 multicentre, randomized, placebo-controlled studies on genetically verified ULD have been performed, but the effect of this drug on action myoclonus was statistically not significant. However, a favourable trend was observed with the 50-mg dose and it was argued that various factors could have negatively influenced the results.

Traditional AEDs used for the treatment of PMEs are valproate, clonazepam, phenobarbital, or primidone. Newer drugs which have been shown to be effective include piracetam, levetiracetam, topiramate, zonisamide, and, possibly, perampanel for LD. Care must be taken to avoid antiepileptic medications that clearly worsen myoclonus, such as vigabatrin, carbamazepine, phenytoin, and gabapentin. Lamotrigine has an unpredictable effect on myoclonus and must be used with caution.

Athough recent advances in molecular genetics have led to the identification of several genes, mutations, and proteins involved in the pathogenesis of PME disorders, therapy targeting the underlying aetiology remains in the experimental phase and results, to date, have not been encouraging. It is expected, however, that future treatments with gene therapy and enzyme replacement, or the identification of drugs that interact with new targets and mechanisms, may help to modify and improve the course of these progressive disorders.

Conflicts of interest: none.

References

Aberg, L., Kirveskari, E. & Santavuori, P. (1999): Lamotrigine therapy in juvenile neuronal ceroid lipofuscinosis. *Epilepsia* **40**, 796–799.

Awaad, Y. & Fish, I. (1995): Baclofen in the treatment of polymyoclonus in a patient with Unverricht-Lundborg disease. *J. Child Neurol.* **10**, 68–70.

Aykutlu, E., Baykan, B., Gurses, C., Bebek, N., Buyukbabani, N. & Gokyigit, A. (2005): Add-on therapy with topiramate in progressive myoclonic epilepsy. *Epilepsy Behav.* **6**, 260–263.

Berkovic, S.F., Andermann, F., Carpenter, S. & Wolfe, L.S. (1986): Progressive myoclonus epilepsies: specific causes and diagnosis. *N. Engl. J. Med.* **315**, 296–305.

Cardinali, S., Canafoglia, L., Bertoli, S., et al. (2006): A pilot study of a ketogenic diet in patients with Lafora body disease. *Epilepsy Res.* **69**, 129–134.

Costello, D.J. & Sims, K.B. (2009): Efficacy of lamotrigine in a patient with a mtDNA A3243 G mutation. *Neurology* **72**, 1279–1280.

Crest, C., Dupont, S., Leguern, E., Adam, C. & Baulac, M. (2004): Levetiracetam in progressive myoclonic epilepsy: an exploratory study in 9 patients. *Neurology* **62**, 640–643.

Demir, C.F., Ozdemir, H.H. & Mungen, B. (2013): Efficacy of topiramamte as add-on therapy in two different types of progressive myoclonic epilepsy. *Acta Medica* **56**, 36–38.

Di Mauro, S. & Mancuso, M. (2007): Mitochondrial diseases: therapeutic approaches. *Biosci. Rep.* **27**, 125–137.

Dibbens, L.M., Michelucci, R., Gambardella, A., et al. (2009): SCARB2 mutations in progressive myoclonus epilepsy (PME) without renal failure. *Ann. Neurol.* **66**, 532–536.

Dirani, M., Nasreddine, W., Abdulla, F. & Beydoun, A. (2014): Seizure control and improvement of neurological dysfunction in Lafora disease with perampanel. *Epilepsy Behav. Case Rep.* **2**, 164–166.

Elridge, R., Iivanainen, M., Stern, R., Koerber, I. & Wilder, B.J. (1983): 'Baltic' myoclonus epilepsy: hereditary disorder of childhood made worse by phenytoin. *Lancet* **2**, 838–842.

Fedi, M., Reutens, D., Dubeau, F., Andermann, E., D'Agostino, D. & Andermann, F. (2001): Long-term efficacy and safety of piracetam in the treatment of progressive myoclonus epilepsies. *Arch. Neurol.* **58**, 781–786.

Fernandez-Baca Vaca, G., Lenz, T., Pestana Knight, E.M. & Tuxhorn, I. (2012): Gaucher disease: successful treatment of myoclonic status epilepticus with levetiracetam. *Epileptic Disord.* **14**, 155–158.

Franceschetti, S., Michelucci, R., Canafoglia, L., et al. (2014): Progressive myoclonus epilepsies - definitive and still undetermined causes. *Neurology* **82**, 405–411.

French, J.A., Krauss, G.L., Biton, V., et al. (2012): Adjunctive perampanel for refractory partial-onset seizures: randomized phase III, study 304. *Neurology* **79**, 589–596.

Frucht, S.J., Louis, E.D., Chuang, C. & Fahn, S. (2001): A pilot tolerability and efficacy study of levetiracetam in patients with chronic myoclonus. *Neurology* **57**, 1112–1114.

Genton, P. & Guerrini, R. (1990): Antimyoclonic effects of alcohol in progressive myoclonus epilepsy. *Neurology* **40**, 1412–1416.

Genton, P. & Gelisse, P. (2000): Antimyoclonic effect of levetiracetam. *Epileptic Disord.* **2**, 209–212.

Genton, P., Guerrini, R. & Remy, C. (1999): Piracetam in the treatment of cortical myoclonus. *Pharmacopsychiatry* **32**, 49–53.

Genton, P., Gelisse, P. & Crespel, A. (2006): Lack of efficacy and potential aggravation of myoclonus with lamotrigine in Unverricht-Lundborg disease. *Epilepsia* **47**, 2083–2085.

Guerrini, R., Dravet, C., Genton, P., Belmonte, A., Kaminska, A. & Dulac, O. (1998): Lamotrigine and seizure aggravation in severe myoclonic epilepsy. *Epilepsia* **39**, 508–512.

Henry, T.R., Leppik, I.E., Gumnit, R.J. & Jacobs, M. (1988): Progressive myoclonus epilepsy treated with zonisamide. *Neurology* **38**, 928–931.

Hurd, R.W., Wilder, B.J., Helveston, W.R. & Uthman, B.M. (1996): Treatment of four siblings with progressive myoclonus epilepsy of the Unverricht Lundborg type with N acetylcysteine. *Neurology* **47**, 1264–1268.

Iivanainen, M. & Himberg, J.J. (1982): Valproate and clonazepam in the treatment of severe progressive myoclonus epilepsy. *Arch. Neurol.* **39**, 236–238.

Ikeda, A., Shibasaki, H., Tashiro, K., Mizuno, Y. & Kimura, J. (1996): Clinical trial of piracetam in patients with myoclonus: nationwide multiinstitution study in Japan. *Mov. Disord.* **11**, 691–700.

Italiano, D., Pezzella, M., Coppola, A., et al. (2011): A pilot open-label trial of zonisamide in Unverricht-Lundborg disease. *Mov. Disord.* **26**, 341–343.

Kälviäinen, R., Khyuppenen, J., Koskenkorva, P., Eriksson, K., Vanninen, R. & Mervaala, E. (2008): Clinical picture of EPM1-Unverricht-Lundborg disease. *Epilepsia* **49**, 549–556.

Kälviäinen, R., Genton, P., Andermann, E., et al. (2016): Brivaracetam in patients with Unverricht-Lundborg disease: results from two randomized, placebo-controlled, double-blind studies. *Epilepsia* **57**, 210–221.

Karvonen, M.K., Kaasinen, V., Korja, M. & Marttila, R.J. (2010): Ropirinole diminishes myoclonus and improves writing and postural balance in an ULD patient. *Mov. Disord.* **25**, 520–521.

Kasteleijn-Nolst Trenité, D.G., Genton, P., Parain, D., et al. (2007): Evaluation of brivaracetam, a novel SV2 A ligand, in the photosensitivity model. *Neurology* **69**, 1027–1034.

Kinrions, P., Ibrahim, N., Murphy, K., Lehesjoki, A.E., Jarvela, I. & Delanty, N. (2003): Efficacy of levetiracetam in a patient with Unverricht-Lundborg progressive myoclonus epilepsy. *Neurology* **60**, 1934–1935.

Koskiniemi, M., Hyyppa, M., Sainio, K., Salmi, T., Sarna, S. & Uotila, L. (1980): Transient effect of L-tryptophan in progressive myoclonus epilepsy without Lafora bodies: clinical and electrophysiological study. *Epilepsia* **21**, 351–357.

Koskiniemi, M., Van Vleymen, B., Hakamies, L., Lamusuo, S. & Taalas, J. (1998): Piracetam relieves symptoms in progressive myoclonus epilepsy: a multicentre, randomized, double blind, crossover study comparing the efficacy and safety of three dosages of oral piracetam vs placebo. *J. Neurol. Neurosurg. Psychiatry* **64**, 344–348.

Krauss, G.L., Serratosa, J.M., Villanueva, V., et al. (2012): Randomized phase III study 306, adjunctive perampanel for refractory partial-onset seizures. *Neurology* **78**, 1408–1415.

Kyllerman, M. & Ben-Menachem, E. (1998): Zonisamide for progressive myoclonus epilepsy: long term observations in seven cases. *Epilepsy Res.* **29**, 109–114.

Lam, C.W., Lau, C.H., Williams, J.C., Chan, Y.W. & Wong, L.J. (1997): Mitochondrial myopathy, encephalopathy, lactic acidosis and stroke-like episodes (MELAS) triggered by valproate therapy. *Eur. J. Pediatr.* **156**, 562–564.

Leino, E., MacDonald, E., Airaksinen, M.M., Riekkinen, P.J. & Salo, H. (1981): L-tryptophan-carbidopa trial in patients with long-standing progressive myoclonus epilepsy. *Acta Neurol. Scand.* **64**, 132–141.

Lim, L.L. & Ahmed, A. (2005): Limited efficacy of levetiracetam on myoclonus of different etiologies. *Parkinsonism Relat. Disord.* **11**, 135–137.

Magaudda, A., Gelisse, P. & Genton, P. (2004): Antimyoclonc effect of levetiracetam in 13 patients with Unverricht-Lundborg disease: clinical observations. *Epilepsia* **45**, 678–681.

Mancuso, M., Galli, R., Pizzanelli, C., Filosto, M., Siciliano, G. & Murri, L. (2006): Antimyoclonic effect of levetiracetam in MERRF syndrome. *J. Neurol. Sci.* **243**, 97–99.

Marseille Consensus Group (1990): classification of progressive myoclonus epilepsies and related disorders. *Ann. Neurol.* **28**, 113–116.

Medina, M.T., Martinez-Juarez, I.E., Duron, R.M., et al. (2005): Treatment of myoclonic epilepsies of childhood, adolescence, and adulthood. *Adv. Neurol.* **95**, 307–323.

Michelucci, R., Serratosa, J.M., Genton, P. & Tassinari, C.A. (2002): Seizures, myoclonus and cerebellar dysfunction in progressive myoclonus epilepsies. In: *Epilepsy and Movement Disorders*, eds. R. Guerrini, J. Aicardi, F. Andermann & M. Hallett. pp. 227–249. Cambridge: Cambridge University Press.

Michelucci, R., Pasini, E. & Tassinari, C.A. (2009): Phenobarbital, primidone and other barbiturates. In: *The Treatment of Epilepsy, 3rd ed*, eds. S.D. Shorvon, E. Perucca. & J. Engel. pp. 585–603. Oxford: Blackwell Publishing.

Miyahara, A., Saito, Y., Sugai, K., *et al.* (2009): Reassessment of phenytoin for treatment of late stage progressive myoclonus epilepsy complicated with status epilepticus. *Epilepsy Res.* **84**, 801–809.

Muona, M., Berkovic, S.F., Dibbens, L.M., *et al.* (2015): A recurrent *de novo* mutation in *KCNC1* causes progressive myoclonus epilepsy. *Nat. Genet.* **47**, 39–46.

Nanda, R.N., Johnson, R.H., Keogh, H.J., Lambie, D.G. & Melville, I.D. (1977): Treatment of epilepsy with clonazepam and its effect on other anticonvulsants. *J. Neurol. Neurosurg. Psychiatry* **40**, 538–543.

Obeid, T. & Panayiotopoulos, C.P. (1989): Clonazepam in juvenile myoclonic epilepsy. *Epilepsia* **30**, 603–606.

Obeso, J.A. (1995): Therapy of myoclonus. *Clin. Neurosci.* **3**, 253–257.

Papacostas, S., Kholou, E. & Papathanasiou, E. (2007): Levetiracetam in three cases of progressive myoclonus epilepsy. *Pharm. World Sci.* **29**, 164–166.

Pedersen, B.A., Turnbull, J., Epp, J.R., *et al.* (2013): Inhibiting glycogen synthesis prevents Lafora disease in a mouse model. *Ann. Neurol.* **74**, 297–300.

Pranzatelli, M.R., Tate, E., Huang, Y., *et al.* (1995): Neuropharmacology of progressive myoclonus epilepsy: response to 5-hydroxy-L-tryptophan. *Epilepsia* **36**, 783–791.

Riguzzi, P., Michelucci, R., Magaudda, A., *et al.* (1997): Epileptic motor status in progressive myoclonus epilepsy: efficacy of iv phenytoin. *Epilepsia* **38**, 70.

Schorlemmer, K., Bauer, S., Belke, M., *et al.* (2013): Sustained seizure remission on perampanel in progressive myoclonic epilepsy (Lafora disease). *Epilepsy Behav. Case Rep.* **1**, 118–121.

Shahwan, A., Farrell, M. & Delanty, N. (2005): Progressive myoclonus epilepsies: a review of genetic and therapeutic aspects. *Lancet Neurol.* **4**, 239–248.

Smith, B., Shatz, R., Elisevich, K., Bespalova, I.N. & Burmeister, M. (2000): Effects of vagus nerve stimulation on progressive myoclonus epilepsy of Unverricht Lundborg type. *Epilepsia* **41**, 1046–1048.

Tai, K.K. & Truong, D.D. (2007): Brivaracetam is superior to levetiracetam in a rat model of post-hypoxic myoclonus. *J. Neural Transm.* **114**, 1547–1551.

Tassinari, C.A., Michelucci, R., Riguzzi, P., *et al.* (1998a): The use of diazepam and clonazepam in epilepsy. *Epilepsia* **39**, S7–S14.

Tassinari, C.A., Rubboli, G. & Shibasaki, H. (1998b): Neurophysiology of positive and negative myoclonus. *Electroencephalogr. Clin. Neurophysiol.* **107**, 181–195.

Tassinari, C.A., Riguzzi, P., Volpi, L., *et al.* (1999): Zonisamide in the treatment of action myoclonus in progressive myoclonus epilepsies. *Epilepsia* **40**(2), 242.

Tein, I., Di Mauro, S., Xie, Z.W. & De Vivo, D.C. (1993): Valproic acid impairs carnitine uptake in cultured human skin fibroblasts: an *in vitro* model for pathogenesis for valproic-acid associated carnitine deficiency. *Pediatr. Res.* **34**, 281–287.

Uldall, P. & Buchholt, J.M. (1999): Clinical experiences with topiramate in children with intractable epilepsy. *Eur. J. Ped. Neurol.* **3**, 105–111.

Uthman, B.M. & Reichl, A. (2002): Progressive myoclonus epilepsies. *Curr. Treat. Options Neurol.* **4**, 3–17.

Vesper, J., Steinhoff, B., Rona, S., *et al.* (2007): Chronic high-frequency deep brain stimulation of the STN/SNr for progressive myoclonic epilepsy. *Epilepsia* **48**, 1984–1989.

Vossler, D.G., Conry, J.A., Murphy, J.V. & the ZNS-502/505 PME, Study Group (2008): Zonisamide for the treatment of myoclonic seizures in progressive myoclonus epilepsy: an open label study. *Epileptic Disord.* **10**, 31–34.

Wallace, S.J. (1998): Myoclonus and epilepsy in childhood: a review of treatment with valproate, ethosuximide, lamotrigine and zonisamide. *Epilepsy Res.* **29**, 147–154.

Wille, C., Steinhoff, B.J., Altenmuller, D.M., *et al.* (2011): Chronic high-frequency deep-brain stimulation in progressive myoclonic epilepsy in adulthood - report of five cases. *Epilepsia* **52**, 489–496.

Yoshimura, I., Kaneko, S., Yoshimura, N. & Murakami, T. (2001): Long-term observations of two siblings with Lafora disease treated with zonisamide. *Epilepsy Res.* **46**, 283–287.

Chapter 17

Post-modern therapeutic approaches for progressive myoclonus epilepsy

Berge A. Minassian

The Hospital for Sick Children, Division of Neurology,
555 University Avenue, Toronto, Ontario, M5G 1X8, Canada
berge.minassian@sickkids.ca

Summary

By and large, progressive myoclonus epilepsies (PMEs) described in this textbook are devastating and lethal. However, most are monogenic, rendering them much more amenable to future therapies relative to other complex diseases, for two reasons; firstly, the pathophysiology is easier to understand, and secondly, therapy may be targeted to a single gene, function, or pathway. In this chapter, some of the cutting-edge therapeutic modalities applicable to monogenic brain diseases is reviewed. In each case, one example is provided, simply as an illustration. It is not possible to provide a comprehensive review since even as this book is being published, discoveries are being made regarding new molecular targeting and delivery systems.

Small molecules

We are accustomed to therapy in the form of a pill ingested daily, the active compound of which travels through the gut and blood, crosses the blood-brain barrier (BBB), and enters cells to impart therapeutic change. The size of small molecules is their abiding therapeutic advantage for PMEs and other brain diseases, and size matters regarding passage through the BBB, but of course, small size is not all it takes. For example, the presence of a monoester (phosphate) bound to a small molecule prevents it from not only crossing the BBB, but even cell membranes.

However, a small molecule will not replace a gene function, but could, as a chaperone, stabilize a gene product which is present but simply misfolded and thus non-functional. In other words, for diseases where at least one of the mutations is a missense mutation that deconvolutes or otherwise destabilizes the tertiary structure of a disease gene product, a small chaperone molecule may stabilize the structure to a sufficient extent to render it functional, effectively above a clinical threshold. Tay-Sachs disease is a neurodegenerative disease due to mutations in the hexosaminidase A (*HEXA*) gene. In its classic form, it is an infantile disease that is fatal by age 2 or 3. However, some 'mild' mutations are associated with a milder neurodegenerative course. The FDA-approved antimalarial BBB-penetrant agent, pyrimethamine, was shown to

199

stabilize certain *HEXA* missense mutants in fibroblasts of patients with late-onset Tay-Sachs disease, and raise enzymatic activity threefold (Maegawa *et al.*, 2007). This led to a pilot clinical study in 4 patients in whom HEXA activity rose 2.24 fold. The rise was unfortunately not sustained and the study was clinically unsuccessful (Osher *et al.*, 2015), but nonetheless this was a start for an otherwise intractable disease.

While small molecules cannot replace gene functions, they can very well affect other parts of a disease pathway, whether metabolic or not, or a second messenger. Often, the absence of a gene causes the activity of a downstream protein to be up or down-regulated, which when corrected through interference by a small molecule, even partially, may revert disease pathogenesis and be therapeutic. mTOR pathway interference with rapamycin and its analogues is a case in point. Tuberous sclerosis and several other epilepsies are caused by genetic disruptions of this pathway, leading to focal or more widespread dysplasias and tumours (usually benign), which drive epilepsy. This therapy, which partially regulates the pathway and presents an entirely novel, more direct mechanism, therefore provides intrinsic support as treatment for these epilepsies (Ricos *et al.*, 2015).

Identifying a small molecule drug commonly requires establishment of *in vitro* assays; *in vitro* (biochemical) and/or cell culture assays. These assays are based on the associated molecular or biochemical disease pathway(s) which are investigated through standard gene function-based research. The assays are used to screen ever-expanding libraries of small molecules in order to identify, by chance, one or more that may affect the assay in the desired way. Huge amounts of work follow in translating 'hits' to something useful. This involves establishing safety and efficacy in animal models, mouse and larger animals, BBB passage, and other pharmacological aspects. Usually, the initial 'hit' is less than optimal, and a prolonged process of medicinal chemistry towards optimization follows, until eventually a drug can be ready for testing in human subjects. This type of work is long and expensive. However, the infrastructure is increasingly in place in many universities, and even more so in pharmaceutical companies. The latter appear to be moving very much in the direction of developing drugs for orphan diseases. These are usually so devastating that families and societies will incur the costs of these drugs which will always be priced high, in part, to recover the large investment of development.

While 'chance' through high-throughput screening is the common and strongest approach to identify interfering molecules, the vast expansion of crystal structures of proteins available as well as the bioinformatics tools to study these structures and their functions, are allowing intelligent drug design, *e.g. in silico* development of chemicals that might fit an enzyme's active site. This is presently in its infancy, but clearly holds much promise. One of the biggest problems with small molecules is their usual incomplete selectivity, *i.e.* their interference with other targets, leading to side effects. This too could partially be managed in the future with complete understanding of protein structures and even stronger informatics tools. Clearly, oral drugs are the most desired therapeutic approach due to non-invasiveness, but drugs are neither permanent solutions, nor, for the moment, easy to tailor to ensure a high degree of target specificity. As such, other approaches are needed, as discussed below. Some are invasive, but this is mitigated by the huge need for them, given the devastating nature of the PMEs.

Targeting RNA

As well as targeting proteins, it is possible to target messenger RNA (mRNA). The same general principles hold, in that it is generally much easier to downregulate mRNA than increase it, and the same issues regarding BBB passage exist. There are a number of anti-RNA approaches, the most advanced of which is the use of antisense oligonucleotides (ASOs). These oligonucleotides are designed to interfere with an mRNA and downregulate it. One of these is already on the market as a drug for familial hyperlipidaemia (Phillips *et al.*, 2015). There are currently many ASOs in clinical trials for various neurological diseases (*e.g.* Huntington disease and spinocerebellar ataxia [Keiser *et al.*, 2015]), but all share the same problem in that they do not cross the BBB and require intra-cerebrospinal fluid administration. This problem is mitigated by specific chemical properties that allow their longevity, and the patient does not require an injection more than once every two months. This is clearly still far from ideal, but for the moment, is the best available treatment. Interestingly, it has been reported that ASOs can actually activate a function which has been lost. The most common cause of spinal muscular atrophy (SMA) is loss-of-function mutation of the *SMN1* gene. It so happens that evolution has led to the *SMN1* gene being located adjacent to the *SMN2* gene. In SMA, *SMN2* is also generally inactive due to a sequence that leads to skipping over exon 7. ASOs have been designed to interfere with this skipping of exon 7 splicing, and thus lead to inclusion of this exon, thus rendering *SMN2* functional. This 'drug' is presently in an advanced clinical trial (Faravelli *et al.*, 2015).

Targeting DNA

Bacteria, of course have an immune system; how else would they survive the onslaught of viruses over millions of years? This immunity consists of generating guide RNAs that specifically target enzymes (*e.g.* Cas9) to viral genomes. The Cas9 then nicks and inactivates the viral DNA. Impressive recent studies have addressed the following questions. Could Cas9 cut human DNA? The answer is yes. Could Cas9 be directed by specific guide RNA sequences to specific sites in the human genome to cut specific genes? Yes. Would the human genome be able to mend itself after being cut? Yes. Does this correction maintain the coding frame of a target gene? No. *In toto*, this CRISPR (which refers to the guide RNA)/Cas9 system can specifically target a desired gene and break it, causing the cell's DNA repair system to mend the chromosomal break, however, usually not in-frame, *i.e.* the targeted gene is knocked out, but the chromosome is otherwise untouched (Ran *et al.*, 2015). The major advantage of this genome editing approach is that it is permanent. Presently, the system only knocks out genes. If a disease pathway is identified in which a protein function in the pathway is increased, and its elimination would correct pathogenesis, then CRISPR/Cas9 could be utilized to remove this protein and treat the disease. The greatest therapeutic promise of the system, however, is in future possibilities. If the system can be targeted to a mutant gene, specifically to the mutation site, such that the mutation is removed and replaced with normal sequence, then the disease would be corrected at the source.

There are countless difficulties to overcome before the CRISPR system delivers. Firstly, Cas9 and guide RNA have to be delivered to the brain, no small feat as this is a large protein. It would be possible to deliver CRISPR/Cas9 through viral gene therapy, but the gene for the commonly used Cas9, from *Strep. viridans*, is too large to fit in the AAV viral vectors that have the greatest promise for gene therapy. This problem, though, appears to have been solved with the identification of a smaller, but equally effective, Cas9 gene from *Staph. aureus*, which does fit in AAV particles (Ran *et al.*, 2015). Another problem is the need to deliver to large numbers of neurons, *i.e.* 'edit' most neurons, which is a limitation, though perhaps not serious, of present viral vectors (see next section). Then there is the likely immunogenicity of Cas9 delivered to humans. However, Cas9 will not need to be delivered many times, because its effect would be permanent. As such, the patient could be immunosuppressed during the treatment. Another problem is the risks associated with off-target nicking. While bioinformatics is used to design specific CRISPRs against specific sequences, the genome is vast enough that there is at least the risk of off-target cutting, with potential for 'side-effects', including oncogenesis. Off-target effects, however, from most recent data, appear to be not nearly as concerning as initially thought (Iyer et al., 2015). In addition, there is, of course, the looming issue that gene deletion as a therapeutic approach would be useful in only very few situations. What is desired is mutation correction, and the CRISPR system is not quite there yet. There have been successes, but correction of gene mutation remains inefficient and much work is required to optimize it. However, if this system proves to be successful, it would allow, as mentioned, correction of the root of the problem in essentially all the diseases described in this book. An important step forward has been taken recently in this endeavour. Yet another bacterial DNA nickase has been identified, which, unlike Cas9, cleaves DNA via a staggered cut, leading to overhanging ends, which should make the replacement of a deleted segment by a corrected sequence much easier (Zetsche et al., 2015).

Gene therapy

Most of the conditions described in this book are autosomal recessive diseases caused by a loss of function of single genes. As such, they can potentially be remedied by replacing the gene function. Gene replacement therapy stalled for a long time in the 1990s due to premature use of immunogenic viruses for gene delivery with subsequent harm to patients. However, gradual careful work has brought to the fore the adeno-associated viruses, in particular AAV9 and AAVrh10, which have superb properties. These viruses are normally present in the human brain, implying natural BBB passage capability and low immunogenicity. However, low immunogenicity does not mean no immunogenicity. The high load of virus that needs to be given generates immune reactions in animal models, although, presumably, this problem can be averted by immunosuppression during treatment. AAV viruses can package genes of average size, which means they are useful, potentially, for most diseases. The DNA vectors are not silenced, leading to persistent expression. Their DNA does not integrate into the human genome, i.e. there is low to no risk of interfering with genomic DNA, including tumour suppressor genes. Finally, AAV9 is capable of delivering its cargo to a large proportion of cells, in particular, when injected in the CSF (Meyer et al., 2015).

Gene therapy is indeed in resurgence and it is hoped the technical difficulties will continue to be overcome, to allow gene replacement, and, as discussed above, gene correction. In fact, clinical trials are ongoing for multiple diseases, including some neuronal ceroid lipofuscinoses reviewed in this book, as well as SMA, as mentioned above. While the ASO approach for SMA aims at activating *SMN2*, the AAV-delivered gene therapy approach aims to replace under-expressed *SMN1*. Over a dozen babies with this fatal disease have been injected so far with virus carrying *SMN1*, and they are doing well (B. Kaspar, *personal communication*); publication of this major potential therapeutic success by the group which has been working on it for many years is anticipated (Mandel, Kaspar and colleagues).

While gene therapy mostly utilizes viruses, it must be noted that there are other approaches. These include packaging the gene of interest in liposomes, which merge with membranes and can potentially make their way through the BBB to neurons. Immunoliposomes are another development on this concept. Here, the liposome membrane contains an antibody that allows it to bind to membrane receptors that are then internalized, thus supporting transduction into the brain.

Protein replacement therapy

In this last section, we touch on the possibility of directly replacing the missing protein, instead of its gene. Multiple approaches are used. This relies, as for immunoliposomes, on antibodies against the transferrin receptor or other proteins. The antibody is covalently bound to the protein to be delivered, and once it interacts with its target, it and the protein are internalized into vesicles, which then merge with lysosomes. As such, this type of therapy would be useful for lysosomal diseases, which make up a large part of PME.

Another exciting possibility is the use of diphtheria toxin. This toxin binds a receptor on the endothelial cell membrane and is internalized into a vesicle into the endothelial cells that make up the BBB. This vesicle translocates to the other side of the cells and releases the toxin into the CSF space. The toxin then binds to its receptor at the surface of neurons, is again internalized into a vesicle, but this time it is injected out of the vesicle into the neuronal cytoplasm, where it blocks protein synthesis and kills the neuron. It was shown that the toxicity of this toxin can be completely eliminated by a point mutation, whilst retaining its translocation properties. Finally, it was shown that a cargo protein, almost of any size, can be attached to this toxin and co-delivered to cells (so far in cell culture experiments only) with maintained function of the delivered protein (Auger *et al.*, 2015).

There are other post-genetic era therapeutic approaches in the works, and indeed a lot of excitement that the expression of certain genes will follow Mendelian genetics. For example, for Lafora disease, one of the prototypical PMEs described in an earlier chapter of this book, progress in understanding the disease has allowed us to 'cure' Lafora mice simply by reducing the amount of glycogen synthase (GS), the enzyme that gives rise to the neurotoxic Lafora bodies that underlie the disease. As such, we are presently applying almost all the methods above to attempt to find a therapy for this horrendous condition. This involves screening for small molecule inhibitors of GS, using ASOs against GS and its activator protein PTG, experimenting with CRISPRs against the latter two proteins, using AAV9 to replace the two respective disease-causing genes, and using inactivated diphtheria toxin-mediated delivery of amylase to mouse brain. Amylase is the only enzyme known to digest Lafora bodies. We have already shown that we are able to deliver amylase to cells in culture in this fashion and that amylase remains functional after crossing the cell membrane (Auger *et al.*, 2015). This disease, which we are particularly familiar with, exemplifies the immense possibilities ahead for all our patients with any form of PME.

Conflicts of interest: none.

References

Auger, A., Park, M., Nitschke, F., *et al.* (2015): Efficient delivery of structurally diverse protein cargo into mammalian cells by a bacterial toxin. *Mol. Pharm.* **12,** 2962–29671.

Faravelli, I., Nizzardo, M., Comi, G.P. & Corti, S. (2015): Spinal muscular atrophy-recent therapeutic advances for an old challenge. *Nat. Rev. Neurol.* **11,** 351–359.

Iyer, V., Shen, B., Zhang, W., *et al.* (2015): Off-target mutations are rare in Cas9-modified mice. *Nat. Methods* **12,** 479.

Keiser, M.S., Kordasiewicz, H.B. & McBride, J.L. (2015): Gene suppression strategies for dominantly inherited neurodegenerative diseases: lessons from Huntington's disease and spinocerebellar ataxia. *Hum. Mol. Genet.* **25**(R1): R53–64.

Maegawa, G.H., Tropak, M., Buttner, J., *et al.* (2007): Pyrimethamine as a potential pharmacological chaperone for late-onset forms of GM2 gangliosidosis. *J. Biol. Chem.* **282,** 9150–9161.

Meyer, K., Ferraiuolo, L., Schmelzer, L., *et al.* (2015): Improving single injection CSF delivery of AAV9-mediated gene therapy for SMA: a dose-response study in mice and nonhuman primates. *Mol. Ther.* **23,** 477–487.

Osher, E., Fattal-Valevski, A., Sagie, L., *et al.* (2015): Effect of cyclic, low dose pyrimethamine treatment in patients with Late Onset Tay Sachs: an open label, extended pilot study. *Orphanet J. Rare Dis.* **10,** 45.

Phillips, M.I., Costales, J., Lee, R.J., Oliveira, E. & Burns, A.B. (2015): Antisense therapy for cardiovascular diseases. *Curr. Pharm. Des.* **21,** 4417–4426.

Ran, F.A., Cong, L., Yan, W.X., *et al.* (2015): *In vivo* genome editing using Staphylococcus aureus Cas9. *Nature* **520,** 186–191.

Ricos, M.G., Hodgson, B.L., Pippucci, T., *et al.* (2015): Mutations in the mTOR pathway regulators NPRL2 and NPRL3 cause focal epilepsy. *Ann. Neurol.* **79,** 120–131.

Zetsche, B., Gootenberg, J.S., Abudayyeh, O.O., *et al.* (2015): Cpf1 is a single RNA-guided endonuclease of a class 2 CRISPR-Cas system. *Cell* **163,** 759–771.

Mariani Foundation
Paediatric Neurology Series

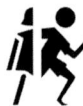

1: Occipital Seizures and Epilepsies in Children
Edited by: *F. Andermann, A. Beaumanoir, L. Mira, J. Roger and C.A. Tassinari*

2: Motor Development in Children
Edited by: *E. Fedrizzi, G. Avanzini and P. Crenna*

3: Continuous Spikes and Waves during Slow Sleep – Electrical Status Epilepticus during Slow Sleep
Edited by: *A. Beaumanoir, M. Bureau, T. Deonna, L. Mira and C.A. Tassinari*

4: Metabolic Encephalopathies: Therapy and Prognosis
Edited by: *S. Di Donato, R. Parini and G. Uziel*

5: Neuromuscular Diseases during Development
Edited by: *F. Cornelio, G. Lanzi and E. Fedrizzi*

6: Falls in Epileptic and Non-Epileptic Seizures during Childhood
Edited by: *A. Beaumanoir, F. Andermann, G. Avanzini and L. Mira*

7: Abnormal Cortical Development and Epilepsy – From Basic to Clinical Science
Edited by: *R. Spreafico, G. Avanzini and F. Andermann*

8: Limbic Seizures in Children
Edited by: *G. Avanzini, A. Beaumanoir and L. Mira*

9: Localization of Brain Lesions and Developmental Functions
Edited by: *D. Riva and A. Benton*

10: Immune-Mediated Disorders of the Central Nervous System in Children
Edited by: *L. Angelini, M. Bardare and A. Martini*

11: Frontal Lobe Seizures and Epilepsies in Children
Edited by: *A. Beaumanoir, F. Andermann, P. Chauvel, L. Mira and B. Zifkin*

12: Hereditary Leukoencephalopathies and Demyelinating Neuropathies in Children
Edited by: *G. Uziel, F. Taroni*

13: Neurodevelopmental Disorders: Cognitive/Behavioural Phenotypes
Edited by: *D. Riva, U. Bellugi and M.B. Denckla*

14: Autistic Spectrum Disorders
Edited by: *D. Riva and I. Rapin*